Health Assessment of the Older Adult

Second Edition

Charlotte Eliopoulos, RNC, MPH
Consultant and Lecturer in Geriatric Care Services
Glen Arm, Maryland

Addison-Wesley Nursing
A Division of The Benjamin/Cummings Publishing Company, Inc.
Redwood City, California • Fort Collins, Colorado • Menlo Park, California
Reading, Massachusetts • New York • Don Mills, Ontario • Wokingham, U.K.
Amsterdam • Bonn • Sydney • Singapore • Tokyo • Madrid • San Juan

Sponsoring Editor: Debra Hunter
Production Coordinator: John Walker
Copy Editor: Jenny Pulsipher
Text and Cover Design: Betty Gee, Side by Side Studios
Illustrators: Jane McCreary
Composition and Film: Polyglot Pte Ltd
Photographer: William Thompson, RN

Copyright © 1984, 1990 by Addison-Wesley Nursing,
A Division of The Benjamin/Cummings Publishing Company, Inc.

Library of Congress Cataloging-in-Publication Data

Eliopoulos, Charlotte.
    Health assessment of the older adult / Charlotte Eliopoulos. — 2nd ed.
        p.   cm.
    ISBN 0-201-06674-2
    1. Geriatric nursing.   2. Nursing assessment.   I. Title.
    RC954.E46   1990
    618.97′075 — dc20   89-28529
                                                                                          CIP

ISBN 0-201-06674-2

ABCDEFGHIJK-MA- 93210

Addison-Wesley Nursing
A Division of The Benjamin/Cummings Publishing Company, Inc.
390 Bridge Parkway
Redwood City, CA 94065

Dedicated to Marge and Lou . . . for being very special parents.

EDITOR

Charlotte Eliopoulos, RNC, MPH
Consultant and Lecturer in
Geriatric Care Services
Glen Arm, Maryland

CONTRIBUTING AUTHORS

Jamie Caplis, BA, MS
Consultant on Aging Services
Associate Professor, University
of Baltimore
Baltimore, Maryland

Nina Glomski, RNC, MA
Director of Nursing
Levindale Geriatric Center
and Hospital
Baltimore, Maryland

Erick Larson, PT
Chief of Physical Therapy
St. Agnes Hospital
Baltimore, Maryland
Consultant in Home Health Care

Mary Jane Lucas-Blaustein
Psychiatric Liaison Nurse
Instructor in Psychiatry
Johns Hopkins University
Baltimore, Maryland

Constance Joan Meyd, RN, MS
Nurse Practitioner
Consultant in Nursing
Baltimore, Maryland

Sandra E. Orem, RN, MSN
Director
Oasis Health Systems Baltimore
Baltimore, Maryland

**Hilary D. Sigmon, RN, MSN,
CCRN**
Nursing Director
Medical Shock Trauma Acute
Resuscitation Unit
Washington Hospital Center
Washington, D.C.

Peggy Yen, RD, MPH
Nutrition Consultant
Aging and Chronic Illness
Administration
Maryland Department of Health
Baltimore, Maryland

Preface

ASSESSMENT: THE ESSENTIAL FIRST STEP

Astute assessment skills are prerequisites for competent nursing practice. A sound assessment provides the foundation for individualized care planning and delivery. Assessment findings can aid in identifying risks and preventing occurrences that could jeopardize the health and well-being of the client. With the current concern about the escalating costs of health care, assessing needs and prioritizing needs promote the effective, efficient use of resources.

In gerontologic nursing, the practice of expert assessment is especially important and particularly challenging. Older adults experience a variety of unique physical, mental, and social problems that often coexist and are interrelated. Age-related changes that alter norms and unique symptomatology may both accompany illness, thereby increasing the difficulty in differentiating normal from abnormal findings. In addition, poor memory, stress, or the effects of illness may interfere with older adults' recall of significant health history.

Proper assessment demands that nurses possess knowledge and skills in interviewing, observation, and physical assessment techniques. In addition, assessment of older adults requires nurses to understand changes associated with the aging process, the aged's unique presentation of illness, altered norms, response to therapy, and the wide range of health and social services available to aging individuals. As the number of older adults in society continues to increase, nurses in virtually every practice setting will be practicing gerontological nursing. Further, as more elderly individuals survive to their eighth decade and beyond—the time of life in which health and social problems tend to increase—nurses will need to possess a strong foundation in gerontologic and geriatric nursing to meet the needs of their elderly clients competently.

CONTENT

Health Assessment of the Older Adult, Second Edition, is a resource to nurses who perform a basic but comprehensive assessment of older persons. Organized for the most part by body systems, this book includes descriptions of anatomical and physiological changes resulting from the aging process, to assist the reader in differentiating normal from abnormal characteristics in the older client. Accompanying these descriptions are instructions for fundamental examination techniques to enrich the assessment process. Characteristics of common disorders and potential problems are presented to alert the reader to clues that can promote early detection and management.

In addition to body systems, assessment of other significant aspects of the older adult are reviewed, including social function, mental status, nutrition, sexuality, and functional independence.

OBJECTIVES

Reading this book will not qualify the reader to function as an advanced practitioner of assessment skills. Nor does the book intend to imply that the reader will no longer require assessment input from other disciplines in the health team. This book's objectives are to help the reader (1) conduct a basic, comprehensive assessment of the older adult; (2) understand the dynamics and interrelationship among physical, mental, and social function; (3) recognize the need for referrals to other providers; and (4) interpret the assessments and care plans of other team members.

NURSING DIAGNOSIS

Assessment is not an independent activity, but rather an interdependent part of the total nursing process. The purpose of assessment is to identify nursing diagnoses that warrant nursing actions. This book discusses in a practical manner how assessment findings are translated into nursing diagnosis statements. Each chapter summary includes a list of related nursing diagnoses to guide the reader in developing nursing diagnoses for clients. This revised edition incorporates the recent diagnoses accepted by the North America Nursing Diagnosis Association.

FEATURES

Many effective learning tools enhance this book and successfully help the reader understand and retain the content. Such features include:

- Numerous photos and illustrations clearly presenting important assessment techniques.
- Informative charts and tables that synthesize material for greater accessibility and understanding.
- Chapter summaries for quick reference and review.
- A case study at the end of the book for integrating and applying skills and knowledge.
- Appendices that include sample assessment tools, references for laboratory values, audiovisual resources, and literature references for further readings in gerontology and assessment.

AUDIENCE

Although primarily addressed to nurses and nursing students, this book can benefit all health professionals who interact with older adults by allowing more realistic and effective planning and care delivery and by enhancing interdisciplinary communication and collaboration. This book complements the reader's existing knowledge and skills in physical assessment, basic nursing, and the rudiments of anatomy and physiology.

Throughout the text, "he" or "she" is used when referring to either the client or the nurse, to avoid the confusion often resulting from the use of combined pronouns. This is not intended, in any way, to suggest sexual role discrimination.

ACKNOWLEDGMENTS

Many individuals participated in this book's development. The fine chapters by Jamie Caplis, Nina Glomski, Erick Larson, Jane Lucas, Connie Meyd, Sandy Orem, Heidi Sigmon, and Peggy Yen give this text the depth and scope that only specialists can contribute. Appreciation is expressed to the following reviewers who helped to smooth out many rough edges: Mary L. Nowotny, RN, PhD; Margaret McMahon, RN, MS; Gail Harkness, RN, PhD; and Ruth Ouimette, RN, MSN.

Charlotte Eliopoulos

REVIEWERS

Carol J. Bear
St. Louis Community College at
Florrisant Valley
St. Louis, Missourri

Dorothy Booth, PhD, RN
Wayne State University
Detroit, Michigan

Kathleen P. Conlon
University of Tennessee at
Knoxville
Knoxville, Tennessee

Diana Coyle
Villanova University
Villanova, Pennsylvania

D. Karl Davis, PhD
Hunter College
Bellevue School of Nursing
New York, New York

Patricia Hall
Lake Michigan College
Benton Harbor, Michigan

E. Gail Harkness, RN, PhD
Associate Professor
The University of Kansas Medical
Center
Kansas City, Kansas

Carolyn F. Hickox
La Grange College
La Grange, Georgia

Margaret McMahon
Assistant Professor
University of Nebraska
Omaha, Nebraska

Professor W. Morse
University of Wisconsin, Eau Claire
Eau Claire, Wisconsin

Mary Nowotny, RN, PhD
Assistant Professor
Baylor University
Waco/Dallas, Texas

Ruth Ouimette, MSN, RN
University of North Carolina at
Chapel Hill
Chapel Hill, North Carolina

Muriel B. Ryden, PhD
University of Minnesota
Minneapolis, Minnesota

Lillian M. Simms
University of Michigan
Ann Arbor, Michigan

Nancy Smith
University of Colorado Health
Sciences Center
Denver, Colorado

Contents

1

Introduction to Assessment

Charlotte Eliopoulos, RNC, MPH

Assessment is the process by which data are collected and analyzed in an orderly, systematic manner. An evaluation of the anatomic normality and functional capacity of an individual is derived through assessment. Health assessment appraises not only the status of various systems within the human organism but also the status of the individual within the family, community, and society.

All facets of care are built on the strong foundation of a thorough, competent assessment. Knowledge of the client's preferences, habits, problems, strengths, and weaknesses can guide you in planning and delivering realistic, effective, and individualized care. The outcome is customized care tailored to meet the needs of the individual; the potential benefits are improved client compliance, appropriate service usage, additional provider protection, and less waste of health care dollars.

As defined, assessment is a *process*. Optimally it occurs with every client–nurse interaction and is not solely confined to isolated activities intended for data collection, such as interviews and physical examinations. During an exchange about the weather, you can observe if there is something different about the client's coloring, posture, breathing, or mood. As medications are administered, you can judge if the client is able to recall the names of the drugs, manipulate the tablets and the water glass, and swallow with ease. While assisting with bathing activities, you can determine if a new medication has caused a rash, if mobility has changed, or if pain is present. Every encounter with the client, no matter how brief, can yield valuable information regarding the changing status of the client, the effectiveness of the care plan, and the development of new problems. With the rapidly changing and/or fluctuating status of many older adults, dynamic continuous assessment is an integral part of gerontologic care.

The nurse collects both objective and subjective data in the health assessment. Objective data are those signs and characteristics that you can observe and measure, such as a rash or contents of a urine sample. Subjective data are symptoms and perceptions that the client describes and confirms, such as pain or blurred vision. Both types of data are essential in compiling a complete data base. Objective and subjective data can be obtained from many sources, including the following: the client, the client's family and friends, physical examinations, laboratory tests, previous health records, and other providers. To develop a complete picture of the client, you should not overlook any source of information.

METHODS OF ASSESSING

The complexity and wealth of information each individual possesses demand that you use multiple techniques in the assessment process. Most of these techniques can be categorized under three major methods of assessing clients: *interview, observation,* and *examination.* Variations of these methods are used in assessing virtually every aspect of the client's anatomy and function. Although specific cognitive and psychomotor skills related to particular areas of assessment will be provided throughout this book, the following general overview of assessment methods will assist in the reader's overall orientation to health assessment.

Interview

The interview is a structured, directed verbal exchange between the nurse and the client. Although its major purpose is to gather information, the interview also serves to give information and lay the foundation for the nurse–client relationship.

Prior to initiating the interview it is important to assure that the environment facilitates rather than hinders the exchange of information. Privacy is one important consideration. Older adults may not have had the exposure to surveys or interviews that younger generations have had and may be uncomfortable sharing personal information. Conducting the interview in a busy waiting room or with another client present in the same room will compound the uneasiness of sharing personal data and could prohibit a full sharing of information. A private room with the door closed will be advantageous. Noise that staff may have learned to block, such as paging systems, ringing telephones, or noisy patients, may be extremely distracting to the older client and may compound communication problems associated with any existing hearing deficits. Sensitivity to glare, secondary to cataracts, can cause older eyes to be uncomfortable and less functional in areas where bright fluorescent lights are used or direct sunlight shines. Room temperatures that are comfortable for active, young staff may be too cold for elderly persons, who commonly have lower body temperatures; eagerness to leave the cold environment may cause the client to limit conversation. Positioning should also be considered; even without arthritic joints clients may find long periods of sitting unsupported on a hard examining table to be difficult.

The initial phase of the interview is the establishment of rapport. The validity and depth of information the client is willing to provide strongly depend on the client's degree of trust in the nurse and the quality of their relationship. The client should feel relaxed and at ease. Seating should be comfortable with a distance of approximately 4 feet between you and the client (Figure 1-1). This is close enough to allow for easy communication yet distant enough to provide for normal social distance.

Inform the client how long the interview is expected to last. The client's understanding of why the information is being sought and how it will be used is important. Understandably, a client may wonder why a medication history

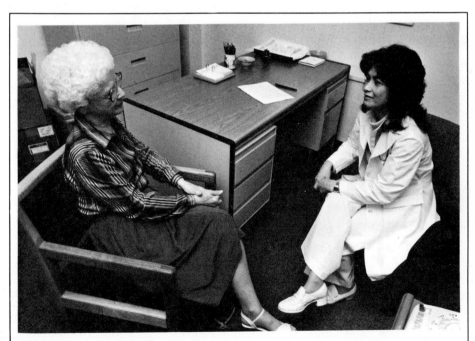

Figure 1-1
Arranging the seating to allow approximately 4 feet between you and the client creates a more comfortable and productive interviewing environment.

is being requested when the purpose of the visit is to have hearing screened. He may also be reluctant to inform you that he shares his home with a friend if he thinks this information will be forwarded to the caseworker who manages his financial aid. Comments such as "I want to see if there is anything else occurring that is related to this problem" and "While you're here I'd like to examine you completely to ensure that no problems are starting to develop" give clear, basic explanations of the rationale for data collection. Many older adults have had limited experience with interviews and have been socialized to keep personal matters, including health-related information, to themselves. Thus, they may be particularly uncomfortable with sharing their personal lives with "strangers." If the assessment will be shared with other providers or if it is being conducted for a specific purpose such as to determine competency to continue employment, inform the client of this at the outset. It must be stated, emphasized, and honored that *the client has the right to refuse to participate in the entire assessment or in any of its components.*

Use language appropriate to the client. Obvious language barriers may exist, such as the client's limited ability to speak English. Bilingual persons may resort to their native tongue when confronted with a stressful situation— for instance, when being examined by health personnel. Other language problems may prevail also. Clients may be unfamiliar with health jargon or know only slang terms for certain anatomy and physiology vocabulary. They may describe their health using terminology that has lost popularity with younger generations. Examples of this are consumption (tuberculosis), rheumatism (arthritis), curse or monthly (menstruation), fits or falling out (seizure), runs (diarrhea), cleaning out (use of a laxative or an enema), and haven't moved (constipation). Every effort must be made to clarify terms and ensure that both you and the client understand the information communicated.

Effective questioning will provide the bulk of information derived during the interview. Plan questions well, in terms of both content and style. When you wish to collect concise, nonexplanatory information, *closed questions* are beneficial. Closed questions are direct and prompt short responses: "Where do you live?" "Did you get your prescription refilled?" "What are your sources of income?" These differ from *open-ended questions*, which encourage discussion and often yield information and insight into the client's thinking and behavior that you may have otherwise missed. Examples of open-ended questions include the following: "Tell me about how your neighbors bother you." "How would you describe your pain?" "What do you believe your problem is?" How you phrase the questions can also determine the accuracy and quality of information provided. By asking the question "Do you take laxatives often?" you may receive a negative response. However, by rephrasing the question to "How often do you take laxatives?" you may learn that the client uses laxatives two to three times a week. Perhaps the client did not think two to three times a week was often, or maybe the client answered according to what he or she thought was proper. Similarly, the question "Can you describe your eating habits to me?" will yield more information than "Do you eat well?" Carefully planned questions are crucial to meaningful data collection.

Listening is also an important assessment skill. Clues to problems may be woven among the threads of responses and comments. Statements such as "No, I don't have any money problems, my husband left me well off . . . but I sure am lonely without him" and "I took the bus here today because I gave up driving" can be accepted at face value or explored further to detect other messages they may be communicating.

Not only what is said, but how it is said is relevant. The client may respond that he or she is doing well but may say so in a manner conveying that he or she is not doing well at all. The client may respond in a tone inappropriate for the content. For example, the client may matter-of-factly state that her daughter is urging her to sell her home and enter a long-term care facility. The loudness of the client's voice can indicate many things, ranging from conviction of feeling about the topic to hearing deficits.

The interview can also serve to identify problems. You may note that, although the client denies a hearing deficit, he or she relies heavily on lip reading and doesn't consistently acknowledge verbal messages. The client may frequently cough and wheeze but tell you that he or she has no respiratory difficulties. The client may reveal specific memory deficits, such as forgetting the name of the clinic he is currently visiting, but may name the physician who operated on his leg during the war. Energy level, attention span, mental clarity, and physical mobility are among the many factors to assess during the interview.

At the close of the interview, you should summarize the experience, validate significant data, and state the next sequence of events that the client can expect. Provide ample time for the client to develop and ask questions.

You must recognize that more time is required to interview older adults than younger adults because of older adults' slower functioning, reduced energy levels, poorer memory, greater volume of problems, and longer history to review. Several interviews with the older adult may be necessary to compile a data base that you might otherwise achieve in one interview for a younger client.

Observation

Observation refers to the conscious, deliberate use of all the senses to gather information. Through skillful observation, you can obtain valuable data to enhance the assessment of your client. The experienced nurse learns to observe the client intentionally during every contact for clues to problems that may not be reported verbally.

Although it is not the sole means of observation, a visual evaluation of the client can yield important information (Figure 1-2). General appearance can reveal much about the client's self-concept, interest in and ability to carry out self-care, eccentricities, and cultural practices. Indications of health problems can be reflected in the client's coloring, breathing pattern, posture, and speed and freedom of body movements. Fidgeting and excessive activity can give clues to the client's anxiety, as well as to neurologic disorders, pain, and other problems. The client's comfort during the interview can be assessed through the degree of eye contact and other forms of body language.

Useful assessment data can also be derived from sounds. The voice's

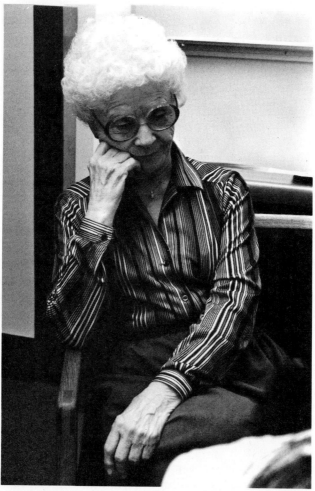

Figure 1-2
Just by visually inspecting the client, you can note physical findings that signal deterioration, improvement, or new revelations in the client's health status.

quality, loudness, and pitch can be altered by general health status and various sensory–motor disorders. You can hear indications of a dry oral cavity and poorly fitting dentures as the client speaks. You may also detect wheezes associated with respiratory disorders and gurgling arising from intestinal activity. Using the stethoscope, as described later in the chapter, can enhance these observations that are possible through your ears.

You can gain data when greeting the client with a handshake. By refusing to shake hands, the client may reveal depression, fear, or hostility. Or the client's cultural norms may dictate that physical contact between strangers (such as the client and the nurse) is highly improper. The grip of the handshake may also help you to detect weakness and musculoskeletal problems. You can derive a gross estimate of body temperature through touch. As you touch different areas of the client's body during the physical examination, you can identify edema, masses, inflammation, and other abnormalities.

You can assess a great deal through odors emitted from the client. Excessive use of cologne and perfume can be associated with the client's poor sense of smell; this is a common finding in the older adult and should raise concern over safety hazards resulting from the inability to smell gas leaks and smoke. The individual with poor olfactory function also may be unaware of body odors that are offensive to others. You should also recognize that foul body odor may not only be attributed to inadequate hygiene practices but may also be caused by systemic problems, such as anemia.

Breath odor is a significant health index as well. Poor oral hygiene, tobacco, certain foods, lung abscesses, and infections of the oral cavity may cause halitosis. A sweet, fruit-like breath odor usually results from increased acetone levels associated with diabetic acidosis. Uremic acidosis gives the breath an odor of stale urine; liver failure gives the breath a smell similar to newly mown clover. Of course, alcohol and other odorous substances yield distinctive odors attributed with their ingestion.

Be aware of other odors throughout the examination. Foul smelling nasal discharge may be due to sinusitis or to crusts or foreign objects blocking the nasal passage. Vaginal odors are often associated with vaginal infections or poor hygiene, and fecal odors may indicate abscesses, fistulas, wound infections, or poor hygienic practices. Although poor hygiene can contribute to foot odors, they can also be caused by fungal infections, which have a high incidence among older adults. Thus, through skillful use of your senses, you can identify many problems that the client has described or perhaps is not even aware of.

Physical Examination

Nurses, as well as physicians, are able to assess health through physical examination. Although your examination may not be as complex as the physician's, it can yield useful information beneficial to early problem recognition and the objective evaluation of care.

Physical examination consists of collecting data through inspection, auscultation, percussion, and palpation. These are defined as follows:

Inspection: Visualizing the body for normality of structure and function (Figure 1-2)

Auscultation: Using a stethoscope to hear sounds within the body (Figure 1-3)

Percussion: Determining the intensity, pitch, quality, and duration of sounds created by tapping the body surface (Figure 1-4)

Palpation: Touching and manipulating body parts for their size, temperature, texture, and mobility (Figure 1-5)

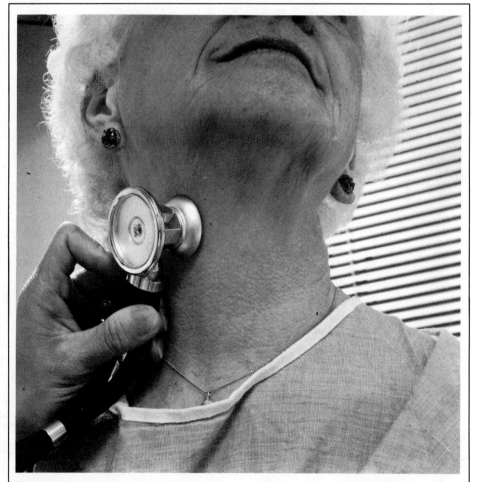

Figure 1-3
Use the bell portion of the stethoscope to perform auscultation of vascular sounds.

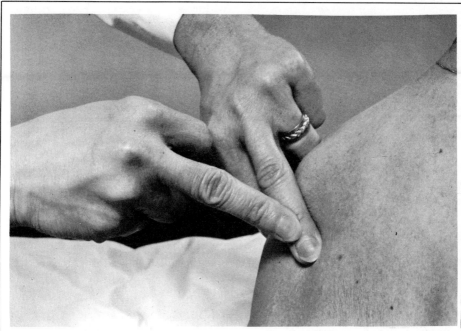

Figure 1-4
Proper position of the hands for percussion.

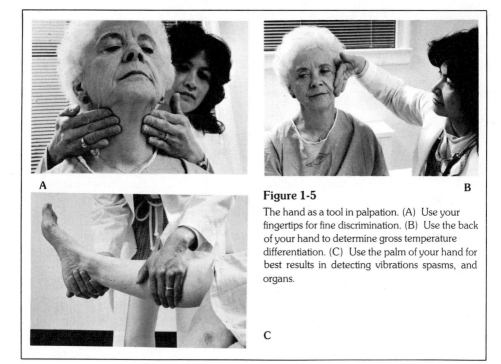

A

B

C

Figure 1-5
The hand as a tool in palpation. (A) Use your fingertips for fine discrimination. (B) Use the back of your hand to determine gross temperature differentiation. (C) Use the palm of your hand for best results in detecting vibrations spasms, and organs.

A more thorough review of these skills, as they apply to various body systems, will be provided throughout this book.

COLLABORATION

The nurse does not work in isolation. To understand completely the various facets of each individual, you must use multiple resources. For instance, when prescribing a special diet for a client, the physician should be aware of the following: the laboratory's evaluation of the client's blood chemistry; the social worker's determination of socioeconomic factors that will influence compliance to the prescribed diet; the nurse's assessment of the functional ability of the client to follow, ingest, and tolerate the diet; the pharmacist's impression of how the prescribed diet and prescribed medications will interact; and the family's judgment of how the prescribed diet will impose on family life. Of course, aides, occupational therapists, nutritionists, physical therapists, speech therapists, psychologists, and many other health team members, all with their unique insights into the client, may also have meaningful input into the plan for the client's special diet. Because of the great quantity and complexity of problems often identified in older adults, collaborative efforts by a diverse health team are essential to good care.

ORGANIZING DATA COLLECTION

The conscientious nurse understands that a large number of data must be collected to evaluate the client thoroughly and to direct effective care. These data, however, can be overwhelming and difficult to manage and use if not well organized. Unorganized data risk being excluded from care planning and delivery, thus creating a tremendous loss to both you and the client.

To ensure optimal use of data, you must record skillfully. Overall, you should document the assessment as concisely as possible. Short documentation can be difficult when the client is old and possesses a lengthy history and set of problems. Remember, however, that busy health team members lack the time to read through voluminous records. Selectivity must be employed in collecting and recording data (for example, unless relevant to current problems, it would not be necessary to review the older client's childhood diseases, friendships with classmates, courtships, and early sibling relationships).

The recorded data must be easily retrievable for all those who need to use it and therefore commands a logical organization of the assessment. A useful approach is to begin with a general profile of the client and progress to a more specific description of individual aspects of anatomy and function. You will find that employing a standard technique in collecting data will provide order to the assessment and reduce the potential for certain data being omitted.

A variety of assessment forms have been developed to serve as a guide for data collection and as a means of easy documentation. (Examples of some geriatric assessment tools are presented in Appendix A.) An effective and efficient assessment form not only considers the client's needs, but also the characteristics and needs of the agency using the form. A form that is ideal in one setting may be inappropriate in another. After reviewing a variety of existing assessment forms, you should select one that is appropriate for use, or design one if necessary. The following is a recommended framework for organizing the assessment with specific suggestions to help obtain the desired data.

Suggested Assessment Framework

Client Profile

Name	
Sex	
Race	
Date of birth	After asking date of birth, follow with a question such as "That makes you how old?" not only to validate data but to gain insight into short- and long-term memory capacity.
Address, telephone	It may be convenient to review some of the items under the Life-style section at this time.
Languages spoken	Under stressful conditions, bilingual persons may resort to their native tongue; thus, it is useful to know that language. Also, the client may be useful as an interpreter for others if this talent is identified.
Religion	Not only the religious category, but the specific name of the church or synagogue and relationship to it are useful. Often, religious organizations provide assistance to older adults that helps keep them functional in the community setting. Special diets and practices consistent with religious or cultural beliefs should be explored.
Education	Even more important than the client's formal education is the client's functional ability. Clues can be gained by asking questions such as "Do you read the daily papers?" "What type of reading do you enjoy?" "Was the insurance application difficult to understand?"

(Continued)

Contact person — A contact person may include next of kin or a significant other who may have more regular contact or live closer to the client.

Employment status — Determine if current employed or unemployed status is due to preference or necessity. Job history is useful for identifying occupation-related diseases, as well as for gaining insight into the client's talents and interests.

Budget — Determine all sources of income and expenses. Review a typical monthly budget to gain insight into priorities and financial management.

Health insurance — Obtain type and policy number.

Family Profile

Marital status — If the client has a spouse, ask about length of marriage, relationship, and spouse's age, health, and occupation. If widowed, discuss when death occurred, resulting life-style adjustments, and current feelings related to death.

Children — Obtain children's names, locations, and ages. The children's health status may yield insight into their dependency on or capacity to assist the client and give clues to familial diseases. Discussion of relationships with children can help determine the extent to which they serve as a resource or a problem for the client.

Support systems — Ask about relatives, friends, neighbors, or professionals who play a significant role in the client's life.

Coping ability — Discover how the client manages problems. It may be helpful to relate questions to real situations in the client's life, for example, "What do you do when your money runs out before the end of the month?" and "How do you manage when your husband has to be hospitalized?"

Life-style

Dwelling — Review the client's housing. Ask specifically about the age and construction of the

	building, number of levels the client uses for daily activities, number of stairs required to climb each day, presence of kitchen facilities, source of heat, location of bathroom, and number of persons sharing the entire dwelling and the client's bedroom. Determining the location of the nearest telephone and the nearest neighbor may be helpful. A discussion of the neighborhood should uncover information pertaining to the proximity of stores and services, and the real and perceived safety of the community.
Living arrangements	Explore the role and responsibilities of others who share the client's household or with whom the client lives. Information may be elicited through questions such as "Do you provide any assistance to your son's family in return for living with him?" and "What type of arrangement do you have with your cousin who shares your apartment?"
Household responsibilities	Review the typical tasks for which the client is responsible. It may be useful to review the pattern of activities for an entire day.
Pets	The companionship and stimulation provided by pets can be significant to an older client. Also, the client's contact with pets can give clues to the origin of specific problems, for example, asthma attacks, parasites, and skin breaks. Determine types of animals with which the client has contact, ability to care for a pet (physically and economically), and role of the pet in client's life.
Social/leisure activities	Ask about all forms of activities in which the client engages, formally or informally, actively or passively, and individually or in groups.
Significant relationships	Question as to who is a close friend or special person in the client's life and the nature of the relationship, for example, a neighbor with whom problems can be discussed or a pastor who visits weekly.

(Continued)

Ability to engage in activities of daily living (ADL)	There may be little correlation between the client's illness or disability and the degree to which routine functions can be accomplished. Ask about each specific ADL. For example, "Are you able to prepare your own meals?" or "How much help do you need getting dressed?"
Ethnic/religious practices	Review specific ethnic or religious practices that may affect activities, dress code, diet, relationships, and health care beliefs. Be aware that adherence to such practices may cause the client to refuse treatments and medications, to fast, to resort to complete bedrest for any illness, to wear garlic or pouches of herbs to cure problems, to dress in excessive clothing in even the warmest temperatures, or to demonstrate other behaviors and attitudes that may impact health status and care.
Typical day	Outline all the routines of the client, from morning to night. Be alert to uneven distribution of activities, length of time between meals, sleep and rest requirements, and routines unique to the client (for example, attending morning mass and drinking several beers at the corner bar after dinner). Explore if there has been any change from previous patterns.
Goals	Ask the client what he or she hopes to accomplish and what he or she feels is most important to preserve. Responses such as "To remain in my own home and not live with my children," "To get my illness under control so that I can visit my sister in Europe," and "To die naturally without using medications or machines" give insights that may assist in care planning and delivery.

Health history

Self-appraisal of health	Ask the client to give a statement of his or her perception of health status, for example, "Tell me your feelings or evaluation of your health." Explore how well the client understands existing health problems. The

correlation between perceived and real health status may give clues as to the need for education or explanations, acceptance or denial of health problems, potential compliance with care plan, and health expectations. The client should also be questioned for specific concerns related to health status.

Health practices	Discuss the client's measures to stay healthy, including diet, vitamins, exercise, regular check-ups, and adequate sleep. Find out how the client usually manages health problems (for example, goes directly to physician, self-medicates, prays). Also, explore the use of fads and unconventional practices.
Changes	In addition to asking about any general changes noted in physical or mental status, ask about specific changes in weight, bowel or bladder habits, appetite, sleep patterns, activity tolerance, pain, sexual function, cough, moles, memory, mood, and personality.
Allergies	Give the client specific clues to trigger memory of allergies: skin rashes or hives; nausea or vomiting; headaches; dizziness; fainting; and specific food, drug, material, plant, animal, or environmental allergies.
Known diseases	Ask the client what diseases or health problems he or she has, how, when, and by whom they were diagnosed, and the related treatment. It may be useful to name major illnesses to ensure that the client hasn't become so accustomed to having the illness that he or she no longer thinks of it as a prominent problem, for example, "Do you have any history of a heart problem, asthma, arthritis, hiatus hernia, diabetes, etc?"
Past problems	Obtain specific information pertaining to nature, cause, time, and outcome of past hospitalizations, surgeries, fractures, and extended health problems.

(Continued)

Resources used	List all health and social resources used, including nature and frequency of contact. This may be the time to obtain the client's written permissions for release of information from these other providers.
Health goals	Ask the client what he or she would like to accomplish in reference to health status. "Control my diabetes so that I can return to work," "Keep the fact that I'm diabetic from my friends and family," and "Find a drug or doctor to get rid of my diabetes" are very different client goals for a similar health problem and each requires a different primary intervention.

Medication History

Drugs used	List the names of all prescription and nonprescription drugs used, how, why, and where obtained, dosage prescribed and actually taken, how and when administered, client's knowledge and understanding of each medication, and side effects experienced. Medication allergies can again be explored at this time.

Physical Status

Temperature	State if obtained via oral, rectal, or axillary route.
Pulse	State if radial or apical and note regularity. Recognize that stress associated with an interview and an examination may cause a more rapid heart beat than may be normal for the client.
Respirations	Give rate, depth, and rhythm.
Height and weight	Describe current measurements and how they compare to earlier years.
Blood pressure	Obtain in sitting, standing, and lying positions. State which arm used.
Skin condition	Describe turgor, breaks, dryness, rashes, discoloration, wounds, moles, warts, scars, and unusual markings.
Hair condition	Describe cleanliness, grooming, texture, baldness, and scalp condition.

Nail condition	Describe apparent circulation, thickness, care, and signs of fungal infections.
Hygiene	Describe apparent cleanliness. Note frequency of baths and general hygienic practices.
Mobility	Note ability to ambulate, climb stairs, and transfer. Question as to specific limitations.
Extremities	Observe for pain, proper function, strength, spasms, and deformities.
Respiratory status	Ask questions pertaining to orthopnea, dyspnea, shortness of breath and cough, for example, "How many pillows do you sleep with?" and "How much can you do before getting short of breath?" Note characteristics of sputum.
Smoking history	Explore current and past practices. (The client may not smoke now but may reveal that she quit last year, after having smoked two packs of nonfiltered cigarettes for 35 years.)
Circulation	Note equality of pulses, skin temperature and color, chest pain, edema, dizziness, and cramping or pain in extremities. Ask specific questions, such as "Do your ring and shoes feel tight as the day goes on?" and "Do your legs begin to throb when you're standing or walking for a long time?"
Oral cavity	Observe for condition and number of teeth. If client is edentulous, ask how and when teeth were lost. If client has dentures, examine for fit and condition and ask how old they are. Examine gums and mucosa for color, moisture, lesions, and infections. Determine date of last dental examination and routine oral hygiene. Ask about ability to chew and swallow.
Digestion	Ask about specific problems, for example, "Do you ever have to use antacids?" or "Do you have difficulty digesting fried foods, large meals, vegetables?"
Usual meal pattern	List how and when the client eats, and the type and amount of food ingested.

(Continued)

Appetite	Ask about the client's appetite as compared to previous years and in relation to others. Review measures used by the client to stimulate or reduce appetite.
Food preferences and restrictions	Determine reasons for preferences and restrictions, for example, cultural or religious practices, affordability, preparation, taste, digestibility, interactions with medications, etc.
Alcohol use	Explore frequency, type, and amount of alcoholic beverages consumed.
Voiding pattern	Describe frequency, amount, and any problems associated with urination. Ask specifically about presence of and any factors associated with incontinence.
Urinary tract symptoms	Question specifically about hesitancy, burning, urgency, and hematuria.
Urine sample	Evaluate for specific gravity and presence of glucose and acetone. If necessary, collect a sample for microscopic examination.
Bowel elimination	Describe frequency, pattern, and characteristics of bowel movements. Question as to the use of laxatives, suppositories, and enemas. Explore if there have been any changes in characteristics of or pattern of bowel movements. Ask about the presence of and any factors associated with incontinence.
Hemorrhoids	Describe characteristics of and client's management of hemorrhoids.
Stool specimen	Note characteristics; perform guaiac test.
Ears	Question as to discharge, tinnitus, and earaches. Examine for cerumen impaction. Describe existing hearing problems. If hearing aid is used, determine how, why, when, and where it was obtained. Note the date of the last audiometric examination.
Eyes	Note symmetry, pupil reaction, discharge, irritation, movement, and lacrimation. Evaluate general sight, depth perception, and color, night, and peripheral vision. If

	corrective lenses are used, determine how, why, when, and where they were obtained. Note the date of last ophthalmologic examination.
Nose	Examine for patency, irritation, discharge, and olfaction.
Speech	Describe clarity, organization, tone, and any apparent disorders.
Sensation	Evaluate client's ability to detect pressure, pain, and temperature differences.
Sleep pattern	Ascertain client's bed time and rising time. Describe sleep pattern and ask about specific interruptions to sleep, for example, "How many times do you go to the bathroom during the night?" and "Are you ever awakened from sleep due to breathing difficulties, your spouse, leg cramps, hunger, hot flushes, etc?" Determine if any sleep inducers are used, for example, drugs or alcohol.
Naps	Describe number, length, and pattern of naps.
Genitalia	Examine for general condition, discharges, lesions, and masses. Note date of last gynecologic or prostatic examination.
Breasts	Examine for masses, discharge, and pain. Evaluate client's knowledge and regular performance of self-examination of the breasts.
Sexual history	Inquire about sexual interest, function, problems, and perceptions.
Physical problems	Describe real and perceived limitations resulting from physical problems. Also, ask client how he or she manages and copes with physical problems.

Mental Status

Consciousness	Describe level of consciousness and orientation to person, place, and time.
Affect	Describe the client's emotional tone.
Memory	Evaluate long- and short-term memory. Pose

(Continued)

	questions such as the following. "Do you remember the name of the physician I mentioned earlier?", "Do you easily forget things?", and "What do you remember best, events that occurred within the past few days or events that occurred long ago?"
Personality	State your impression of the client's personality. Ask the client if there has been any personality change noticed by self or others.
Response and reaction time	Describe unusual delays, for example, "Client took 30 seconds to state his name and took longer to answer other questions."
Emotional status	Describe how client appears to you, for example, depressed, anxious, suspicious, etc. Also, ask client for his or her self-perception.
Mental health history	Ask the client if he or she has ever had a mental illness or mental hospital admission. Elicit the client's perspective on his or her mental health history. Ask if client has ever thought about suicide.
Self-concept	Note how the client presents and feels about himself or herself. Ask specifically, "What do you think of yourself?" and "What kind of person do you believe yourself to be?"
Coping ability	Ask the client how crises and daily problems are managed, for example, "How do you deal with your children's problems?" and "What do you do when several problems confront you at once?"
Mental problems	Describe real and perceived limitations resulting from problems.

Other Data

Describe any other significant information.

Chapter 16 provides a case example of an assessment conducted with an older adult. The key elements of a good assessment are accuracy, organization, and completeness. The crucial role that proper documentation plays, not only in facilitating good care, but in licensure and accreditation of the facility, reimbursement for services, and legal liability cannot be overstated.

The documented assessment, like all parts of the client's record, is confidential information. Although the agency providing care to the client can appropriately regard the record as its property, the client has the legal right to the information within the record and to determine who shall have access to that information. As helpful and benign as it may seem, you should not share the contents of the client's record with other health care agencies, employers, or family members without the client's permission. The agency and the individual provider can be held liable if client information is not kept confidential.

NURSING DIAGNOSIS

The purpose of the assessment is not to collect a thorough description of the client so that the pages of a chart can be filled, but rather to learn the unique capacities and limitations of the client so that effective, individualized nursing care can be delivered. In order for the data collected during the assessment process to be translated into care planning and delivery, it must be analyzed, sorted, and clearly defined. For instance, a client may have a poor appetite. By analyzing all the collected data, you may be able to ascertain that this poor appetite is related to decayed teeth or inflamed gums. Knowing the etiology certainly gives clearer direction to the intervention required by the client. The process used to analyze and define assessed problems is that of nursing diagnosis. This process bridges the collected client data with nursing care. It is used to identify problems or conditions (altered health states) that could benefit from nursing intervention. It is a "statement of a potential or actual altered health status of a client which is derived from nursing assessment and which requires intervention from the domain of nursing" (Carlson et al 1982).

Each professional member of the health team will use a diagnostic process in analyzing data to plan care strategies. In fact, several disciplines may interpret and treat the same diagnosis in different ways. For example, a client may be demonstrating depression related to the physical limitations imposed by arthritis. The physician may treat this problem with an antidepressant medication; the social worker may plan to increase opportunities for socialization; and the nurse may intervene by instructing the client in alternative self-care methods. This is not to imply that different disciplines couldn't perceive a problem in a similar fashion. They could, and it is quite appropriate for all to employ a similar treatment plan. However, it should be remembered that nursing diagnoses are those problems or conditions that can benefit from *nursing* intervention; to tread on areas beyond the scope of nursing would be professionally inappropriate.

The term nursing diagnosis has gained popularity in recent years, although it was coined in the early 1950s. Interest in nursing diagnosis was renewed in 1973 when the American Nurses' Association published *Standards of Nursing Practice*, which emphasized the importance of nursing diagnosis in professional nursing care. That same year, the first National Conference on the Classification of Nursing Diagnoses was held to develop a list of health problems that appropriately fell within the realm of nursing practice. Future national conferences refined and expanded this list of acceptable nursing diagnoses (Table 1-1). Numerous articles, books, conferences, research activities, and a national clearinghouse exist specifically for nursing diagnoses. These efforts have clarified what constitutes nursing practice and identified independent nursing actions that go beyond the realm of "following physicians' orders." The terminology used in nursing diagnosis clearly defines the problem and enables nurses to communicate in a specific, standardized manner. Less confusion exists regarding what the nursing action is addressing, so care can be specific to the client's particular problem. Such specificity will

Table 1-1 NANDA Approved Nursing Diagnostic Categories

PATTERN 1: EXCHANGING

Altered nutrition: more than body requirements
Altered nutrition: less than body requirements
Altered nutrition: potential for more than body requirements
Potential for infection
Potential altered body temperature
Hypothermia
Hyperthermia
Ineffective thermoregulation
Dysreflexia
Constipation
Perceived constipation
Colonic constipation
Diarrhea
Bowel incontinence
Altered patterns of urinary elimination
Stress incontinence
Reflex incontinence
Urge incontinence
Functional incontinence
Total incontinence
Urinary retention
Altered (specify type) tissue perfusion (renal, cerebral, cardiopulmonary, gastro-intestinal, peripheral)

Table 1-1 (*Continued*)

Fluid volume excess
Fluid volume deficit
Potential fluid volume deficit
Decreased cardiac output
Impaired gas exchange
Ineffective airway clearance
Ineffective breathing pattern
Potential for injury
Potential for suffocation
Potential for poisoning
Potential for trauma
Potential for aspiration
Potential for disuse syndrome
Impaired tissue integrity
Altered oral mucous membrane
Impaired skin integrity
Potential impaired skin integrity

PATTERN 2: COMMUNICATING

Impaired verbal communication

PATTERN 3: RELATING

Impaired social interaction
Social isolation
Altered role performance
Altered parenting
Potential altered parenting
Sexual dysfunction
Altered family processes
Parental role conflict
Altered sexual patterns

PATTERN 4: VALUING

Spiritual distress (distress of the human spirit)

PATTERN 5: CHOOSING

Ineffective individual coping
Impaired adjustment
Defensive coping
Ineffective denial
Ineffective family coping: disabling
Ineffective family coping: compromised
Family coping: potential for growth
Noncompliance (specify)
Decisional conflict (specify)
Health seeking behaviors (specify)

Table 1-1 *(Continued)*

PATTERN 6: MOVING

Impaired physical mobility
Activity intolerance
Fatigue
Potential activity intolerance
Sleep pattern disturbance
Diversional activity deficit
Impaired home maintenance management
Altered health maintenance
Feeding self care deficit
Impaired swallowing
Ineffective breastfeeding
Bathing/hygiene self care deficit
Dressing/grooming self care deficit
Toileting self care deficit
Altered growth and development

PATTERN 7: PERCEIVING

Body image disturbance
Self esteem disturbance
Chronic low self esteem
Situational low self esteem
Personal identity disturbance
Sensory/perceptual alterations (specify) (visual, auditory, kinesthetic, gustatory, tactile, olfactory)
Unilateral neglect
Hopelessness
Powerlessness

PATTERN 8: KNOWING

Knowledge deficit (specify)
Altered thought processes

PATTERN 9: FEELING

Pain
Chronic pain
Dysfunctional grieving
Anticipatory grieving
Potential for violence: self-directed or directed at others
Post-trauma response
Rape-trauma syndrome
Rape-trauma syndrome: compound reaction
Rape-trauma syndrome: silent reaction
Anxiety
Fear

---

increase nursing's accountability for its practice and demonstrate nursing's unique contribution to the client's care. Nursing diagnoses can also provide a more refined basis for theory and research development that will enhance a *science* of nursing. Many benefits to clients, nurses, and the nursing profession as a whole can be derived through nursing diagnosis.

Nursing diagnosis is a process requiring considerable knowledge and problem-solving capabilities. Several intellectual processes are necessary to derive a nursing diagnosis. First, keen assessment skills are required to gather a range of data on the individual client. From the wealth of information collected, relevant data is sorted out. Patterns or related data are grouped and then analyzed. Problems or potential problems can be identified after this analysis to form nursing diagnoses. Numerous diagnoses may be present and must be prioritized realistically. (Prioritization should be done with respect to both the urgency of need for intervention and the risks associated with not intervening immediately.) Diagnostic-specific interventions are developed and implemented. Most experienced professional nurses progress through these stages automatically, using advanced cognitive and psychomotor skills to deliver individualized care efficiently and effectively.

A nursing diagnosis describes a set of signs and symptoms that nurses are prepared and licensed to treat, such as potential footdrop related to bedrest. A problem, not a need, is described by the nursing diagnosis, and the problem can indicate an actual or *potential* health problem. A nursing diagnosis differs from a medical diagnosis, which demands medical intervention. Of course there are areas of overlap, such as obesity, in which a problem can be successfully managed by either nursing or medicine.

To formulate a nursing diagnosis note the problems, signs, or symptoms of the client that can benefit from nursing intervention and are within the realm of nursing practice to independently manage, such as:

- Inability to feed self
- Inability to self-inject insulin
- Confusion, disorientation
- Fatigue

Next, review the list of nursing diagnoses for the diagnostic term that best describes the problem, sign, or symptom:

- Feeding self-care deficit
- Knowledge deficit
- Altered thought processes
- Activity intolerance

To complete the full diagnostic statement identify the cause or contributing factor to the problem and link it to the stem of the diagnosis using the term "related to," for example:

- Feeding self care deficit related to cognitive inability to know what to do with food
- Knowledge deficit related to new requirement of having to self inject insulin
- Altered thought processes related to Alzheimer's disease
- Activity intolerance related to effects of cardiac disease

Skill in writing nursing diagnoses comes with experience. However, there are some common pitfalls, such as the following, that you should be careful to avoid as you learn to use nursing diagnoses:

1. *Stating the diagnosis in medical terms.* Sick sinus syndrome, rheumatoid arthritis, and chronic renal failure may be legitimate diagnoses of the client, but they are medical, not nursing diagnoses. Anxiety related to newly diagnosed sick sinus syndrome, hygiene self care deficit related to limitations imposed by arthritic hands, and dysfunctional grieving related to prognosis for chronic renal failure express the client's diagnoses in nursing terms and give specific direction to nursing actions.

2. *Making the diagnosis too broad.* The diagnosis should describe the factors contributing to the problem as specifically as possible. For example, disturbance of body image related to loss of teeth communicates significantly more information than poor body image related to losses.

3. *Combining unrelated problems.* For efficiency, you may mistakenly attempt to join two problems that seem to have similar outcomes. Body image disturbance and grieving related to losses is an inappropriate diagnosis if the loss causing the disturbance in body image is hair, and the loss causing the grief is death of a spouse.

4. *Using unnecessarily complex terminology.* Avoid jargon and sophisticated-sounding phrases. Aim for effective communication of the problem, not demonstration of your eloquence. The diagnosis should be clear enough to be easily understood.

5. *Including value judgments or legally troublesome terms.* Nursing diagnoses are part of the client's record, and that record is a legal document. Opinions, accusations, and moral judgments have no place in the diagnostic statement. Avoid diagnoses such as hygiene self care deficit related to insufficient nursing care, and diversional activity deficit related to lazy disposition.

6. *Describing the nursing intervention rather than the client's problem.* You may be tempted to identify the act you will need to perform

rather than the problem the client presents, for instance, protocol II wound care related to skin breakdown or need for increased socialization at meal time related to anorexia. The diagnosis should describe the *client's* problem and the factor that contributes to the problem. After this information is provided, nursing plans can then be developed specific to the problem and its unique contributing factors.

Each chapter's summary section ends with a list of nursing diagnoses associated with the area being assessed. These can be used to stimulate thinking about diagnoses applicable to individual clients. To these diagnostic stems the unique causes or contributing factors discovered in the individual client can be added. For example, the diagnosis "sexual dysfunction" can be related to a variety of factors, including poor self-concept, impotency secondary to antihypertensive medication, dry vaginal canal, fear of causing another heart attack, or institutionalization of spouse. You will discover that by specifically identifying the cause or contributing factor to which the diagnosis is related, the necessary nursing actions will more easily surface.

Using published nursing diagnoses may be helpful because they are universal, and they eliminate having to develop your own. However, these diagnoses may not be individualized enough to reflect the unique problems associated with a specific client. You may find published diagnoses useful as a general guide but should not feel prohibited from developing diagnoses that best describe an individual client. Clearly defined nursing diagnoses form a strong foundation for effective, competent professional care.

READINGS AND REFERENCES

Agan RD. Intuitive knowing as a dimension of nursing. *ANS* October 1987; 10(1):63–70.

Bates B. *A Guide to Physical Examination*, 4th ed. Philadelphia: Lippincott, 1987.

Campbell C. *Nursing Diagnosis and Intervention in Nursing Practice*. New York: Wiley, 1978.

Carlson JH, Croft CA, McGuire AD. *Nursing Diagnosis*. Philadelphia: Saunders, 1982.

Carotenuto R, Bullock J. *Physical Assessment of the Gerontologic Client*. Philadelphia: Davis, 1981.

Carpenito LJ. *Nursing Diagnosis: Application to Clinical Practice*, 2nd ed. Philadelphia: Lippincott, 1987.

Eggland ET. How to take a meaningful nursing history. *Nursing 77* July 1977; 7(7):22–30.

Eliopoulos C. *A Guide to the Nursing of the Aging*. Baltimore: Williams and Wilkens, 1987.

Gotto AM Jr. The family history in health care evaluation. *Health Values*. March/April 1987; 11(2):25–29.

Hillman R. *Clinical Skills: Interviewing, History Taking, and Physical Diagnosis.* New York: McGraw-Hill, 1981.

Lindsley JM. Guidelines for nursing diagnosis . . . medical record documentation. *Nursing Homes* January/February 1987; 36(1):42–44.

Malasanos L et al. *Health Assessment,* 3rd ed. St. Louis: Mosby, 1986.

McVan B. What the nose knows—odors. *Nursing 77* April 1977; 7(4):46–49.

Reichel W (editor). *Clinical Aspects of Aging,* 2nd ed. Baltimore: Williams and Wilkens, 1983.

Rogers JC. Advocacy: The key to assessing the older client. *Journal of Gerontological Nursing* January 1980; 6:33–36.

Seidel H et al. *Mosby's Guide to Physical Examination.* St. Louis: Mosby, 1987.

Steel K. Evaluation of the geriatric patient. In: *Clinical Aspects of Aging,* 2nd ed. Reichel W (editor). Baltimore: Williams and Wilkens, 1983.

Tanner CA et al. Diagnostic reasoning strategies of nurses and nursing students. *Nursing Research* November/December 1987; 36(6):358–363.

Wolanin MO, Phillips LRP. *Confusion.* St. Louis: Mosby, 1981.

2 Assessment of Social Function

Jamie Caplis, BA, MS

PURPOSE OF SOCIAL ASSESSMENT

A social assessment should be an integral component of any comprehensive assessment of an older adult. Since you can only obtain accurate diagnoses by evaluating the "total" individual, that is, the client's social situation as well as physical and mental health, you must use a multidisciplinary assessment tool. Only through careful completion of such assessments can you develop effective and appropriate treatment plans.

The interrelationship of physical health, mental health, and social situation is particularly evident in the older adult. For example, an older adult may be severely arthritic (physical condition) causing depression (mental state) and isolation from friends and the community (social problem). The arthritic condition may limit mobility as well as ability to use regular modes of transportation. An effective social assessment will evaluate the individual's degree of autonomy and independence. This consideration is particularly important for older adults because aging usually implies increased dependency on family and local support services. Living on a limited income may also prohibit the older adult from using more costly and/or specialized transportation. Furthermore, arthritis makes the older adult an easy target for crime, particularly if the person lives in an urban environment. All of these factors reduce opportunities for socialization, and thus contribute to loneliness and isolation.

On completion of a comprehensive assessment, the older adult's needs will become evident. The treatment plan should include all physical health, mental health, and social service resources necessary to minimize the individual's deficits while simultaneously maximizing his or her capabilities. Your ability to accomplish this task effectively will enhance the older adult's quality of life.

BACKGROUND ON PSYCHOSOCIAL ASSESSMENT

Demographic analyses indicate a tremendous surge in the number of older American citizens: persons 65 and older represent 11% of the population (US Bureau of Census 1986). Studies reveal that not only is the number of older adults growing faster than any other age group, but within the older population two new subgroups are emerging—the "young old" and the "old old." Persons generally considered to be members of the younger group are 55 to 74 years of age and are relatively healthy, active individuals. Persons considered to be members of the "old old" group are generally 75 and over and are more likely to be infirm and socially confined.

The growth in number of older adults and in projections for the future have grave social implications in terms of quality of life. Advanced medical technology, enabling more persons to live longer, having the option of retirement, and other factors may cause more persons to live a greater portion of their lives in retirement. This will necessitate new approaches to coping with the social problems inherent in a nonworking existence.

As people age, they experience various psychosocial changes. The impact of such changes on life-style depends on the individual's flexibility and coping mechanisms. "Old age" can be characterized as a period of gains and losses. The advantages of living longer can be seen in the new freedoms the individual experiences. Suddenly persons are free from homemaking and child-rearing responsibilities. Through retirement, many persons are free from an intolerable job situation. With this freedom, persons can travel and explore talents, interests, and hobbies that they were before unable to pursue. Newly found leisure encourages one to become creative, to go back to school, to begin a second career, or to volunteer to help others. As persons age, however, they also experience many personal losses (Table 2-1). Retirement results in decreased income, making it difficult for individuals to cover the rising costs of such essentials as food, clothing, medical care, and transportation. Furthermore, the effect of reduced purchasing power, combined with the impact of inflation, makes it increasingly difficult for older adults to pursue leisure activities.

In addition to the financial consequences of retirement, the individual often undergoes various psychologic changes. If not properly prepared, many persons have difficulty adjusting to a life without work.

On retirement, the person ceases to perform a professional working role. Since many persons view their work as a central life task and source of self-

Table 2-1 Personal Losses Prompted by Change in Age

50–65	65–75	75–85	85+
Begin to prepare for retirement; children leave household	Loss of job, spouse, friends, income, and some body image	Increased loss of sensory activity, health, strength, and independence	Serious loss of health and independence

Source: Pastalan and Carson, 1970, as adapted by Regnier. In: *Aging: Scientific Perspectives and Social Issues.* Woodruff and Birren (editors). New York: Van Nostrand Reinhold, 1975, p 298.

identity, it is easy to comprehend the retiree's reduced self-image. No longer the provider and no longer associating daily with co-workers (often a main source of friendships), the individual may experience a loss of social and occupational status. If working previously fulfilled needs for prestige, recognition, achievement, competition, and belonging, retirement may leave these needs largely unmet.

For the poorly adjusted retiree, the loss of a daily employment routine results in a loss of "order" to life. Older adults may also have difficulty accepting their new retirement status since it negates the prevailing work ethic that measures persons according to the work they produce. The work ethic further influences the retiree's ability to enjoy his or her leisure since society has not yet accepted the pursuit of leisure interests as a legitimate use of time.

In addition to the losses associated with retirement, other changes are experienced that may profoundly affect the individual's life-style. Aside from the obvious physiologic and psychologic impact of poor health, illness limits an individual's psychosocial world. As a result of sickness, the ability to interact with others becomes limited because of effects on personal stamina, social activity, and mobility. Furthermore, body image (physical strength, appearance, and performance) may become more negative as illness and disability increase. This may cause the individual to retreat from his or her social world, thus compounding feelings of isolation and loneliness.

As people age, the family structure is likely to change. When both spouses retire, the husband-and-wife relationship is altered due to the unaccustomed quantity of time together. Resentment may develop if either spouse believes the other partner is invading his or her special realm of activities. Retirement, therefore, necessitates a major readjustment in marital relationships. The domestic situation is further strained if one partner becomes ill. Under such circumstances, the healthy spouse is forced to take on the added responsibility of caretaker. Again resentment may develop between the spouses, further complicating the marital relationship. The death of a spouse also requires a major readjustment for the surviving spouse. Widowhood is a role for which there is no adequate emotional preparation.

Older persons also experience a change in relationship with their adult offspring. Traditionally called on for advice and guidance, the older person may no longer be sought for help by the children. When illness strikes the older adult, the family may become emotionally as well as financially drained. The once independent, self-sufficient parent may become dependent on others in terms of decision making and daily care.

The losses and gains experienced by older adults may result in various role changes. Specifically, older adults may experience such transformations as from worker to retiree, from independent to dependent person, from married person to widow or widower, from healthy to ill or disabled individual, and from socially active to lonely and isolated person.

The role changes experienced by the older adult require orientation to the individual's psychosocial environment. The degree to which the individual is flexible and can cope with the role realignments will determine the success with which problems are averted and social behavior is positively influenced.

SOCIAL ASSESSMENT

Role changes, resulting from the older adult's losses or gains, have tremendous effects on his or her life-style (see Table 2-2). You are responsible for determining the impact of these changes on the everyday affairs of the older

Table 2-2 Age-related Environmental Changes and Personal Losses

50–65	65–75	75–85	85+
Loss of relationships to younger friends and acquaintances of children. Loss of neighborhood role to schools and youth. Home is too large, but mortgage payments are low and equity high.	Loss in relation to work environment. Loss of mobility due to lessened income. Dissolving of professional work associations and friendships. Move to apartment, smaller home, or struggle with increased maintenance costs of larger home.	Loss of ability to drive independently. Must rely on bus or relatives and friends. Connections with community associations slowly severed. Move to more supportive housing, such as apartments with meals and maid service. Maintenance costs for single-family house unmanageable.	Loss of abilities to navigate in the environment. Loss of strong connections with outside neighborhood. Dependence on supportive services. Move to supportive environment necessary, such as nursing home, home for the aged, or siblings' home.

Source: National Center for Housing Management, 1974, as adapted by Regnier. In: *Aging: Scientific Perspectives and Social Issues.* Woodruff and Birren (editors). New York: Van Nostrand Reinhold, 1974, p 299.

adult. The purpose of the social assessment is to determine the individual's competence in his or her social world.

In addition to obtaining the name, address, and phone number of the individual, you should inquire about the person's age, marital status, and whether the individual has Medicare, Medical Assistance, or other third-party insurance. You should also request the name, address, and phone number of the next of kin or other "caring" person who might play a role in the treatment plan. Finally, ascertain whether the individual has had previous contact with other health and social service agencies. This information is important because the treatment plan may refer the individual to the original agency for further assistance, thus eliminating the need to open a new case with another agency.

ECONOMIC WELFARE

To assess the older adult's financial status, you must determine whether the older adult is receiving all entitled financial and social benefits. Accomplish this by asking the approximate amount of monthly or annual income obtained from such sources as social security, supplemental security income, Veterans Administration, public and/or private pensions, and investments. Inquiring whether the individual receives food stamps or other forms of government assistance (such as rent subsidy or welfare) also will determine the individual's financial status.

Another mode of questioning to assess the older adult's financial status is to inquire whether or not (a) assets and financial resources are sufficient to meet emergencies; (b) expenses are so heavy that he or she cannot meet or can barely meet payments; (c) the financial situation is such that additional assistance is needed; (d) the individual feels he or she has enough for future needs (Pfeiffer 1975a).

ENVIRONMENTAL ISSUES

An examination of the environment is critical to understanding the social behavior of the older adult. Because physical losses often accompany old age, the individual's environment should allow him or her to feel safe and secure. In an assessment of the environment, necessary subjects to inquire about include the following: (a) the older adult's living arrangements, (b) the residence, (c) the individual's proximity and/or access to essential services, and (d) the safety of the neighborhood. The responses to these questions will indicate how the environment affects the older adult's social functioning. Specific problem areas that affect the individual's quality of life may be revealed.

You must inquire about the older adult's current living situation and determine whether the individual lives in a room, regular apartment house, foster care home, senior citizen apartment, domiciliary care facility, sheltered or congregate housing, and/or long-term care facility. Inquiries as to whether the individual lives alone, with a spouse, relatives, and/or friends are important. If the older adult lives with someone, you should ask whether that person could care for the individual if necessary. This information enables you to determine whether a social support system is immediately available.

You should pose certain key questions to determine whether the individual's physical residence is conducive to maintaining independent living. Although a home visit is probably the best method for assessing the physical environment, any assessment must address the following:

1. Proximity of neighboring homes
2. General condition of the home
3. Need to climb stairs to enter the home and manage within the home
4. Availability and location of a bathroom, kitchen, and bedroom
5. Availability of a telephone
6. Presence of unstable furniture, scatter rugs, or other potential safety hazards
7. Room, hall, and doorway accommodations for wheelchairs, walkers, or other special equipment if necessary

Closely related to the condition of the physical residence is the home's proximity to essential services. The older adult's access to transportation, food and drug stores, medical care, laundry services, restaurants, neighbors, churches, banks, libraries, and social centers will, in large measure, determine his or her social realm. An inability to participate in these functions because of their locations may cause loneliness and isolation for the older adult. Therefore, you should inquire whether these services are in close proximity and what mode of transportation is used to and from the destination (walking, public transportation, cabs, specialized transportation, friends, and/or family). You should also ask about the frequency of visits, for example, how many times a week the visit is made.

Finally, in assessing the older adult's environment, pose questions concerning the security of the area in which the person is living. All too often older adults become prisoners in their own home for fear of becoming victims of criminal attacks. This fear factor tremendously limits social participation. You should elicit whether fear of crime is a problem for the older adult and if the individual is aware of crime prevention education programs available in the area.

HEALTH ISSUES

As previously stated, the older adult's physical and mental condition affects the ability to participate in the social world. In order to develop a treatment plan aimed at minimizing these problems, discover which daily functions are hindered by the individual's physical and mental status.

In determining the older adult's ability to perform daily functions, you may wish to develop a scale for evaluation. For example, evaluations may be made based on the following performance scale: performs independently, needs minor assistance, needs moderate assistance, needs extensive assistance, or cannot perform regardless of assistance.

Specifically, you should provide a functional evaluation of the individual that includes such areas as the ability to see, hear, speak, ambulate, toilet self, bathe, groom, dress, and feed self. The responses to these questions indicate the individual's capacity for physical self-maintenance. These responses will also direct you to include in the treatment plan all support necessary to enable the individual to remain successfully in his or her home.

In addition to obtaining a functional assessment at the physical level, you should evaluate the impact of physical and mental status on the ability to perform activities of daily living. Again, a scale should be used to determine the degree to which these activities are affected. The areas to be investigated include the ability to prepare meals, perform housekeeping, do laundry, use the telephone, take medications, handle finances, travel, shop, write, and read. It is important to ascertain the level of functioning in these areas because the treatment plan might include, for example, escort and chore aides to alleviate some of these problems. Again, the ability to coordinate and implement community resources vis-à-vis the treatment plan will enhance the older adult's quality of life.

SOCIAL/RECREATIONAL FUNCTIONING

The ability to function in the social/recreational world is largely determined and influenced by the older adult's economic, housing, transportation, physical safety, and health status. Any assessment of social/recreational interaction, however, must also include an examination of the individual's "life space," the environment over which he or she has control. It is important to note the effect of role changes (for example, from married person to widow(er) or from worker to retiree) on an individual's social world as part of this process.

The essential key to assessing social/recreational functioning is determining the amount and frequency of social participation. You should develop a form that lists all activities and the frequency with which each is performed. Specifically, the list should include the following: shopping, performing chores, reading, watching the television, listening to the radio, engaging in one's hobby, writing, visiting, walking, riding, traveling, as well as attending sporting events, church activities, senior centers, the library, meetings, movies, or theater.

In order to determine further the level of social activity, inquire about (a) the number of people the individual knows well enough to visit in their homes, (b) the number of times the individual talked on the phone in the past week, and (c) the number of times during the past week the individual engaged in an activity with someone who did not live in the same house (Pfeiffer 1975b).

Additionally, you should ask what prohibits the individual from more active participation. The responses should indicate what social intervention should be included in the treatment plan. For example, if transportation cost is a key factor, the plan might include the provision of a reduced fare transit card. Similarly, if lack of motivation is the cause of inactivity, counseling may be necessary.

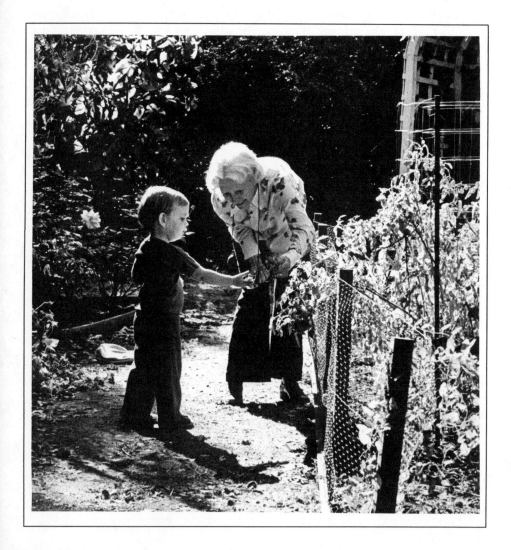

Also included as part of an individual's social functioning is the ability to handle his or her administrative, financial, legal, and protective affairs. To determine the performance level in these areas, inquire whether the individual takes complete responsibility for these matters, needs little assistance, much assistance, or cannot take care of them at all.

Finally, a comprehensive assessment of social status should include a statement from the older adult as to his or her perceived problems and needs. The older adult's description, plus your own observations, should provide enough information to develop an appropriate treatment plan.

As mentioned, the purpose of a social assessment is to determine the individual's degree of autonomy and independence. Many times the evaluation will reveal a particular problem for which there is help. Consequently, you must be knowledgeable enough about community resources to incorporate them into the treatment plan. In order to enhance the quality of life, you must recognize the older adult's needs. The gap between health and social services must be bridged if the person is to receive the best possible care.

2 Chapter Summary

I. Age-related changes
  A. More time spent in retirement
    1. Reduced income
    2. Loss of social and occupational status
    3. Reduced self-image
    4. Isolation from former co-workers
    5. Loss of daily, structured routine
    6. Difficulty accepting leisure time in presence of prevailing work ethic
  B. Altered family structure
    1. Readjustment in marital relationship
    2. Potential widowhood
    3. Increased dependence on adult offspring
  C. Limited social activity and mobility due to poor health
    1. Possible altered life-style due to physical strength, appearance, and performance
    2. Potential disengagement

II. Assessment
  A. Purpose: to determine competence of individual in his or her social world
  B. Preliminary identifying information
    1. Name
    2. Address
    3. Telephone number
    4. Age
    5. Marital status
    6. Insurance
    7. Name, address, and phone number of contact person
    8. Previous contact with health and social service agencies
  C. Economic welfare
    1. Financial and social benefits
    2. Income

3. Assets
4. Expenses
D. Environmental issues
1. Living arrangements
2. Physical residence
3. Proximity and access to essential services
4. Physical safety of neighborhood
E. Health issues
1. Capacity for self-maintenance
2. Physical and mental status
3. Level of functioning
F. Social/recreational functioning
1. Impact of economy, housing, transportation, physical safety, and health status
2. Life space
3. Amount and frequency of social participation
4. Activities
5. Number and frequency of contacts with others
6. Factors prohibiting active participation
7. Ability to manage administrative, financial, legal, and protective affairs
G. Perceived problems and needs
III. Disorders and problems
A. Isolation
B. Loneliness
C. Loss of purpose
D. Limited finances
E. Poor acceptance of retirement
F. Inability to enjoy leisure
G. Negative body image and self-concept
H. Disengagement
I. Marital problems
J. Widowhood
K. Increased dependency
L. Shrinking social world
M. Decreased ability to manage financial, legal, and protective affairs
IV. Related nursing diagnoses
A. Anxiety
B. Impaired verbal communication
C. Ineffective individual coping
D. Ineffective family coping
E. Diversional activity deficit
F. Altered family processes
G. Fear
H. Grieving
I. Impaired home maintenance management
J. Knowledge deficit
K. Noncompliance
L. Powerlessness
M. Personal identity disturbance
N. Impaired social interaction
O. Social isolation
P. Spiritual distress
Q. Potential for violence

READINGS AND REFERENCES

Barckley V. How to eat on $1.18 per day . . . an elderly woman who was living below the poverty level. *Geriatric Nursing* May/June 1980; 1:50–51.

Brock AM. From wife to widowhood: A changing life style. *Journal of Gerontological Nursing* 1984; 10(4):8–15.

Brower HT. Social organization and nurses' attitudes towards older perons. *Journal of Gerontological Nursing* May 1981; 7(5):293–298.

Cassels CS, Eckstein AM, Fortinosh KM. Retirement aspects response and nursing implications. *Journal of Gerontological Nursing* June 1981; 7(6):355–359.

Dobrof R (editor). *Gerontological Social Work with Families*. New York: Haworth Press, 1987.

Gelein JL. The aged American female: Relationships between social support and health. *Journal of Gerontological Nursing* February 1980; 6:69–73.

George LK. *Role Transitions in Later Life*. Monterey, CA: Brooks/Cole Publishers, 1980.

Lee GT et al. Societal literacy and the status of the aged. *International Journal of Aging and Human Development* 1980–1981; 12(3):221–234.

Lohmann N. A factor analysis of life satisfaction, adjustment and morale measures with elderly adults. *International Journal of Aging and Human Development* 1980; 11(1):35–43.

Mauksch IG. Transportation. How do senior citizens get around? *Geriatric Nursing* July/August 1980; 1:136–137.

Pfeiffer E (editor). Multidimensional functional assessment: The OARS Methodology. Durham: Duke University, Center for the Study of Aging and Human Development, 1975. (a) adapted from questions 21, 22, 23, 24, and 30; (b) adapted from questions 8, 9, 10.

Rauckhorst LM, Stokes SA, Mezey MD. Community and home assessment. *Journal of Gerontological Nursing* June 1980; 6:319–327.

US Bureau of Census. Table no. 178. Population by age. *Statistical Abstracts of the United States* (105th edition). Washington, DC, 1986, p 111.

3

Assessment of the Family System

Charlotte Eliopoulos, RNC, MPH

Each individual is a product of some form of family unit. From the family, the individual gains status and identity, and learns values, beliefs, and attitudes. The manner in which an individual interprets, approaches, and copes with the world is influenced by the family. The family can be a source of strong support or chronic stress; it can nurture or destroy; it can promote wellness or illness. The health of the family unit is significant to the health status of the individual; thus, the profile and dynamics of the family must be understood for an adequate insight into the individual client. To assess the individual out of the context of the family unit is as limiting as attempting to understand the status of one body system in isolation from the rest. Effective assessment, care planning, and care delivery rests on the recognition that *the family is the client*.

IDENTIFYING THE FAMILY SYSTEM

Members

The initial task in assessing the family is to establish who constitutes the family. The family is an adaptive unit that takes many forms. It may be the traditional unit of either a nuclear family consisting of parents and their offspring or of an extended family that has more than two generations of blood relatives. However, other combinations may form the family unit, including single parent and offspring, siblings, unmarried couples, homosexual couples, homosexual couples and children, or a group of unrelated individuals. When compiling a family profile, you should inquire not only about the living spouse, parents, children, and siblings, but also about significant others, important relationships, and the household's composition.

Roles

Once you determine the primary figures of the family, explore their roles within the family system. Some of the potential roles may be as follows:

- *Caregiver*: This individual assumes responsibility for daily care activities or supervision of a frail, dependent, or ill relative. Typically a daughter or daughter-in-law fills this role.
- *Decision maker*: This individual makes important decisions, through granted or assumed authority. This person may be geographically distant or uninvolved in daily activities but will still be sought to make decisions.
- *Deviant*: This individual is the "problem child" of the family, who has strayed from the family's norms. The family may use the deviant as a scapegoat, as an excuse for the total family's problems, or as a source of humor. The family may reward this role, as exemplified by the jobless, alcoholic adult who is supported by the parents.
- *Dependent*: This individual does not assume responsibility for his or her own life, but rather, relinquishes his or her rights and responsibilities to the family.
- *Victim*: This individual forfeits his or her legitimate rights and may be physically, emotionally, socially, or economically abused within the family unit.

Although not all inclusive, these roles give insight into the family's dynamics. These roles are a product of the family's history of interaction and usually are accepted by the individual family member and the total family unit. The cultural background and tradition of the family may influence adherence to certain roles, such as the oldest son being the decision maker or the wife being the victim. An understanding of the roles played by family members can be enhanced by tracing the roles played by family members of older generations.

Dynamics

After determining the individual roles of each family member, examine the dynamics of the family as a whole. Considerations to explore include:

- *Emotional climate*: Is the tone of the family cheerful, serious, sarcastic, unhappy? Are members nurturing and supporting each other? Does the family unit supply stability, security, and respite, or is it a source of tension and conflict?

- *Communication*: Do members give clear messages? What is the nature and frequency of their communication? Are feelings expressed? How are satisfaction, anger, displeasure communicated?
- *Lines of authority*: Who holds the power within the family? How are decisions made? What control do authority figures exercise over the entire family?
- *Division of labor*: Who holds what responsibilities in the family? Are traditional roles adhered to (for example, father as breadwinner, mother as homemaker)? What are family members' reactions to their responsibilities?
- *Attitudes, values, beliefs*: What themes guide the family? What are family members' expectations and goals?
- *Flexibility*: What is the family's capacity for change? Is the family a unit that can grow, develop, and learn? Can members exchange roles and functions?
- *Problem solving*: Does the family solve problems within their structure or seek outside intervention? Do crises strengthen or threaten the family unit? How are problems managed?
- *Relationship to community*: Does the family see itself as an integral part of the community, or as outsiders? What is the quality and quantity of the family's interaction with the community? Is community approval important to the family? How similar is the family to the community?

From this data, you can understand the family's personality and gain valuable insight into the strengths, conflicts, expectations, and needs of the total family system.

ETHNICITY

Ethnicity is a major influence on the older adult's role within the family system. Settlers and immigrants who came to America brought with them the attitudes toward older adults that prevailed in their former countries. Establishing and living in ethnic communities in America helped to perpetuate these attitudes. For instance, immigrants from Ireland, England, Russia, Greece, and Poland tend to adhere to family unity and respect the older adults in their families. You can anticipate a variety of ethnic-related attitudes and practices as you intervene in the health care of older adults.

Chinese and Japanese families have a long tradition of extended families that shows tremendous respect and concern for their elders. Until recently, the eldest son had the major responsibility for caring and providing for his parents. The responsibility for parents now rests on all children, not just the eldest son. Chinese and Japanese women also have become less subordinate

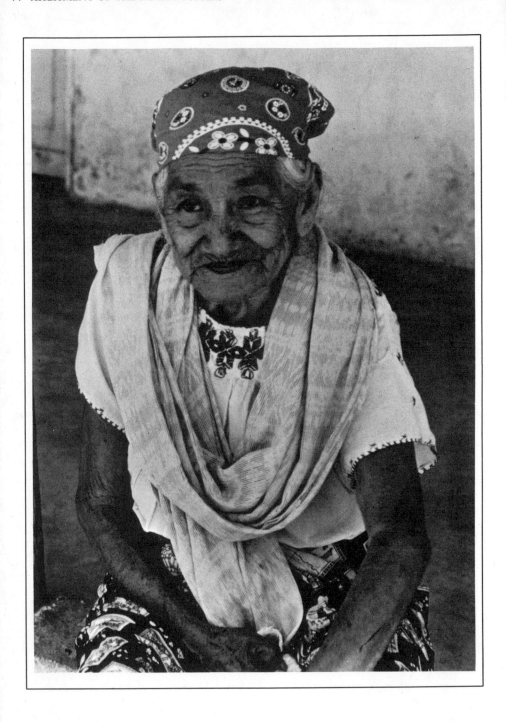

and are less apt to care for and follow the commands of their husbands' parents. These families are also more willing to allow government services to provide assistance to older family members. These changes, however, have not removed Chinese and Japanese older adults from high status in their families (Martinson 1982).

Black Americans demonstrate strong family ties. The black older adult typically has less income and more health problems than the white older adult but is able to depend on his or her children for assistance more than the white older adult (Vital Statistics of the US 1986). Extended families exist, particularly in urban areas, and may take the form of multigenerational households or several relatives living in the same neighborhood.

American Indians have a history of treating their elders with respect and viewing them as important as long as they are able to fulfill their roles. If an Indian older adult was ill and dependent, he or she was viewed negatively. Health and independence gave older Indians high status, and high status gave the individual family support and admiration. Programs facilitated by the Bureau of Indian Affairs have improved conditions for older American Indians. Although American Indians have depended on the Bureau for essential services, they also have resented and distrusted this government intervention. This ambivalence may be transferred to other public services and create barriers to the establishment of trust in the nurse–client relationship (First National Indian Conference on Aging 1978).

Filipino older adults are unique in that men outnumber women four to one (Bureau of Census 1979). This relatively new group in America has not developed the strong ethnic communities similar to other groups, thus strong bonds between Filipinos may be lacking. Customarily, Filipino families provide assistance to their older adults, and this may cause difficulty for the Filipino older adult when offered assistance from other sources.

Hispanics are a relatively poor group in America, having twice the incidence of poverty as Caucasians (Vital Statistics of the US 1986). Children are still viewed as a parent's source of security for old age, and it is not uncommon to encounter older Hispanic women who have borne children in the fifth decade of their lives. Family ties remain strong in these families.

Jews and Mormons, although very different groups, share both a belief in families caring for their own and a history of discrimination. Both of these groups reacted by developing their own sophisticated network of health and social services. When the family is unable to fulfill all of its older members' needs, this network is an acceptable resource. The continued strong support of these networks by new generations of Jews and Mormons testifies to people's strong ties to their roots.

A client's ethnic background can influence health practices, diet, illness management, perception of symptoms, acceptance of assistance, reaction to institutionalization, and a host of other factors that affect health status and the nurse–client relationship. Rather than force the client into the health system's mold, adjust nursing care to conform to the client's ethnic background as much as possible. Such consideration for ethnicity promotes individualized care, facilitates compliance, and conveys that you appreciate the client's heritage.

THE FAMILY AS A HELPING UNIT

Most families do not neglect their elder members. They do not abandon their older relatives, nor do they desire to see them institutionalized. Most families still provide intergenerational assistance when able (Hendricks and Hendricks 1981a, Brody 1985). A majority of older adults live within one hour's distance from their children and interact with them regularly. One in ten older women and one in twenty older men live with their children and grandchildren (Hendricks and Hendricks 1981b). Most older adults live alone and prefer that arrangement. Eighty to 90% of all older adults with health problems receive assistance from family members (Shanas 1979, Brody 1985), and most of this assistance comes from female family members. The family remains a major source of support and assistance to most older adults.

The existence of a family does not guarantee that it will be a resource to the older adult. One obvious reason may be that the older adult's family members live too far away to be closely involved. Relatives may be financially limited and unable to provide economic assistance. Family members may suffer physical or mental illnesses that prohibit them from assisting; this may be particularly significant for the "old-old" whose children may be "young-old" with their own set of problems.

More subtle factors may exist that prevent the family from assisting their elder members. Aiding an older-adult parent can drain time, energy, and money from the children's family. A spouse who was never liked by the in-laws may resent carrying the burden of assisting these in-laws when they become old. Middle-aged children may not welcome the responsibility of caring for their parents at a time when they desire enjoying the freedom granted by their own children's departure. One relative may feel that other family members are not contributing equally and may refuse to assist.

Another significant factor that may be difficult for adult offspring is that they actually may not like their parent. The parent–child relationship may have been very weak. Children may have been neglected, deserted, embarrassed, or abused by the parent and may not feel compelled to help now that the parent is in need. Rather than a sweet, pleasant, rosy-cheeked grandparent figure, the older adult may be an irritable, demanding person who is difficult to be with. Even when the older parent and child love each other and wish to help, personality clashes may stand in the way of a supportive relationship.

Society sends strong messages fostering the belief that children should love, honor, respect, and care for their parents. Thus, an adult offspring may have difficulty admitting an unwillingness or inability to assist the parent. During the assessment process, you must be perceptive to clues indicating the offspring's capabilities rather than assume the offspring will be a willing resource. Comments such as "my house is too small," "I'm a sick person myself," "I'm afraid I can't give her what she needs," and "I'll do it for a while, but I think my brother ought to be helping" may be communicating a reluctance to care for the older adult. You must be sensitive to this and not be judgmental or attempt to force the relationship.

RECOGNIZING FAMILY DYSFUNCTION

Ideally, the family is a nurturing, supportive system that guides its members through the trials and tribulations of life; it is the pinnacle of strength and pride; it offers respite, security, and stability in an unpredictable world; it is the optimum source and object of love. This ideal profile is highly desirable but is frequently inapplicable to many real families. A family is composed of individuals, each with a personal set of strengths, capabilities, conflicts, and needs. Combining individuals into a family system can create a strength and wholeness unachievable by members separately, or the combination can compound and exacerbate problems and inadequacies. A decrease in the physical, emotional, or social health of the family system can cause dysfunctional behavior symptoms to appear.

Manipulation

One such problem that may be observed in the family is the manipulation by one member of one or more others. Illness may be used as a means of manipulation. An older parent may claim to become ill when his daughter leaves him temporarily in someone else's care, or he may comment to his family, "I may not be alive when you return from your vacation," even though he may not be in any danger. The guilt such behavior elicits in the older adult's relatives may cause them to concede to his wishes of remaining by his side. Money may also be used to manipulate relatives by buying gifts, supplementing the relatives' budget, or promising to remember them in a will. Unnecessary dependency and flattery may also be used to manipulate family members into desired actions.

Older Adult Abuse

Another serious family problem that has recently gained visibility and public concern is older adult abuse. This abuse can take many forms besides the infliction of pain or injury. Abuse may include withholding food, money, medications, or services. Confinement may constitute abuse, as can the intentional mismanagement of the older adult's funds. It may also take the form of sexual abuse. Important to remember is that the *threat* of these actions is considered an abuse of the older adult due to the fear and anguish that the threat may cause (Bergman et al 1979, Hickey and Douglass 1981).

Abuse exists among all ethnic groups. It occurs within private homes and institutional settings, among rich and poor. No older adult is immune to the risk of abuse. Studies have shown, however, that a majority of abused older adults are likely to be (Bergman et al 1979, Block and Sinnott 1979, Select Committee on Aging 1981):

- Very old (75 years and older)
- Female
- Disabled
- Living with a relative (children and spouses make up the leading categories of abusers)
- Physically, socially, or financially dependent

Be particularly sensitive to clues indicating abuse since the victim may not readily reveal this problem. Fear of additional harm from the abuser may make the older victim reluctant to discuss the problem. Shame that others will know that their relative abuses them may also prevent abused older adults from admitting to the problem. The older adult may also feel that, although abused, her current situation is preferable to any alternative; that is, staying at home with a daughter who beats and threatens her may seem better than entering an institution. Convey to the client that you will respect confidentialities and withhold judgments. Several meetings with the client may need to occur before the client feels enough trust to discuss an abusive situation openly with you.

On identifying abuse, you must manage the situation tactfully and sensitively. Your primary concern should be to safeguard the older adult victim from future abuse. Strategies to deal with the problem may include seeking placement for the older adult, arranging respite care, or providing family counseling. Selected actions will depend on the individual circumstances.

A major contribution that you can make in assessing the family is to identify dysfunctions and problems that can potentially lead to abuse and to assist the family in seeking interventions that are appropriate. Situations that should signal special concern include the following:

1. Alcohol or drug abuse by any family member
2. Lack of respite for a family caring for a dependent older adult

3. Unequal sharing of responsibility resulting in one family member carrying all burdens

4. Financial strain on family caused by the older adult

5. Inability or lack of opportunity to communicate feelings and frustrations

6. Marital conflict among children of the older adult

7. Significant change in family life-style to accommodate the older relative

8. Emotional instability of family members

9. Verbalization of feeling overwhelmed with a caregiving situation

Recognizing and guiding the family to assistance with these problems reduces family stress and averts abuse.

3 Chapter Summary

I. Family system

  A. Family structure may vary
1. Nuclear
2. Extended
3. Single parent–child
4. Siblings
5. Unmarried couple
6. Homosexual couple
7. Homosexual couple–children
8. Group of unrelated individuals

  B. Each member plays a different role in family
1. Caregiver
2. Decision maker
3. Deviant
4. Dependent
5. Victim

  C. Family dynamics
1. Emotional climate
2. Communication
3. Lines of authority
4. Division of labor
5. Attitudes, values, and beliefs
6. Flexibility
7. Problem solving
8. Relationship to community

II. Ethnicity

  A. Ethnic background influences role and function of older family members

  B. Acceptance of interventions by extra family source can be influenced by ethnic group

III. Family as a resource

  A. Families do feel a sense of responsibility toward and maintain regular contact with their older members
1. Eighty to 90% of older adults with health problems are aided by families
2. Majority of older adults live within one hour's distance of children
3. Older adults prefer to live alone; only 10% of older women and 5% of older men live with offspring

  B. Existence of a family does not guarantee family will be a resource
1. Geographic distances
2. Financial limitations

3. Poor health status
4. Marital conflicts
5. Infringement on life-style
6. Poor relationships

IV. Family dysfunctions
  A. Manipulation of entire family unit by older relative
  B. Elder abuse
     1. Includes actual or threatened infliction of pain or injury; withholding food, money, medications, or services; confinement
     2. Occurs most frequently to females, the old-old, disabled, and those who are physically, socially, or financially dependent
     3. Most frequently, the abusers are children and spouse with whom the older adult lives
     4. Intervention with entire family unit is necessary

V. Related nursing diagnoses
  A. Anxiety
  B. Impaired verbal communication
  C. Ineffective individual coping
  D. Ineffective family coping
  E. Altered family processes
  F. Grieving
  G. Altered health maintenance
  H. Impaired home maintenance management
  I. Potential for injury
  J. Knowledge deficit
  K. Noncompliance
  L. Powerlessness
  M. Self care deficit
  N. Personal identity disturbance
  O. Sexual dysfunction
  P. Sleep pattern disturbance
  Q. Impaired social interaction
  R. Social isolation
  S. Spiritual distress
  T. Potential for violence

READINGS AND REFERENCES

Aging and the family. 33rd Annual Scientific Meeting of the Gerontological Society of America, San Diego, California, 1980. Abstracts. November 1980. *Gerontologist* 20(5):1–292.

Anderson CL. Abuse and neglect among the elderly. *Journal of Gerontological Nursing* February 1981; 7(2):77–85.

Archbold PG. Impact of parent caring in middle-aged offspring. *Journal of Gerontological Nursing* February 1980; 6:78–85.

Bergman J et al. Elder abuse in Massachusetts: A survey of professionals and paraprofessionals. Boston: Legal Research and Services for the Elderly, 1979.

Block MR, Sinnott JD. The battered elder syndrome. An exploratory study. College Park, Maryland: University of Maryland, Center on Aging, 1979.

Botwinick J. *Aging and Behavior.* New York: Springer, 1978.

Brody EM. *Long-Term Care of Older People. A Practical Guide.* New York: Human Sciences Press, 1977.

Brody EM. Parent care as a normative stress. *Gerontologist* 1985; 25(1):19–29.

Bureau of Census, US Dept. of Commerce. Ancestry and language in the United States. *Current Population Reports Series* November 1979; (116):323.

Dobrof R (editor). *Gerontological Social Work with Families.* New York: Haworth Press, 1987.

Ebersole P, Hess P. *Toward Healthy Aging. Human Needs and Nursing Response*, 2nd ed. St. Louis: Mosby, 1985.

First National Indian Conference on Aging: The Indian Elder, a Forgotten American. Albuquerque: Adobe Press, 1978.

Gaitz CM. Aged patients, their families and physicians. In: *Aging: The Process and the People.* Usdin G, Hofling C (editors). New York: Brunner/Mazel, 1978.

Gelfand DE, Kutzik AJ. *Ethnicity and Aging. Theory, Research, and Policy.* New York: Springer, 1979.

Hendricks J, Hendricks-Davis C. *Aging in Mass Society. Myths and Realities*, 2nd ed. Massachusetts: Winthrop Publishers, 1981, (a) p 306, (b) p 72.

Hickey T, Douglass RI. Mistreatment of the elderly in the domestic setting: An exploratory study. *American Journal of Public Health* May 1981; 71(5):506–507.

Johnson D. Abuse of the elderly. *Nursing Practitioner* January/February 1981; 6(1):29–34.

King D. Elder abuse. *Perspectives* 1986; Winter 10(4):13–15.

Lesnoff-Caravaglia G. *Health Care of the Elderly.* New York: Human Sciences Press, 1980.

Martinson IM. Does China really have the solution? *Journal of Gerontological Nursing* May 1982; 8(5):263–264.

Mitchell J. An exploration of family interaction with the elderly by race, socioeconomic status, and residence. *Gerontologist* 1984; 24(1):48–54.

Select Committee on Aging. US House of Representatives Ninety-Seventh Congress. April 3, 1981. *Elder Abuse: An Examination of a Hidden Problem.* Committee Publication No. 97–277.

Shanas E. The family as a social support system in old age. *The Gerontologist* 1979; 19(2):169–174.

Vital Statistics of the United States, P-60, No. 144. Washington, DC: US National Center for Health Statistics, 1986.

Weeks JR, Cuellar JB. The role of family members in the helping network of older people. *Gerontologist* August 1981; 21(4):388–394.

Woodruff DS, Birren JE. *Aging. Scientific Perspectives and Social Issues.* New York: Van Nostrand Reinhold, 1975.

4

Assessment of Functional Independence

Nina Glomski, RNC, MA

An important part of the client's overall assessment is the assessment of functional independence: the ability to perform activities that permit a person to be independent in daily living. Functional independence extends to bed mobility, transfer, locomotion, hygiene, eating, dressing, dexterity, and use of braces and prostheses. It also includes a less tangible aspect: the client's psychologic state, which affects achievement of the highest potential of functional ability. Part of a care plan for helping the client reach maximum independence in activities of daily living is addressing the psychologic factors that will promote this goal.

Functional assessment begins at the time of initial contact with the client. It is an ongoing process because not all the information can be gathered at one time or by one person. In an institutional setting, all three shifts play an important role. For example, the client may require assistance in putting on a shirt in the morning but is perfectly capable of removing it without assistance at the end of the day. Another client may be very alert in the morning but totally fatigued and helpless in the evening. These same problems can exist with the client at home, and several visits at different times of the day may be necessary to assess him or her accurately.

No client should be denied the right to function at his or her highest level. Do not wash a client out of a misguided sense of speed or efficiency rather than letting the client wash himself or herself. Instead, give a face cloth and an encouraging word to the client and have patience. Similarly, it is easier to give a bedpan than to help a client out of the bed and into the bathroom. In giving the bedpan, you are causing the client to lose the muscle strength and coordination maintained or gained from ambulation. You also lessen the client's self-respect and dignity, along with the motivation to remain independent. Moving at the client's pace promotes independence rather than dependence. This is especially true with the older client, for whom it is generally easier to rush through a procedure than to wait for him or her to accomplish the task.

SELF-MOTIVATION

The nurse working with the older adult knows from professional experience the possible permanent effects of a specific chronic illness. The nurse knows what goals are realistic in terms of the restorative and rehabilitative process following that illness. He or she knows what is possible and what is necessary to achieve and maintain that goal. One objective of nursing care is to enable the patient to formulate the same objective assessment of the illness, and, most importantly, to assume personal responsibility for the restorative and rehabilitative process. In other words, a goal of nursing care is the fostering of self-motivation in the client.

Fostering of self-motivation is a continual process that encompasses assessment of the client's perception of reality, client education to enable him or her to perceive accurately the illness, identification of realistic goals, and reinforcement of those personal patterns of behavior that contribute to self-motivation.

LACK OF SELF-MOTIVATION

The client who fails to assume personal responsibility for the healing and rehabilitative process after an illness presents one of the most difficult challenges to a nurse. This client is frequently labeled as lacking in self-motivation or as unmotivated. This client might follow the most rigorous of routines while in the hospital or under the constant guidance and supervision of the health care staff, but once he or she leaves the hospital environment, regression is inevitable due to lack of self-motivation.

Lack of motivation, however, is not a phenomenon unique to the ill. It is a common characteristic of many people and may particularly plague older adults due to the many disruptions to their physical, emotional, and social homeostasis brought about by aging. For instance, older retirees may feel no need to maintain attractive appearances and keep abreast of current events; widowed persons may have no desire to prepare and eat nutritious meals just for themselves; depressed, lonely individuals may lack the emotional energy to engage in self-care activities; and older adults in physical decline may be inhibited or prohibited from interacting with a larger social world. Disappointments, hopes permanently shattered, apparent loss of a meaningful and necessary role in society, failing health . . . these and other factors can cause the older adult to slip into inactivity. When that same adult is stricken with illness, the compounded effect of lack of self-motivation can permanently obstruct the road to recovery and rehabilitation.

PERCEPTIONS OF REALITY AND GOALS

What is self-motivation, that quality that enables one to take control of and be responsible for one's life? Self-motivation is contingent on the interaction of two dynamic factors: perceptions of reality and personal goals. Perceptions of reality include a myriad of issues, such as the following: the mental ability to perceive reality accurately; creativity and imagination; accuracy of perceptions of how people behave or of what other people expect of us; self-perception of how one relates towards family, authority figures, peers, and subordinates. From the perceptions of reality, the individual selects a cluster of personal goals. These goals are "drives" or "needs" that at times are noble, such as independence, affection, altruism, and loyalty. Other drives or needs are less noble, for example, dominance, vengeance, or greed.

IMPACT OF ILLNESS ON SELF-MOTIVATION

Through life-long experiences, perceptions of reality, and the selection and internalization of goals, the mature adult develops a pattern of self-motivation. That same adult, however, may suddenly be at a loss when he or she becomes the victim of illness, either acute or chronic. Illness can do violence to both the real and the personal world that the client perceives and to the goals that he or she has internalized. The net impact on self-motivation can be debilitating, if not totally paralyzing.

Throughout the assessment process, therefore, you must constantly address and provide appropriately for the psychologic impact of the illness. Give specific attention to the illness's effect on self-motivation. Within this framework you can proceed with the physical assessment of the client's functional capabilities.

IDENTIFYING THE CLIENT'S STRENGTHS

The first objective of an assessment of functional independence, as the term implies, is to identify those areas in which the client can perform activity or movement independently. Your intent is to help the client claim as his or her own any independent activity, regardless of how minimal it might be. For example, if the only movement that the client can perform is to move from side to side in bed, this level of independence must be identified—explicitly, for both you and the client—and maintained. The casual or nonprofessional observer may perceive such an activity as simple. On the contrary, it is rather complex and affects the musculoskeletal, integumentary, respiratory, gastrointestinal, and cardiovascular systems. For the client, such an activity can represent a major achievement and should be acknowledged as such.

THE CLIENT'S SPECIAL CONDITIONS

In assessing the client's functional independence, always keep in mind any special conditions brought out in the physical assessment. Is the client blind, deaf, aphasic, confused, depressed, or agitated? Is he or she incontinent of bowel or bladder? Does the client have a poor cardiac status? Such information is essential in assessing specific and overall functional independence and in identifying what intervention is necessary for helping the client maintain and develop a level of independence. For example, a confused and agitated client might have the ability to wash his or her face only if he or she is constantly encouraged or brought to the sink. For the blind person, whether or not his or her belongings are consistently put in the same place will affect his or her independence. If the client has a poor cardiac status, watch for signs of fatigue and take the pulse at regular intervals. If the client is incontinent, establish a training routine. If the client is deaf or aphasic, keep a communication board or paper and pencil within his or her reach.

INDEPENDENCE–DEPENDENCE SCALE

The assessment of functional independence is not done by a question-and-answer process, but by observation during actual performance of an activity and by active involvement with the client in the activity itself. Suggest, encourage, and even demonstrate how an activity might be performed. Evaluate each activity during the client's performance according to the following scale of independence–dependence:

1. Independent: The client can perform a specific function without any assistance.
2. Minimal assistance: The client needs supervision or contact guarding.
3. Moderate assistance: The client needs assistance from one person.
4. Maximum assistance: The client needs assistance from two or more persons.
5. Dependent: The client cannot help herself or himself at all.

Rate each area that you assess from 1 to 5, according to how much assistance the client needs. For example, a client with left hemiparesis may be independent (a rating of 1) in washing the face, neck, trunk, left hand, and arm, but needs someone's assistance (a rating of 3) to wash the right arm and underarm. A transfer activity, from bed to chair, might be assessed as requiring maximum assistance (a rating of 4) if the client is obese. In the case of a client with muscular contractures of all extremities, a rating of 5 would probably be indicated for most activities.

LIST OF ACTIVITIES

The following is a recommended list of activities to assess, including suggestions to facilitate the assessment of a specific activity or aspects for which you should be alert.

Bed Activities

Moving from place to place in bed	Ask client, as he is lying in bed on his back, to roll from one side of the bed to the other. Grabbing a raised bed rail may give leverage needed to roll or move over.
	Ask client to turn onto his abdomen, and then roll back onto his back.
	Have client sit up erect in bed, and then swing his legs over the side of the bed.
	Place some objects on the night table, and see if client can reach them.
	For each action (and for all other activities you assess) note how much assistance client needs to complete the action.

Elevations

Bed to standing	Make certain the bed is in the lowest position. Have client sit on the edge of the bed; ask her to stand.
Standing to bed	As client stands next to the bed, have her sit on the edge of the bed, then ask her to raise her legs up onto the bed.
In and out of a chair	Observe client's balance when moving in or out of an armless chair, or a hard arm chair. In the latter case, observe how she uses the upper extremities to push up from the chair, using the hard arms of the chair.

In and out of a couch or upholstered chair	Observe balance. Note the use of feet and legs to move to the back or edge of the couch or chair.
Standing to toilet, and toilet to standing	Note the use of the wall or of the seat to move onto or off the toilet.

Transfers

Bed to wheelchair or other chair; chair to bed; chair to auto; auto to chair; in and out of bathtub	Make certain that the surface client is leaving and the one to which he is transferring are firmly in place. If a wheelchair is involved, the wheels should be checked to see that they are locked in place. If client uses another type of chair, wedge it against the wall or bed, or have someone hold it in place. This might be the only assistance client needs. Observe balance. Does client fall to the right or the left? For entering or leaving a bathtub, have client sit on the edge and then swing his feet into or out of the tub. Are there nonskid pads in the tub? Is contact guarding necessary?

Wheelchair Mobility

Raise and lower foot rests	Foot rests need to be adjusted so that they do not obstruct transfer in or out of chair.
Manipulate brakes	Are brakes functioning properly? Does client have the hand strength to operate the brakes?
Propel wheelchair	Observe upper extremity strength and coordination.
Turn corners	Observe coordination and perception.

Ambulation

Walking; maneuvering stairs; support while walking	Observe balance. Observe the carpeting. Thick carpeting can be a hazard since client might not be able to raise his feet sufficiently when walking. Do area rugs, especially at home, slide? Is hand rail needed to maneuver stairs? Does client lean on wall when walking? Does client hold onto furniture? Is that furniture stable?

Hygiene

Showering; bathing; brushing teeth; combing and brushing hair; washing hands, face, upper and lower extremities; shaving

Observe strength of upper extremities.

Note ability to lift arm to face and head.

Note ability to manage a razor. An electric razor is recommended for older adults.

Place basin of water, soap, and washcloth in reach of client. Note ability to handle soap and washcloth. Can client rinse the cloth?

Use of urinal

Note ability to zip and unzip a zipper.

Observe proper placement of urinal.

Observe ability to remove urinal without spilling contents.

Toilet hygiene

Observe thoroughness in use of toilet paper.

Observe for washing and drying of hands after using toilet.

Insertion of suppository

Observe for dexterity in handling of suppository.

Care of fingernails

Observe for cleanliness, use of clipper or file.

Eating

Eating with knife, fork, and spoon; drinking from cup or glass; use of a straw; use of adaptive equipment

Observe hand grip, coordination, and range of motion.

Observe use of each utensil and the ability to eat "finger" foods.

Does client need someone to prepare her plate by cutting food into bite sizes so that she can feed herself? Determine if adaptive utensils may be necessary to enable client to bring food to her mouth. For persons who have the use of only one hand, combination knife-fork and fork-spoon utensils may be helpful. Unbreakable plates may be in order if client lacks coordination. Client may also need to have her plate stabilized, for example, by placing a wet cloth under it on the table.

Dressing

All clothing, on and off

Assess client's ability to put on and remove all clothing.

Observe dexterity with zippers, buttons, snaps, and shoelaces.

Brassieres present a particular problem for the older woman. A brassiere with a front hook is recommended.

Generally, if the upper extremities are functioning well, the client should have relatively little difficulty with dressing.

Braces and Prosthesis

Leg or arm	Assess ability to put on, remove, and manage artificial limb.
Braces	Assess ability to lock and unlock brace.
	Assess coordination and dexterity of the hand.

Dexterity

Using telephone; reading; writing; putting on and removing eyeglasses; use of smoking equipment; turning faucets; etc.	Observe coordination and ability to perform fine hand movements.
	Observe for potential safety hazards, especially for the smoker.
	Assess ability to handle electrical appliances (such as lights, toaster, or oven).

FAMILY INVOLVEMENT

Family members play an important role in maintaining the client's independence. In an institutional setting, the family should be involved from the beginning in learning how to help the client retain and expand independent activity. Teach the family techniques of transfer, grooming, dressing, and washing, and alert them to safety hazards. Encourage the family to be with the client at any time of the day, observing activities the client can perform independently in the course of a 24-hour routine. Encourage the family to ask questions of the professional staff. The goal is to assure continuity of care when the client returns home; the family will have to pick up where the institutional staff left off.

The institutional involvement does not end abruptly when the client is discharged. Rather, there should be a phase-out process, one that includes home visits to enable you to observe and assess the client in a normal setting. Invariably, you will have to modify portions of the assessment of functional independence. The transition from the temporary setting of the institution to the permanent and familiar environment of the home will have a definite impact on the client's functioning, creating more independence or encouraging regression to more dependency. A home visit is essential to evaluate accurately the interaction between the family and the client, to see how each is coping with new needs and expectations.

ENVIRONMENT

An important role for you is to create and maintain an environment of independence within the institution or the home. This environment encompasses physical facilities, space, and time—all of which influence the client's abilities to function independently. Washing and grooming articles should be within easy reach for the client. If the client is washing in bed, place the necessary articles on an over-bed table in front of him or her. If the client washes in the bathroom, place a chair in front of the sink and have all articles within reach. Facilitate dressing by placing articles of clothing in the order that they are put on.

You should visit the home to assess the environment. Look for steps leading to the home, split levels, the presence of elevators (can someone in a wheelchair reach the buttons?). Scatter rugs are a hazard and should be removed. If carpeting is too thick, the client might not be able to maneuver the wheelchair. Architects often do not consider the possibility of wheelchairs when they design bathroom doors or place bath fixtures. However, some modifications are relatively simple. Grab bars can be installed in the bathroom, tub seats on tubs, and shower chairs in showers. Kitchen equipment can be adjusted for one bound to a wheelchair. A mirror over the stove lets the client in a chair see the contents of pans on the stove. Keep in mind that a person's home is his or her pride. Be tactful in making even the slightest suggestion for modifications. Seek the help of an occupational therapist if necessary.

4 Chapter Summary

I. Independence–dependence scale
  A. Independent
    1. Activity performed without assistance
  B. Minimal assistance
    1. Supervision or contact guarding needed
  C. Moderate assistance
    1. Aid of one person needed
  D. Maximum assistance
    1. Aid of two or more persons needed
  E. Dependent
    1. Unable to help one's self to any degree

II. Assessment activities
  A. Bed activities
  B. Elevations
  C. Transfers
  D. Wheelchair mobility
  E. Ambulation
  F. Hygiene
  G. Eating
  H. Dressing
  I. Braces and prosthesis
  J. Dexterity

III. Related nursing diagnoses
  A. Activity intolerance
  B. Anxiety

C. Pain
D. Impaired verbal communication
E. Ineffective individual coping
F. Diversional activity deficit
G. Altered family processes
H. Fear
I. Dysfunctional grieving
J. Altered health maintenance
K. Impaired home maintenance management
L. Potential for injury
M. Knowledge deficit
N. Impaired physical mobility

O. Noncompliance
P. Powerlessness
Q. Self care deficit
R. Personal identity disturbance
S. Sensory/perceptual alterations
T. Sexual dysfunction
U. Impaired skin integrity
V. Sleep pattern disturbance
W. Impaired social interaction
X. Altered thought processes
Y. Altered patterns of urinary elimination

READINGS AND REFERENCES

Brower HT. The gerontological nurse specialist in rehabilitation settings. *Rehab. Nurs.* 1985; 10(3):20–22.

Christopherson VA, Coulter PP, Wolanin MO. *Rehabilitation Nursing Perspectives and Applications.* New York: McGraw-Hill, 1974.

Coombs J. *Living with the Disabled: You Can Help.* New York: Sterling Press, 1984.

Gardner H. *The Shattered Mind: The Person After Brain Damage.* New York: Vintage Books, 1976.

Lawton EB. *Activities of Daily Living.* New York: McGraw-Hill, 1963.

Lonnerblad L. Exercises to promote independent living in older patients. *Geriatrics* 1984; 39(2):93–101.

Redford JB. Assistive devices for the elderly. Pages 166–174 in: *The Practice of Geriatrics.* Calkins E, Davis PJ, Ford AB (editors). Philadelphia: Saunders, 1986.

Statler, E, Earl L. Help with activities of everyday life. *Gerontologist* 1983; 23(1):64–70.

Stryker R. *Rehabilitative Aspects of Acute and Chronic Nursing Care,* 2nd ed. Philadelphia: Saunders, 1977.

Tobis JS. Rehabilitation of the geriatric patient. Pages 579–589 in: *Clinical Geriatrics,* 3rd ed. Rossman I (editor). Philadelphia: Lippincott, 1986.

5 Assessment of the Integumentary System

Charlotte Eliopoulos, RNC, MPH

The skin is not only the largest, but also one of the most complex organs of the body. It protects the body's internal structures and offers the first line of external defense against infection. Its blood vessels, influenced by the nervous system, provide thermal regulation. Through the nerve endings in the dermis, temperature, touch, and pressure sensations are received. Infection, dehydration, cardiovascular disease, respiratory problems, and other internal changes can be reflected by the skin. Of course, skin also reflects individual appearance and helps to provide personal identity.

REVIEW OF THE INTEGUMENTARY SYSTEM

Skin

The integumentary system consists of the skin and its appendages: the hair, nails, sebaceous glands, and sweat glands. The skin is perforated vertically and stratified horizontally (Figure 5-1). The epidermis is the visible skin and this is comprised of two layers. The horny, outermost layer of the epidermis is the *stratum corneum*; this consists of dead keratinized cells that are continuously shed and replaced by new cells from lower layers. The *stratum germinativum* is the inner layer of the epidermis, where keratin and melanin are formed. Beneath the epidermis lies the dermis, consisting of connective tissue,

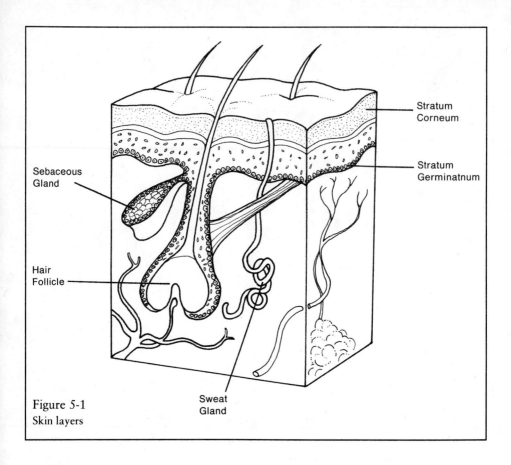

Figure 5-1
Skin layers

sebaceous glands, and some hair follicles. Collagen, a fibrous protein, gives the dermis its firmness. The dermis has a rich supply of blood. Although subcutaneous tissue is not formally categorized as part of the integumentary system, it lies beneath the dermis and contains sweat glands and hair roots, in addition to fat that aids in the body's insulation.

Hair

Hair goes through alternate cycles of growth and rest. Individual hairs do not always go through the same cycles simultaneously, and hair growth varies according to its location on the body and the time of year.

Nails

The nail bed consists of epithelial cells and has a firm, colorless covering called the nail plate (Figure 5-2). The blood supply to the nail bed is reflected by the

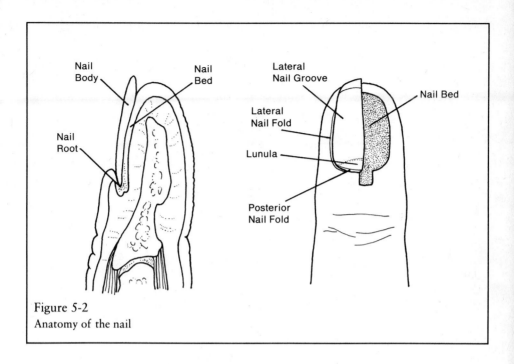

Figure 5-2
Anatomy of the nail

color seen through the nail plate. The semicircular whitish area at the base of the nail, the *lunula*, results from the underlying matrix that forms the nail. The nail plate is characterized by fine longitudinal ridges.

Sebaceous Glands

The sebaceous glands secrete a protective fatty substance, *sebum*, through the path of the hair follicle. Sebaceous glands are present everywhere on the body, with the exception of the soles and palms; the greatest concentrations are on the forehead, the scalp, and the periumbilical, perianal, and scrotal areas. The amount of sebum secreted varies.

Sweat Glands

There are two types of sweat glands. The *eccrine* glands are widely distributed and aid in temperature regulation by secreting a dilute saline solution in response to heat. The *apocrine* glands, located primarily in the axillary and genital areas, secrete an odorless fluid in response to stress; this fluid facilitates decomposition of bacteria on the skin, which produces body odors. Although the eccrine glands begin functioning during the first few months of life, the apocrine glands are nonfunctional until puberty.

AGE-RELATED CHANGES IN THE INTEGUMENTARY SYSTEM

Aging affects all body systems; however, the manifestations of aging within the integumentary system are most obvious to the naked eye. These changes are frequently the focus of more attention and stigma than other body changes, particularly in our youth-oriented society, where the fight against lines, wrinkles, blemishes, baldness, and gray hair is a billion dollar obsession. Integumentary changes are influenced by heredity, environment, diet, activity, emotions, and general health state and consequently will be different in each individual; however, there are some general changes that are associated with the aging process in most individuals.

Skin

The "thinning" of the epidermis associated with aging is actually a flattening due to the loss of papillae. This flattening reduces the contact area between the dermis and epidermis, creating a greater risk of peeling of the epidermis in the presence of a shearing force. The epidermis also decreases in elasticity, strength, and vascularity. Large frecklelike spots on the skin, commonly referred to as age or liver spots, are more prevalent, particularly on areas of the body exposed to sunlight; these result from a clustering of the melanocytes and are not related to disease. There are fewer active basal cells in the epidermis as well.

A loss of cells causes the dermis to thin, especially in females. Collagen is reduced and is stiffer and less soluble. The elastin increases in sun-damaged skin; elastin fibers become thicker and more branched.

A loss of subcutaneous fat contributes to the lines and wrinkles that increasingly appear with age. This loss of fat also contributes to drooping eyelids and the accentuation of nasolabial folds. The decrease in subcutaneous fat also reduces the body's natural insulation.

Small vessels in the skin start to deteriorate. Tactile sensitivity lessens and the reduced acuity of pain perception makes older adults more susceptible to burns and other serious injuries.

Hair

There are fewer hair follicles and the hair on the scalp grays and becomes thinner. Hair in the nose and ears becomes thicker, easily trapping particles. Women may notice the growth of facial hair, particularly on the chin; this tends to be more common in women of Mediterranean descent. Men may develop coarse hairs over the rims of the ears. Hair follicles remain responsive to hormonal stimulation. Graying of the hair usually begins in mid-life.

Nails

Fingernails and toenails develop more exaggerated longitudinal lines and become thicker.

Sebaceous and Sweat Glands

Sebaceous gland activity, related to androgen level, is reduced, resulting in less oil production. Sweat gland activity is also reduced. A longer time is necessary for thermal stimulation to affect the sweat glands; because sweating is delayed, evaporative heat loss is impaired and the risk of heat stroke increases. Body odor becomes less of a problem.

Higher Incidence of Dermatologic Problems

A variety of dermatologic problems increase with age. There is a higher incidence of benign tumors, skin tags, lentigines, seborrheic keratoses, and fungus infections of the feet. A decrease in acute inflammatory skin reactions can delay awareness of problems. Herpes zoster and pemphigus are more prevalent due to impaired cell-mediated immunity. There is delayed wound healing and a greater risk of dehiscence of abdominal wounds, although a wide range of individual variation is present (Kligman et al 1985).

ASSESSMENT OF THE INTEGUMENTARY SYSTEM

General Observation

Evaluation of the status of the integument begins on the first contact with the client. A gross determination of age, self-care capacity, self-concept, nutritional status, and general health can be obtained from a general observation of the skin and hair.

Skin Color

Inspect and palpate the entire skin surface. It is advisable to use nonfluorescent lighting since fluorescent lights can make the detection of fine skin rashes and lesions difficult. Note areas of the skin that differ from the rest in color and describe them in terms of:

Location: total body surface, arms, right side of face, left heel
Color: brown, blue, purple, red, yellow
Size: 0.5 cm, 2″ × 1″
Onset: birthmark, 10 days

Related symptoms: itching, painful

Associated factors: onset coincided with nausea, new pet in household, drug change, use of perfume

Irregular brown patches, similar to large freckles, should be noted. When these appear on areas of the body exposed to sunlight they are usually of no concern; however, when generalized or located at points of pressure or friction, they can be associated with Addison's disease, pituitary tumors, and hyperthyroidism. Brown spots also may be inherited.

Bluish discoloration occurs due to a reduction in hemoglobin associated with hypoxia. Cardiac and respiratory disease, anxiety, or a cold environmental temperature can be the cause. Common areas involved include the nail beds, lips, and oral mucosa.

Increased oxyhemoglobin (which may occur with fever), alcohol intake, and exposure to cold can cause generalized redness of the skin. If a specific body part is exposed to cold, inflamed, or traumatized, only that area will appear red. Care should be taken to differentiate red areas from purple or reddish blue areas; the latter can be petechiae or ecchymoses associated with bleeding outside the vessels.

Yellow discoloration of the sclera, mucous membranes, and skin usually is caused by jaundice from increased bilirubin levels, which occur with liver disease and red blood cell hemolysis. With chronic renal disease there can be a similar yellow coloring, but the sclera and mucous membranes are not affected. Hypothyroidism, diabetes, and an excessively high intake of carotene-containing fruits and vegetables (eg carrots) can cause the face, palms, and soles to take on a yellow-orange color; the sclera and mucous membranes are not affected.

A variety of conditions can cause the skin to pale or lose color. These include albinism, anemic states, shock, fatigue, and vitiligo (a patchy loss of color due to autoimmune or neurologic disorders).

Lesions

Note the skin's integrity and describe lesions that are detected. Lesions are described by their:

Configuration: clustered, linear, annular (Figure 5-3)

Distribution: generalized, specific area

Type: macule, papule, fissure, etc. (Table 5-1)

Moisture

The moisture of the skin should be described, noting excessively dry, sweaty,

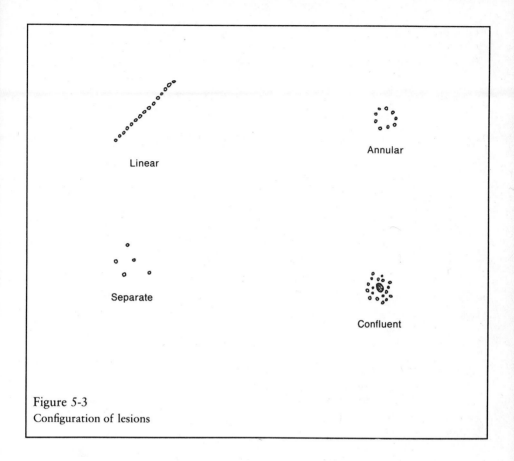

Figure 5-3
Configuration of lesions

or oily areas. Black skin may be dry and flaky, a condition known as "ash"; this is a normal finding and can indicate the need for a moisturizer.

Temperature, Texture, Turgor

Use the back of your hands to determine temperature; note if findings are bilateral. The texture (roughness, smoothness) of the skin should be noted, as well as the turgor. Since decreased skin elasticity is present in advanced age, poor turgor is a common finding; the forehead and sternum tend to be the best sites to assess skin turgor in the elderly.

Nails

The fingernails and toenails also should be examined and palpated. Fungal infections of the toenail (*onychomycosis*) are not uncommon and are characterized by dry, scaly looking material under the toenail. Splitting of the

Table 5-1 Types of Skin Lesions

Macule	Small spot or discoloration on skin surface Nonpalpable Texture similar to surrounding skin
Papule	Discoloration of skin less than 1/2 cm in diameter Palpable elevation Firm
Plaque	Group of papules
Nodule	Lesion 1/2–1 cm in diameter Skin may or may not be discolored Palpable elevation Firm
Tumor	Lesion exceeding 1 cm in diameter Skin may or may not be discolored Palpable elevation Firm
Wheal	Red or white skin discoloration Palpable elevation Variable size
Vesicle	Fluid-containing lesion less than 1/2 cm in diameter Palpable elevation
Bulla	Fluid-containing lesion over 1/2 cm in diameter Palpable elevation
Pustule	Lesion containing purulent fluid Variable size Palpable elevation
Fissure	Groove in skin
Ulcer	Open depression in skin Variable size

nail, or toenails that are loose at the distal portion (*onycholysis*) should be noted.

Normally the angle between the fingernail and nail base is 160 degrees (Figure 5-4) and the nail base feels firm. Poor oxygenation can cause clubbing, in which the angle between the nail and nail base becomes 180 degrees or greater and the nail base becomes springy and swollen. Some persons normally display a convex curve to their nails, which can be mistaken for clubbing; such nails will have a normal angle, however, and the nail base will be firm when palpated.

Transverse ridges across the nail bed are referred to as *furrowing* or *Beau's lines*. This finding is usually associated with severe systemic illness or injury to the nail.

Press on several of the nails to test for blanching. Normally pink color should return to the nail bed. Poor return of color can be associated with anemia or circulatory insufficiency.

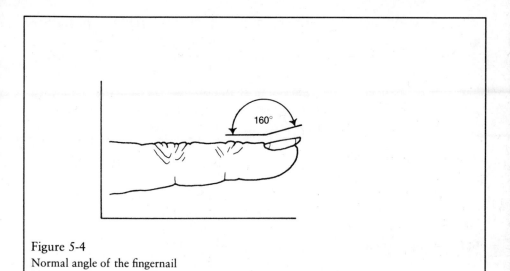

Figure 5-4
Normal angle of the fingernail

Brown, red, or white hairline linear markings under the nail can be caused by trauma, although they have been known to appear for no apparent cause. Brown or black pigmentation of the nails can be a normal finding among black persons.

Hair

Note the grooming of the hair and ask the client about hair care practices. Excessive shampooing and the use of harsh soaps on the scalp are not advisable. Question the client about hair loss, itching and flaking of the scalp, unusual hair growth, and other problems.

Balding is an inherited trait that demonstrates individual patterns. Most men begin to experience some receding of the hairline in their twenties, resulting in various degrees of baldness by old age. Persons of European and Near Eastern ancestry display higher rates of balding than other groups. Balding in women is an unusual finding, associated with disease or severe hair care or coloring measures. Graying usually precedes hair loss.

Use a comb to part the hair into rows for complete examination of the hair and scalp. Note lesions, discolorations, lice, and tender areas. Smooth round nodules can be *sebaceous cysts*. Glossy, nodular, raised growths that bleed easily can be *melanomas* or *basal cell carcinoma*. *Squamous cell carcinoma* can appear as a flesh-colored, wartlike lesion. Reddish patches of dry skin less than 1 cm in diameter that have a scale may be *solar (actinic) keratoses*. Tender, red areas near the hairline accompanied by pulsations of the superficial temporal arteries can reflect *giant cell arteritis*. Abnormal findings should be specifically described and the client should be referred for further evaluation.

Excessively oily hair most often is associated with poor grooming practices, although it can be a finding in persons with Parkinson's disease. Dry hair can be associated with excessive shampooing, use of harsh hair care products, or bleaching or dying of the hair. Dry hair that is coarse and brittle can occur with hypothyroidism. Irregular patches of hair loss are associated most commonly with fungal infections of the scalp, although nervous disorders and syphilis also can be causes. Of course, poor nutrition can influence hair condition.

Less body hair may be observed on older adults, although the amount of hair is largely influenced by racial, genetic, and sex-linked factors. Persons of white European descent tend to be hairier than Asians or blacks; American Indians have little body or face hair (Rossman 1986).

DISORDERS OF THE INTEGUMENTARY SYSTEM

Dermatologic disorders increase with age. It has been estimated that 40% of persons 65–74 years of age have skin problems serious enough to be seen by a dermatologist and that this incidence is even higher in persons over age 75 (Gilcrest 1986). Skin disorders reflect underlying illness. They also can alter self-image, comfort, and function; thus, prompt diagnosis and treatment are important.

Seborrheic Keratosis

Of the many neoplasms that occur with aging, seborrheic keratosis is the most common. These yellow-brown, greasy-looking growths can be flat or wartlike and appear anywhere on the body, although they are most common on the trunk. Sometimes blackheads are seen within the lesions. Although these growths are harmless, removal for cosmetic purposes may be advised. It is important that seborrheic keratosis be differentiated from basal cell epithelioma and nevocarcinoma.

Skin Cancers

Basal cell carcinoma is the most common skin cancer. It is believed to be associated with exposure to ultraviolet light; thus, most are located on the face, extremities, and trunk, areas that have the most exposure to sunlight.

The borders of basal cell carcinomas are well defined. Typically, the lesions are glossy, raised, and the same color as the skin, although occasionally they are brown or black pigmented. Size can range from a few millimeters to over a centimeter. Bleeding and ulceration can occur, followed by crusting of the surface. Although they are painless, slow growing, and rarely metastatic, they should be removed. Recurrence is not uncommon; therefore, follow-up is necessary.

Squamous cell carcinoma commonly occurs on the dorsum of the hands, neck, ears, tongue, and lower lip. This lesion may begin as keratosis or leukoplakia and develop into a nodular area that forms a crusty ulceration. These tumors metastasize rapidly; thus, prompt attention is warranted.

Melanomas are highly malignant and metastasize quickly. They appear as isolated, smooth, irregularly shaped lesions. They may enlarge and darken with time. Any part of the body can be affected, although most melanomas result from preexisting lesions on the feet, hands, legs, back, and trunk.

Contact Dermatitis

Contact dermatitis is caused by irritants or allergens to the skin, which result in redness that leads to vesicle formation, crusting, and scaling. Pruritus is usually present. This dermatitis can be generalized or confined to the specific area that has been in contact with the irritant.

When clinical signs of dermatitis are present, question the client about new cosmetics, soaps, laundry detergents, clothing, jewelry, or other material that may be used or worn. Paints, clay, yarns, and other materials used in group activities should not be overlooked.

Treatment involves removing the cause and applying fluorinated corticosteroid cream.

Seborrhea

Seborrhea is a common, although frequently missed, problem of the aged and can be of three types:

Senile: fine, whitish scaling of the scalp

Cumular: patches of greasy accumulations

Dermatitis: erythematous scaling, primarily involving nasolabial folds, eyebrows, hairline, and scalp, although it may be generalized in severe cases

Seborrhea can easily be confused with psoriasis and contact dermatitis, so astute evaluation is necessary. The condition usually can be corrected with medicated shampoos.

Pruritus

The uncomfortable condition of pruritus can be generalized or confined to a specific area. Typically the skin looks normal, although there may be indications of scratching.

A comprehensive history is important in identifying the cause of pruritus. Approximately one-half of the cases are associated with systemic disease (Gilcrest 1986) such as diabetes and liver disease, so other signs and symptoms must be reviewed. Medications also should be considered a potential cause.

Management of the underlying cause is essential to treatment of pruritus. Topical antipruritic preparations, along with antihistamines and tranquilizers, can be used to control itching. Clients, particularly those with altered mental function, should be prevented from traumatizing their skin by severe scratching.

Pediculosis

Older adults are not immune to lice infestations. Body lice (*pediculosis corporis*) are difficult to detect; small, red, macular lesions and severe itching are the major signs. Head lice (*pediculosis capitis*) can appear as white specks in the hair accompanied by itching; weeping, crusty areas may eventually develop on the scalp. The easiest lice to detect are pubic lice (*pediculosis pubis*), which appear as small gray flecks on pubic hairs. These highly contagious infestations need prompt treatment.

Scabies

Another highly contagious infestation is scabies, caused by itch mites. An indication of this problem is severe itching, commonly at the flexor surface of the wrist, digital web spaces, axilla, nipples, and genitalia. Itching is usually worse at night. Inspection of these areas reveals a whitish-gray linear pattern with a dark dot at the end; lesions may be macular, papular, urticarial, vesicular, or nodular.

Treatment consists of gamma benzene hexachloride (Kwell) applied to the entire body surface and thorough cleaning of all clothing and bed linen.

Herpes Zoster

A reactivation of the varicella virus, which causes chicken pox, is responsible for herpes zoster, commonly called shingles. Incidence of this problem increases with age, making it most common among older adults.

Usually involvement is unilateral, with symptoms following the path of the nerve. Shingles begins with several days of paresthesia or dysesthesia, followed by the appearance of extremely painful vesicles. The vesicles crust approximately two weeks later and can take several months to resolve. The trunk and face are commonly affected areas, although the ophthalmic branch of the trigeminal nerve and other areas also can be involved. Local lymph nodes may be tender and palpable, and malnutrition, secondary infections, and general debilitation may be noted.

Treatment is aimed toward controlling symptoms and preventing or managing secondary infection. Older persons experience a higher incidence of postherpetic neuralgia, in which phantom pain is present for months after the lesions have resolved.

Decubitus Ulcers

Prolonged pressure can impair circulation and cause necrosis to the skin and subcutaneous tissue, resulting in decubitus ulcers, a major health risk to the elderly. In addition to pressure to bony prominences, malnourishment, immobility, and the presence of a shearing force (eg, sitting up in bed) can contribute to skin breakdown.

Inspection will determine the specific stage of the decubitus. The early stage of *hyperemia* is characterized by redness that disappears if the pressure is removed. If pressure has been present for at least several hours *ischemia* will occur, with discoloration and swelling of the area. *Ulceration* is the stage in which an open lesion is present. When dead skin and eschar are present *necrosis* has occurred. The area of the decubitus needs to be carefully examined because looks can be deceiving; some sores may appear small on the skin surface but affect a larger underlying area.

A variety of treatment measures can be employed to debride tissue and promote granulation and epithelialization. Nutritional factors that contribute to decubitus formation should be assessed and corrected. Of course, the prevention of prolonged pressure to the skin is essential.

5 Chapter Summary

I. Age-related changes
   A. Loss of thickness, elasticity, vascularity, and strength of epidermis
   B. Clustering of melanocytes, causing dark "age spots"
   C. Thinning of dermis
   D. Decreased amount, solubility, and flexibility of collagen
   E. Loss of subcutaneous fat, causing lines, wrinkles, drooping eyelids, less natural body insulation
   F. Loss of hair follicles; thinning and graying of scalp hair
   G. Thicker hair in nose and ears
   H. Thicker nails, accentuated longitudinal lines
   I. Less sebaceous and sweat gland activity
   J. Higher incidence of benign and malignant growths, infections, and other dermatologic problems

II. Assessment
   A. Inspection
      1. Skin color
      2. Skin lesions
      3. Skin moisture, temperature, texture, turgor

4. Nail condition, color, firmness, angle, texture
5. Hair cleanliness, distribution, color, texture
6. Scalp condition

B. Palpation
1. Skin masses, lesions
2. Nail firmness

III. Pathologies
A. Seborrheic keratosis
1. Yellow-brown, greasy looking
2. Most common on trunk; can appear anywhere
3. Harmless, usually removed for cosmetic purposes
4. Should be differentiated from skin cancers

B. Skin cancers
1. Basal cell
   a) Most common; believed to be associated with exposure to ultraviolet radiation
   b) Well-defined border; glossy, raised lesion
   c) Painless; slow growing
2. Squamous cell
   a) May begin as keratosis or leukoplakia that develops into nodular area; eventually forms crusty ulceration
   b) Most frequently occurs on dorsum of hands, neck, ears, tongue, lower lip
   c) Metastasizes rapidly
3. Melanomas
   a) Appear as isolated, smooth, irregular-shaped hairy lesions; can enlarge and darken with time
   b) Commonly arise from preexisting lesions on feet, hands, legs, back, and trunk
   c) Highly malignant; metastasize rapidly

C. Contact dermatitis
1. Redness leading to vesicle formation, crusting, scaling; pruritus
2. Caused by irritants or allergens

D. Seborrhea
1. Scaling or patches of greasy accumulations on scalp, eyebrows, hairline, nasolabial folds

E. Pruritus
1. Itching; no change to skin unless secondary from scratching
2. Half of all cases associated with systemic illness
3. Must identify underlying cause

F. Pediculosis
1. Pediculosis corporis (body lice): small red macular lesions with severe itching
2. Pediculosis capitus (head lice): white specks in hair with itching; crusts may develop on scalp
3. Pediculosis pubis (pubic lice): small gray flecks on pubic hair
4. All types contagious

G. Scabies
1. Caused by itch mites
2. Severe itching, worse at night; linear whitish-gray pattern with dark dot at end
3. Common sites are digital web spaces, flexor surface of wrists, axilla, nipples, genitalia
4. Contagious

H. Herpes zoster
1. Caused by reactivation of varicella virus
2. Unilateral symptoms along nerve pathway: paresthesia, dysesthesia followed by extremely painful vesicles

that crust in two weeks and resolve within several months

3. Local lymph glands can be tender and palpable

4. Postherpetic neuralgia more common in older adults

I. Decubitus ulcers
1. Result from prolonged pressure impairing tissue circulation
2. Immobility, malnutrition, shearing forces are contributing factors
3. Stages
   a) Hyperemia: redness, disappears when pressure removed
   b) Ischemia: discoloration, swelling
   c) Ulceration: break in skin, open lesion
   d) Necrosis: dead skin, eschar
4. Must identify and decrease risk factors

IV. Related nursing diagnoses
A. Pain
B. Potential for infection
C. Potential for injury
D. Knowledge deficit
E. Altered oral mucous membrane
F. Self-care deficit
G. Personal identity disturbance
H. Sensory/perceptual alterations
I. Impaired skin integrity
J. Sleep pattern disturbance
K. Social isolation

READINGS AND REFERENCES

Gilcrest BA. Dermatologic disorders in the elderly. Pages 375 and 379 in: *Clinical Geriatrics*, 3rd ed. Rossman I (editor). Philadelphia: Lippincott, 1986.

Kligman AM, Grove GL, Balin AK. Aging of the human skin. Page 837 in: *Handbook of the Biology of Aging*, 2nd ed. Finch CE, Schneider EL (editors). New York: Van Nostrand Reinhold, 1985.

Rossman I. Anatomy of aging. Page 12 in: *Clinical Geriatrics*, 3rd ed. Rossman I (editor). Philadelphia: Lippincott, 1986.

6 Assessment of the Cardiovascular System

Sandra E. Orem, RN, MSN

REVIEW OF THE CARDIOVASCULAR SYSTEM

Perhaps no other single factor is as crucial to our lives as the healthy functioning of the cardiovascular system. The status of this system influences the normality, efficiency, and potential of all physical and mental functions. To conduct a comprehensive assessment that sheds light on the multiple, complex processes of the human organism, your understanding of the composition and dynamics of the cardiovascular system is essential. A review of related anatomy and physiology will provide the basis for future physical examination. Abbreviations for various terms are listed in Table 6-1.

Chest Wall Landmarks

Because an examination of the heart is accomplished chiefly through the anterior chest wall, an understanding of chest wall landmarks is crucial (Figure 6-1). Recording and describing findings using these landmarks is necessary to guide other practitioners in interpreting information from your assessment.

The chest wall landmarks are the midsternal line; the midclavicular line; and the anterior, middle, and posterior axillary lines. The suprasternal notch, ribs, and intercostal spaces are other descriptors used to define findings of

Table 6-1 Abbreviation Guide

ASCVD	Arteriosclerotic cardiovascular disease	MI	Myocardial infarction
		MSL	Midsternal line
AV	Atrioventricular valve	PVD	Peripheral vascular disease
CHF	Congestive heart failure	PMI	Point of maximal impulse (apical impulse)
ECG, EKG	Electrocardiograph		
HBP	Hypertension	RCA	Right coronary artery
IHSS	Idiopathic hypertrophic subaortic stenosis	RICS	Right intercostal space (aortic area)
LAD	Left anterior descending artery	RVH	Right ventricular hypertrophy
LCA	Left circumflex artery	S_1	First heart sound
LVH	Left ventricular hypertrophy	S_2	Second heart sound
LICS	Left intercostal space (pulmonic area)	S_3	Third heart sound
		S_4	Fourth heart sound
LSB	Left sternal border (tricuspid area)	SA	Sinoatrial
		SB	Sternal border
MCL	Midclavicular line		

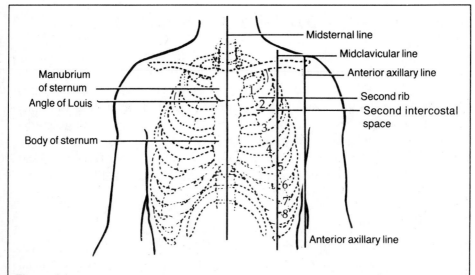

Figure 6-1

Chest wall landmarks. Numbers designate intercostal spaces. Source: Holloway NM. *Nursing the Critically Ill Adult*, 3rd ed. Menlo Park, CA: Addison-Wesley, 1988.

physical examination. The precordium is that area of the chest that overlies the heart and pericardium.

The Heart in the Thorax

The position of the heart within the thorax can vary among individuals based on body build, chest shape, and diaphragm level. The heart is located in the mediastinum in the thoracic cavity and rests on the diaphragm (Figure 6-2). The right atrium is located to the right of the sternum; the right ventricle is directly behind the sternum; the left ventricle is positioned between the sternum and left midclavicular line. The left atrium is located directly behind the other chambers.

A tough double-walled fibrous sac, the pericardium, encases the entire heart. The outer layer of the pericardium is firmly attached to the aorta, esophagus, pleura, diaphragm, and sternum. Several cubic centimeters of fluid separate the two walls of the pericardium to allow easy movement with cardiac muscle activity.

The upper portion of the heart is known as the base and includes the aorta, pulmonary arteries, and great veins. The lower portion is referred to as the cardiac apex. The apex is positioned downward and to the left, and includes the left and right ventricles. The heart is positioned so the right ventricle makes up the greatest anterior aspect. The thrust of the left ventricle at the apex generates what is known as the apical impulse or point of maximal impulse

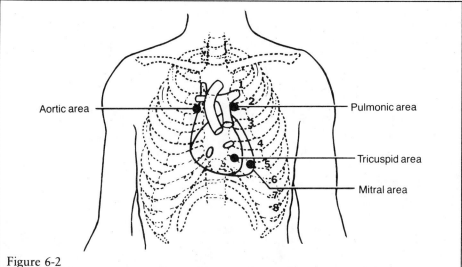

Figure 6-2
Position of the heart in the thorax. Source: Holloway NM. *Nursing the Critically Ill Adult*, 3rd ed. Menlo Park, CA: Addison-Wesley, 1988.

(PMI). The PMI occurs briefly in systole and is found in the fifth intercostal space 7 to 9 cm to the left of the midsternal line.

The Great Vessels

Unoxygenated blood returning to the heart enters the right atrium via the inferior and superior vena cavae. The pulmonary artery carries this unoxygenated blood to the right and left pulmonary arteries and to the right and left lungs. Oxygenated blood from the lungs returns to the left atrium via pulmonary veins, enters the left ventricle, and exits the heart to nourish the body via the aorta. The aorta exits upward from the left ventricle and arches to the left, backward and downward at the level of the sternal angle. (See Figure 6-2.)

Heart Valves and Blood Flow

The diagram in Figure 6-3 illustrates blood flow through the heart and identifies cardiac structures.

Heart Sounds

Valve closure, tension, and vibrations of myocardial structures and blood flow are all believed to contribute to the production of heart sounds. The diagram

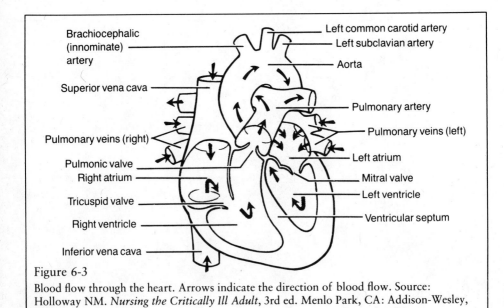

Figure 6-3

Blood flow through the heart. Arrows indicate the direction of blood flow. Source: Holloway NM. *Nursing the Critically Ill Adult*, 3rd ed. Menlo Park, CA: Addison-Wesley, 1988.

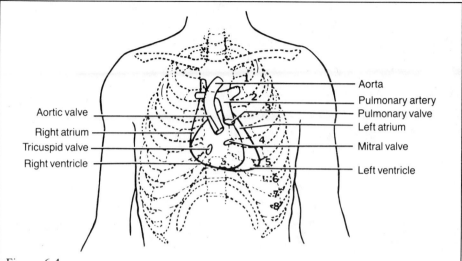

Aorta
Pulmonary artery
Pulmonary valve
Left atrium
Mitral valve
Left ventricle

Aortic valve
Right atrium
Tricuspid valve
Right ventricle

Figure 6-4

Auscultatory areas: location of heart and valves and topographic areas where sounds are best heard. Source: Holloway NM. *Nursing the Critically Ill Adult*, 3rd ed. Menlo Park, CA: Addison-Wesley, 1988.

in Figure 6-4 presents anterior chest wall topographic areas where each heart sound can best be heard. Note that each sound is not heard directly over the valve producing the sound and that valve sounds are transmitted to other areas of the chest wall. The topographic areas include:

- *Mitral area*: mitral valve closure can best be heard at the fifth left intercostal space (LICS) at the midclavicular line (MCL).
- *Tricuspid area*: the tricuspid valve is best heard at the fourth LICS at the sternal border (SB).
- *Pulmonic area*: pulmonic valve activity is heard at the second LICS at the SB
- *Aortic area*: aortic valve sounds are best heard at the second right intercostal space (RICS) at the SB.

A brief description of heart sounds is offered here; cardiovascular medicine texts can offer more extensive descriptions of events in the cardiac cycle and their relationship to heart sounds.

First heart sound (S_1) = ventricular pressure rise causing atrioventricular (AV) valve closure

    Characteristics: Best heard at the apex

                       At base of heart, S_1 is usually louder on the left than on the right

On both sides of the base, S_1 is usually softer than S_2

Both mitral and tricuspid components of S_1 are usually heard as one sound

Occurrence of S_1 can be timed with apical or carotid pulse

Second heart sound (S_2) = vibrations produced by closure of aortic and pulmonic valves

   Characteristics: Usually louder at the base than S_1

Pulmonic component is softer than aortic component and is therefore heard best at the pulmonic area

Transient physiologic splitting of S_2 may be found in normal persons at end of inspiration

Third heart sound (S_3) = ventricular filling sounds due to rapid ventricular filling. Also referred to as ventricular gallop

   Characteristics: Sounded out as the word Ken–tuc'–ky

Low pitched and best heard at apex

Common in children and young adults

Appearance of S_3 in adult with known heart disease is abnormal and usually associated with dilatation of left ventricle

A main diagnostic clue for early congestive heart failure

Occurs after S_2

Fourth heart sound (S_4) Referred to as atrial gallop

   Characteristics: Sounded out as the word Ten'–nes–see

Occurs before S_1

Rarely heard in persons with normal hearts

Occurs often with myocardial infarction and may be early indicator of onset of congestive heart failure

May be associated with hypertensive cardiovascular disease, coronary artery disease, aortic stenosis, severe anemia, or hyperthyroidism

Summation gallop may occur in persons with severe myocardial disease and tachycardia. It is a result of S_3 and S_4 combining.

Other Abnormal Heart Sounds

Murmurs or *bruits* are more prolonged audible sounds during systole or diastole. They are produced by vibrations within the heart or walls of the large vessels. A *thrill* is a palpable vibration. Murmurs, bruits, or thrills are produced by three main factors alone or in combination: (a) increased rate of blood flow across normal valves; (b) forward blood flow through irregular or constricted valves, or into dilated blood vessel or chamber; (c) backward or regurgitant blood flow through an incompetent valve, septal defect, or patent ductus arteriosus.

Pericardial friction rub is caused by inflammation of the pericardial sac in which the two surfaces become roughened and rub against each other. The rub is described as grating, scratching, or rasping as squeaky leather does. This sound occurs during systole and diastole, and may be best heard between the apex and sternum. Pericardial inflammation may be caused by infection, trauma, or myocardial infarction.

Coronary Circulation

The myocardium receives its blood supply via the right and left coronary arteries that originate in the aorta just as it exits the left ventricle. The left coronary artery branches into the left circumflex artery (LCA) and the left anterior descending artery (LAD). The LCA supplies the posterior heart in about 20% of the population. (Usually the right coronary artery [RCA] supplies the posterior right heart.) The LAD artery supplies the anterior and left portion of the heart. In most people, branches of the RCA nourish the sinoatrial node and atrioventricular node in the conduction system and the left coronary artery supplies the interventricular septum. Coronary circulation increases in response to increased heart rate, increased activity, and stimulation of the sympathetic nervous system.

Cardiac Rhythm and Innervation

Cardiac rhythm is influenced by the autonomic nervous system plus the heart's own intrinsic nervous control. Impulse formation and conduction are influenced by spontaneous depolarization of the heart's conduction system plus sympathetic and parasympathetic innervation. Sympathetic stimulation increases impulse formation and conduction as well as strength of contraction. Parasympathetic stimulation, mainly vagus nerve stimulation, slows impulse formation and conduction, and decreases contractile force. Vagal fibers chiefly innervate the (SA) node, atrial tissue, and AV node. Sympathetic fibers innervate all areas of atria and ventricles.

Function of the Cardiovascular System

It is the task of the heart and blood vessels to (a) deliver nutrients, oxygen, hormones, and other materials continuously to all tissues and cells throughout the body; and (b) remove waste materials arising as end products of cellular metabolism. The heart acts as a pump to move oxygen-rich blood into the arterial system where it is delivered to capillaries in body tissues. The heart also functions to collect unoxygenated blood returning from the body's tissues and pump it to the lungs for reoxygenation.

AGE-RELATED CHANGES IN THE CARDIOVASCULAR SYSTEM

Structural Changes

In the past it was believed that the heart size decreased as one aged; however, current research has shown that there is no change in heart size with age. The cardiothoracic ratio may increase because of the decreased thorax width. The valves get thick and rigid, secondary to fibrosis and sclerosis, especially the mitral valve and the base or aortic cusps. There is thickening of the left ventricle in normotensive persons. The endocardium thickens and scleroses, and the amount of subpericardial fat increases. Fibroelastic thickening increases in the region of the SA node. There is calcification of media and elastic proliferation of musculoelastic arteries, including the coronary arteries. As this calcification occurs, the aorta and aortic branches dilate and become tortuous; the carotid arteries may become kinked, a problem more commonly found in women (Rossman 1986); and the superficial vessels of the forehead, neck, and extremities become prominent and tortuous.

Other heart muscle changes that become evident with age also occur. Increased collagen and scarring, decreased elasticity, and increased rigidity lead to difficult contraction and dilation of the cardiac muscle. Amyloid accumulation in the heart is associated with aging and leads to cardiac enlargement with clinical symptoms of arrhythmias and intractable congestive heart failure. A degenerative process of the upper ventricular septum and sclerosis of heart skeleton and bundle of His or branches lead to arrhythmias, including complete heart block.

Hemoglobin is noted to be lower in many older adults. This is secondary to loneliness, poor eating, and atrophic changes in gastric mucosa that may contribute to anemia and result in decreased oxygen transported per liter of cardiac output.

The diaphragm is raised in obese older adults and thereby makes the heart lie in a transverse position. The diaphragm is low in thin persons, especially those with emphysema, and the heart is found in a vertical position. These facts have implications for palpating PMI and determining heart size by palpation and percussion.

Physiological Changes

The heart rate slows with age, ranging anywhere from 44 to 108 beats per minute. Resting heart rate is not altered. The systole prolongs; therefore, a heart rate of 120 or greater is not well tolerated cardiodynamically. Stroke volume decreases and cardiac output decreases about 1% per year below normal of liters/minute, beginning in the mid 20s. Maximum coronary blood flow at age 60 is about 35% less than that occurring in youth.

Cardiovascular stress response is less efficient in the older adult. The heart rate elevation under stress is not as great as when the person was younger, and an elevated heart rate takes longer to return to baseline. To compensate for decreased heart rate elevation, stroke volume may increase. This increase may produce elevated blood pressure, or the blood pressure may stay stable and tachycardia may progress to heart failure in older adults.

Cardiac oxygen usage is less efficient in the older adult. The proportion of oxygen extracted from arterial blood as it passes through tissues decreases with age. Systolic blood pressure rises with aging as an adaptation to the loss of elasticity in peripheral vessels and subsequent increased peripheral resistance. Increased vasopressor lability tends to raise both systolic and diastolic blood pressure.

Recovery of myocardial contractility and irritability is delayed; the heart, therefore, does not tolerate tachycardia well. Tachycardia produced by fever, emotions, exercise, or other conditions may give rise to heart failure in the older adult.

Vasomotor tone decreases and vagal tone increases. Baroreceptor sensitivity decreases. The heart is more sensitive to carotid sinus stimulation and less sensitive to atropine.

Electrocardiogram (EKG) changes may occur secondary to cellular aging changes, fibrosis of the conduction system, and neurogenic effects. These changes include: (a) possible decreased voltage of all waves, (b) slight prolongation of all intervals, and (c) left axis deviation.

Symptoms and Findings in the Older Adult

When assessing the older adult, evaluate symptoms to determine if they represent cardiovascular disease or if they are associated with therapy. Digitalis and diuretic therapy often produce iatrogenic symptoms in the older adult that can make it difficult to evaluate and diagnose the client accurately.

Complaints associated with digitalis and diuretic toxicity include nausea, vomiting, blurred and yellow vision, weakness, apathy, diarrhea, fatigue, arrhythmias, tachycardia, dryness and dehydration, anxiety, and depression.

Other complaints of the older adult that must be assessed with regard to their relationship to cardiovascular disorders include abdominal pain, anorexia, insomnia, easy fatigability, urinary frequency, and nocturia. Abdominal pain may be associated with hepatomegaly from congestion. Insomnia may be related to Cheyne-Stokes respiration that appears in the older adult.

Common complaints generally related to cardiovascular disorders are as follows:

Confusion, dizziness, blackouts, and syncope in the older adult may be secondary to aortic stenosis, decreased carotid flow, inadequate cardiac output in response to exertion, marked vasodilatation of skeletal muscle vessels, water and electrolyte disorders, digitalis toxicity, and digitalis delirium.

Ectopic beats described as palpitations, butterflies, or skipped heartbeats may be benign or pathologic and must be evaluated thoroughly.

Murmurs are common in 60% or more of the older adult population (Malasanos et al 1986). The most common murmur is a soft systolic ejection murmur heard at the base of the heart due to sclerotic changes at the base of the cusps of the aortic valve.

Coughs and wheezes may indicate early left-sided heart failure and are always important symptom complaints to investigate in the older adult.

Hemoptysis may be indicative of heart failure as well as pulmonary embolus in the older adult. Pulmonary embolus has a high occurrence rate in the older adult.

Shortness of breath is a common complaint that may be described as tiredness, fatigue, or breathlessness. Heart disease should be suspected in the older adult who describes shortness of breath after exercise that previously did not bother him or her, or who suddenly awakens with breathlessness. Complaints of shortness of breath or dyspnea may be the chief symptom of acute myocardial infarction.

Edema of the legs may be suggestive of right-sided heart failure.

Chest pains, while commonly thought of as relating to heart disorders, may be associated with a variety of conditions in the older adult. Among these conditions are angina pectoris, myocardial infarction, pericarditis, pleurisy, pulmonary embolism, dissecting aortic aneurysm, and hepatomegaly secondary to heart failure. Other chronic and acute causes of recurrent chest pain in the older adult include spinal arthritis, kyphoscoliosis of the spine, herniated disc, hiatus hernia, esophagitis, peptic ulcer, and gallbladder disease.

ASSESSMENT OF THE CARDIOVASCULAR SYSTEM

History Taking and Physical Examination

The following combination of history taking and physical examination is recommended, whether you are performing an initial assessment or a reassessment of the older adult.

Chief complaint:	Elicit the client's chief complaint at the beginning of the assessment. Watch nonverbal behavior while the older adult talks. Note signs of pain, tension, fear, fatigue, posture, color, and general physical appearance. Elicit complaints of mental status changes, chest pain, dyspnea, orthopnea, syncope, edema,

palpitations, cough, paroxysmal nocturnal dyspnea, and hemoptysis.

History of present illness: Review the onset in chronologic order. For symptoms presented, elicit location, quality, intensity, duration, causes, and known relief measures.

Life-style: A review of daily living activities can yield insight into potential cardiac problems. It is useful to know if the client is unable to shop for groceries, walk to the corner mailbox, or bathe or dress without becoming fatigued and needing several rests during the activity. Some older adults have become accustomed to compensating for their activity intolerance, so they will not acknowledge this as a problem during the interview. To reveal activity tolerance problems, specific questions can be asked such as: "How long does it take you to get dressed in the morning?" "Describe how you shop for and put away your groceries." "What type of activities do you do in your spare time?" "How do you compare your energy and activity with others your age?" "What changes have you noticed in your daily activities in the past ten years . . . the past five years?" Questions pertaining to social activities can indicate if social functions have been decreased due to insufficient energy or other physical limitations.

Physical assessment: Select a systematic approach to physical examination and use it consistently. Cardiovascular assessment will include examination of arterial pulses and arterial blood pressures, venous pulses and pressure, and the heart. As a rule, the four assessment skills used in physical examination are used in the following sequence for assessment of the cardiovascular system: inspection, palpation, percussion, auscultation. Using a head-to-toe approach apply the four assessment skills in sequence as you examine each body part to assess cardiovascular status (Table 6-2).

Table 6-2 Systematic Assessment Approach

	Extremities	Head and Neck	Chest	Abdomen
Inspect	Pulses: compare bilaterally Color of nails, fingers, extremities Venous distention	Temple and carotid pulsations Venous distention, neck and forehead Venous pressure in neck veins Color of face, lips, neck	Surface vein distention Heaves at apex (PMI) Pulsations at apex (PMI) Color	Aortic pulse
Palpate	Peripheral pulses: compare bilaterally Temperature Thrills	Pulses, carotid and temple Thrills	PMI	Aortic pulse
Percuss			Heart size	
Auscultate	Systemic blood pressure	Bruits, neck, and temple	Heart sounds	Bruits Aortic pulse

The Heart

Inspect and palpate systematically while standing on the client's right side. A light shining tangentially across the chest surface facilitates observations of the supine client. Observe the chest, precordium, and epigastrium for size, symmetry, retractions, pulsations, lifts, and heaves. Note the location and timing of all impulses observed. Using either the palm of your hand at the base of your fingers, or your finger pads, systematically palpate the precordium as the client is supine or has his head slightly elevated. Observe and palpate for PMI, thrills, lifts, heaves, or retractions. Retractions are a normal finding when they occur as a slight retraction of the chest wall slightly medial to MSL at 5th LICS. Occurrence of marked retraction of the rib is abnormal, and in such cases this may be an indicator of pericardial disease. Heaves or lifts are associated with forceful work of the right ventricle. They appear as diffuse lifting along the LSB during systole.

Use a systematic approach by either starting at the base of the heart and proceeding to the apex, or vice versa. Select your own approach and practice it consistently. Mentally picture underlying structures and timing in the cardiac cycle as you examine the client (Figure 6-5).

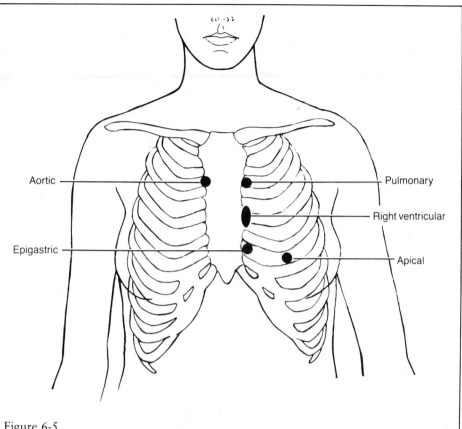

Figure 6-5

Areas of inspection and palpation using systematic approach. Source: Olds SB et al. *Obstetric Nursing*. Menlo Park, CA: Addison-Wesley, 1980.

I. *Apical area*: the left ventricular area located at 5th LICS, at or slightly medial to the MCL.

    A. Observe for and palpate the PMI, sometimes referred to as the apical impulse.

    B. The PMI occurs almost simultaneously with the carotid pulse. Palpate both at the same time to help locate the PMI.

    C. Have the client turn to the left lateral recumbent position to help locate the PMI.

    D. Record and describe impulse location, diameter, duration, amplitude, and timing.

	Normal Findings	Abnormal Findings
Location	5th LICS at MCL	Displaced to left and/or downward. Occurs in left ventricular hypertrophy (LVH).
Diameter	2 cm or smaller	Becomes diffuse, palpable, and observable in more than one interspace.
Duration	About 1/2 second	Sustained lift or heave rather than brief light tap.
Amplitude	Light tap	
Timing	First part of systole	

E. Thrills noted here are related to mitral valve disease.

II. *Right ventricular area*: located at lower left sternal border.

A. Observe and palpate diffuse, lifting systolic impulse, and thrills.

B. Associated abnormal findings:

1. Diffuse, lifting systolic impulse is associated with right ventricular hypertrophy (RVH) related to pulmonary hypertension, COPD, pulmonary valve disease.

2. Thrills noted here are associated with ventricular septal defects.

3. Brief right ventricular impulse is seen with increased metabolic states and increased cardiac output as in anemia, fever, exercise, hyperthyroidism, and pregnancy.

III. *Pulmonary area*: located at the second LICS at the base of the heart.

A. Observe and palpate pulsation, thrill, vibration of pulmonary valve closure.

B. Associated abnormal findings:

1. Thrills related to pulmonic stenosis, felt in 2nd and 3rd LICS.

2. Vibration of pulmonic valve closing accentuated with pulmonary hypertension.

IV. *Aortic area*: located at 2nd RICS.

A. Observe and palpate pulsation, thrill, vibration of aortic valve closure.

   B. Associated abnormal findings:
   1. Thrill associated with aortic stenosis; may be felt in 2nd and
       3rd RICS.
   2. May feel vibration of aortic valve closing if accentuated.
   3. Pulsation of aortic aneurysm.
V. *Epigastric area*:
   A. Observe and palpate pulsations of abdominal aorta.
   B. Associated abnormal findings:
   1. Increased pulsation associated with aneurysm.
   2. RV pulsation associated with RVH.

Following inspection and palpation, *percuss* to outline the left border
of cardiac dullness and to define heart size. Percussion is a supplement to
palpation that more accurately assesses cardiac enlargement. Using a systematic approach, assess the 3rd, 4th, and 5th LICS for cardiac dullness. To
do this, place your pleximeter (middle) finger parallel with each interspace.
Move your finger in a lateral to medial direction about 1 cm at a time and
percuss lightly until you define the border of cardiac dullness at each interspace. Measure the distance between the midsternal line and the border of
dullness at each interspace.

> Usual findings: 3rd LICS— 4 cm
>   4th LICS— 7 cm
>   5th LICS—10 cm

Percussion of RSB should disclose no cardiac dullness beyond RSB. The
successfulness of percussion is influenced by chest shape and size, and the
amount of air and fatty tissue present.

Auscultation demands the use of an adequate stethoscope. The stethoscope should feature snugly fitting ear pieces, appropriately short tubing
(about one foot) to decrease dampening effect of long tubing, bell, and diaphragm. The bell, applied lightly, will bring out low-frequency sounds like
S_3, S_4, and diastolic murmur of mitral stenosis. The diaphragm, applied
firmly, brings out high-frequency sounds like S_1, S_2, and murmurs associated
with aortic and mitral regurgitation, and pericardial friction rub.

The environment should be quiet and warm enough to prevent the
exposed client from shivering. Examine the client in supine, left lateral
recumbent, and sitting positions. Again, a systematic approach is valuable
(Figure 6-6):

   I. Begin either at the apex and proceed to the base, or vice versa.
       Pick your own system and adhere to it consistently.

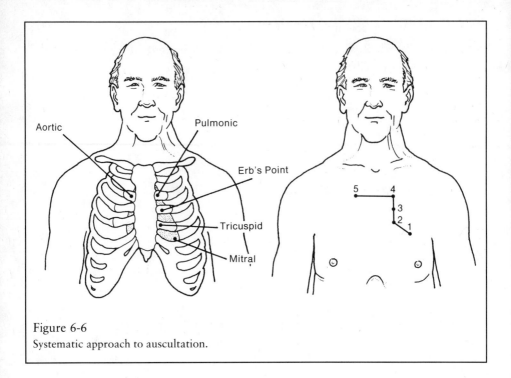

Figure 6-6
Systematic approach to auscultation.

II. Examine areas of sound radiation including carotid arteries and axillary areas.
III. Note rate and rhythm.
IV. At each auscultatory area, selectively listen for and note separately:
   A. S_1—intensity and variations, effects of respiration
   B. S_2—intensity and variations, effects of respiration
   C. Systole—extra sounds and murmurs
   D. Diastole—extra sounds and murmurs
V. Use diaphragm first and move progressively to each auscultatory area by inching the stethoscope along:
   A. Apex (mitral area)—5th LICS, inch medially toward
   B. Left sternal border (LSB) (tricuspid area)—inch upward along LSB to
   C. Erb's Point—3rd LICS at SB (aortic and pulmonic murmurs may be heard here), move to
   D. 2nd LICS (pulmonic area), and then to
   E. 2nd RICS (aortic area)

VI. Complete preceding auscultatory examination using both the diaphragm and bell with client in each of three positions: supine, left lateral recumbent, and sitting up while leaning slightly forward.

VII. Describe findings:

    A. Rhythm: regular/irregular, association with respiration

    B. Extra sounds: note timing, intensity, pitch

    C. Murmurs: note and record the following:

        1. Timing—systole, diastole

        2. Location—number of centimeters from landmark lines

        3. Radiation to other precordial or surrounding areas

        4. Pitch—high, medium, low

        5. Quality—musical, harsh, blowing, rumbling

        6. Grade—1 to 6:

            1—Very faint; may not be heard in all positions

            2—Faint but heard as soon as stethoscope is placed on chest

            3—Moderately loud; no thrill

            4—Loud; thrill may be present

            5—Very loud; often heard with stethoscope slightly off chest; thrill present

            6—Very loud; heard without stethoscope on chest; thrill present

The EKG has long been an essential tool in the evaluation of cardiac function. An EKG should be performed on a regular basis and, certainly, whenever any suspicion of cardiac dysfunction exists. Diagnostic advances such as the Doppler ultrasound, radionuclide imaging, computerized tomography, and magnetic resonance imaging may be used as a means to allow earlier, less invasive detection of heart disease than previous diagnostic techniques.

The Arterial and Venous Pulses and Pressures

Examination of *jugular venous pressure* is an indirect assessment of central venous pressure using inspection. To prepare the client for this procedure, remove the clothing from the client's neck and chest. If venous pressure is normal or slightly elevated, place the client flat; if congestive heart failure (CHF) is present, place the client at a 45° angle. Turn the client's head slightly away from you and shine a light tangentially across the neck to increase

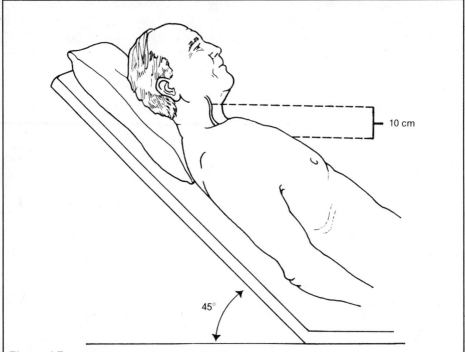

10 cm

45°

Figure 6-7

Measurement of jugular venous pressure. A distance of 10 cm exists between the meniscus of the distended neck veins and the manubrium sterni.

shadows. Examine both sides of the neck. Measure from the manubrium sterni to the level of elevation (Figure 6-7). Describe findings in centimeters and state client's position for that reading. Normal findings are that full neck veins appear when the client is supine. At a 45° angle elevation the venous pulse ascends a few millimeters above the clavicle. Abnormal findings are listed in Table 6-3.

The *hepatojugular reflux* is used to check for right-sided heart failure. This procedure involves applying moderately firm pressure with the palm of the hand for one-half to one minute over the right upper quadrant of the abdomen and noting jugular vein distention. An increase of greater than 1 cm is abnormal. In the absence of right-sided heart failure, neck vein distention will increase as pressure on the right upper quadrant increases venous return to the heart.

Use the techniques of inspection, palpation, and auscultation to examine both *carotid arteries*. Inspect for large, bounding carotid arterial pulses. Place the index and middle fingers on the lower neck at the medial edge of the sternocleidomastoid muscle and palpate gently. Palpate both carotids, one at a time, with the client's head turned slightly toward you. Note rate, rhythm,

Table 6-3 Jugular Veins: Abnormal Findings

Characteristics	Associated Conditions
Neck vein distention, which can reach to angle of jaw, while client is sitting upright or at 45° angle	High pressure on right side of heart
Unilateral neck vein distention	Kinking of left innominate vein
Bilateral neck vein distention	Elevated venous pressure associated with congestive heart failure, pericarditis, and superior vena cava obstruction

equality, contour, and amplitude (size). Palpating one side at a time averts carotid sinus massage, which slows the heart rate. Such heart-rate slowing and decreased cardiac output can produce additional problems for older adults with already compromised circulation. Auscultate both carotids with the stethoscope bell to detect bruits.

Normal pulse characteristics with single positive wave include:

Smooth and rapid upstroke

Dome-shaped summit

Downstroke that is less steep than the stroke

Appearance of a dicrotic notch on downstroke, which is often not palpable

Occurrence of the carotid pulse nearly simultaneously with the S_1

Abnormal findings of the carotid arteries are listed in Table 6-4.

Blood Pressure

To assess blood pressure, position the client comfortably and put him or her at ease. The arm should be free, without restrictive clothing, and positioned so that the brachial artery is approximately at the heart level. Measure blood pressure bilaterally, using brachial and popliteal arteries on first examination. Normal variation of up to 10 mm Hg between arms is acceptable. A normal leg systolic pressure is 10 to 40 mm Hg higher than arm systolic. Observe for interfering conditions such as anxiety and obesity.

To identify the palpatory systolic pressure, apply the cuff over the brachial artery so that the bottom edge is 2 to 3 cm above the antecubital crease (Table 6-5). Inflate the cuff to 30 mm Hg above the point where the palpated radial pulse disappears. Lower cuff pressure and note the point at which the radial pulse is palpable. Fully deflate the cuff.

To auscultate blood pressure, apply the stethoscope over the brachial artery so that it does not touch the cuff or clothing, or rub against itself. Inflate the cuff to 30 mm Hg higher than the palpatory systolic blood pressure and

Table 6-4 Carotid Arteries: Abnormal Findings

	Characteristics	Associated Conditions
Hyperkinetic pulse:	Large, strong, with normal contour, or high rapid upstroke, or, very rapid downstroke	Hyperdynamic conditions: fever, exercise, anxiety, hyperthyroidism, anemia Aortic insufficiency, common in adults Complete heart block with bradycardia and increased stroke volume
Hypokinetic pulse:	Weak pulse with diminished stroke volume	Left ventricular failure secondary to myocardial infarction Constrictive pericarditis Aortic valvular stenosis Other conditions that decrease stroke volume, increase resistance in peripheral vasculature, and/or affect flow across valves
Pulsus biferiens:	Double pulsations instead of usual single pulsation	Combination of aortic stenosis and insufficiency
Pulsus alternans:	Pulse occurs at regular intervals but amplitude varies	Conditions that affect force of contraction of left ventricle, as in cardiomyopathy and failure

Table 6-5 Blood Pressure Cuff Sizes

The size of the cuff bag will influence the accuracy of the blood pressure measurement. It is recommended that the cuff bag be 20% wider than the limb on which it will be used. In general, cuff widths should be as follows:

12–14 cm	Average adult
Narrower cuff	Thin adult
18–20 cm	Obese adult

then deflate slowly. Note and record three auscultatory levels:

1. Level at which you first hear at least two beats
2. Level at which sounds *become* muffled
3. Level at which all sounds disappear

For example: 128/82/74.

Observe for the auscultatory gap. This gap is a silent period between systolic and diastolic blood-pressure levels. It occurs in some persons, especially in the presence of hypertension. The gap is characterized by the onset of sounds, then a silent pause, followed by the return of sounds, then sudden muffling of sounds, and finally the disappearance of all sounds. Record all findings as in this example: 190/100/92 with auscultatory gap from 180 to 172.

DISORDERS OF THE CARDIOVASCULAR SYSTEM

Recognizing disorders, acute or chronic, in older adults is often difficult because of age-related changes they are undergoing. Changes in certain homeostatic processes contribute to altered presentation and perception of signs and symptoms. Age modifies the individual's responses to disease in general. Changing levels of pain threshold, blood pressure, and basal metabolism contribute to easily misinterpreting a clinical picture. Other factors that contribute to the difficulty in recognizing diseases and abnormalities in the older adult include:

1. Persistence of signs and symptoms of previous illnesses with a present illness (for example, changes in EKG from previous myocardial infarction [MI], high blood pressure)
2. Altered responses to drug therapy in older adults
3. Presentation of physical disorders as mental disturbances
4. Psychologic factors in the older adult that contribute to difficulty in evaluating the client. Many older adults become excited easily, resulting in an increase of catecholamine secretion, and hence an increase of stress on the heart

Specific cardiovascular disorders characteristic of this age group have not been defined. Older adults are, however, subject to any cardiovascular disorder. Because of other age-related changes affecting them, clinical manifestations of these disorders may often be aberrant and diagnoses may be difficult. The older adult may be more likely to experience and present cardiovascular disturbances than younger adults based on age-related changes in the cardiovascular system's structure and functions. The following section presents common cardiovascular disorders and their general characteristics, along with special features to consider when they occur in older adults.

Hypertension (HBP) and Hypertensive Heart Disease

The effect of high blood pressure on the body includes impairment of circulation to the heart muscle itself, contributing to the development of atherosclerosis and congestive heart failure. High blood pressure in the older adult is defined as levels greater than 170/95 on repeated measurements over several weeks (Moser and Block 1986). The Department of Health, Education, and Welfare's Joint National Committee on Detection, Evaluation, and Treatment of High Blood Pressure recommends repeated blood pressure measurements:

- Within one month for adults all ages with BP 160/95 or greater
- Within two to three months for adults under age 50 with BP 140/90–160/95
- Within six to nine months for adults over age 50 with BP 140/90–160/95

The Joint National Committee also recommends that treatment be individualized for persons with diastolic blood pressure (BP) 90 to 104, and that antihypertensive therapy is definitely indicated for persons with diastolic BP 105 to 119.

Physical examination should include checking for systemic manifestations of *and* contributors to hypertension. A thorough assessment includes the following:

- Standing and sitting BP
- Funduscopic examination for arteriovenous nicking, and tortuousity, hemorrhages, and papilledema
- Height and weight
- Examination of neck vessels for bruits and distention, and inspection of thyroid size
- Auscultation of lungs
- Evaluation of heart rate, heart size, precordial heave, murmurs, gallops, and arrhythmias
- Inspection of the abdomen for aortic size, aneurysm, and kidney size
- Assessment of extremities for edema, pulses, and neurologic deficits

Selective laboratory tests, useful before and after antihypertensive therapy, include hematocrit; urinalysis for protein, blood, and glucose; creatinine and/or blood urea nitrogen; serum potassium; and electrocardiogram. These baseline tests may evaluate changes in other systems or organs related to hypertension.

Blood pressure does tend to increase with aging. As previously described, this elevation represents an adaptation to structural changes of increased rigidity in arterial vessels. *It is essential to assess the value that blood pressure has for the individual's total systemic functioning.* The body's organs often adapt to the gradually increasing blood pressure that accompanies aging. Brain, kidney, and heart functioning depend on a certain blood flow that is partly maintained by a given blood pressure for the individual. That blood pressure may be elevated according to the usual definition of normal blood pressure. However, decreasing the client's blood pressure to or below this normal cut-off point may produce symptoms of insufficient blood and oxygen supply to the brain, heart, and kidneys. Symptoms of mental changes (disorientation, forgetfulness, short attention span, easy fatigability, dizziness), chest pain, dyspnea, decreased urinary output may suggest that the blood pressure, while at a "normal" level, may be too low to sustain blood flow essential for the individual's body-organ functioning.

Atherosclerosis and Its Manifestations

Atherosclerosis is not synonymous with aging and is not to be considered an inevitable outcome of aging. Atherosclerosis is, however, the most common cause of heart disease in older adults.

Atherosclerotic processes affecting coronary arteries develop rapidly in middle-aged men and postmenopausal women. Manifestations include angina, myocardial infarction, arrhythmias, congestive heart failure, and sudden death.

Angina

Typical angina presentation includes retrosternal pain or distress and radiating pain in the neck, jaw, arms, and back. Exertion, emotional excitement of a positive or negative nature, cold weather, or even meals may bring about angina. Nocturnal angina, occurring after one lies down, may be an indicator of early left-sided heart failure. Careful assessment must be made to distinguish angina from other conditions in the older adult that can produce similar symptoms. These conditions include, but are not limited to, esophagitis, ulcer, gallbladder disease, and hiatus hernia.

Acute Myocardial Infarction (MI)

Acute myocardial infarction is manifested by sudden dyspnea, acute confusion, and congestive heart failure more often in older adults than in younger persons, who present primarily with chest pain. Older adults may present with some angina symptoms, pressure, substernal distress, or pain radiating to left arm, neck, or abdomen. Moist pale skin, decreased blood pressure, and low-grade fever may also be manifested. Acute MI is often accompanied by arrhythmias. Older adults using diuretics may develop electrolyte imbalances, and in the presence of digitalis toxicity, increase the occasion of arrhythmia, especially after MI.

Recovery from a simple MI is generally successful in older adults. Potential complications following MI may include the following: arrhythmias, aneurysm of the myocardial wall; pump failure secondary to the previous two complications; papillary muscle dysfunction or rupture and subsequent cardiac failure; free wall rupture of the myocardium with transmural MIs and leading to cardiac tamponade; and sudden death. These complications of MI may occur more in the older adult because of aging structural changes and because other changes prevent the person from appreciating the signs and symptoms of MI or from reporting them to the physician. Many older adults who experience silent MIs do not enter into treatment early after the infarct and are, therefore, more subject to such complications. In addition, late mortality after the first five days from complications of renal failure, sepsis, and pulmonary and systemic emboli are more common in the older adult.

Peripheral Lesions

In the older adult, peripheral lesions include vascular ulcers and gangrenous lesions. Regular and careful examination of peripheral pulses, condition of nails and skin, plus follow-up for complaints of pain or paresthesias are essential for early detection of potentially ulcerating or gangrenous lesions. Remember that tactile sense and pain perception in the older adult may be diminished, making vital the demand for conscientious physical examination for peripheral lesions.

Mesenteric Arteriosclerosis

This disorder may be manifested with ischemic colitis, hemorrhagic enteropathy, and death. Assessment of the older adult must include thorough examination of all peripheral pulses, complaints of back, hip, and leg pain, changes in mentation, and sensory changes in extremities.

Pulmonary Heart Disease

Acute cor pulmonale usually occurs after pulmonary infarction. There is a high incidence of infarction with the older adult because of the greater tendency toward prolonged immobilization and propensity for thrombophlebitis. Most emboli develop in the lower extremities; a minority originate in the abdominal and pelvic veins, thorax, upper extremities, and head and neck vessels. Pulmonary embolus, chronic congestive heart failure, and atrial fibrillation may also contribute to development of acute cor pulmonale.

Chronic cor pulmonale usually occurs in association with emphysema.

Pulmonary Embolus

This disorder may be manifest by mental status changes of apprehension and confusion, dyspnea, fever, and pneumonitis. Pain may or may not be present based on the person's altered pain perception.

Bacterial Endocarditis

A high incidence of bacterial endocarditis occurs in older adults, attributable to several factors. For instance, the person may have decreased immunologic responses to infection associated with chronic steroid therapy, cancer chemotherapy, and the aging process itself. The increased use of instruments in diagnostic and treatment activities, especially genitourinary examination, increases the opportunities for fungal, staphylococcal, and other infections. Metabolic changes with age and the presence of diseases such as diabetes also contribute to the development of this condition.

Bacterial endocarditis, often difficult to diagnose, can originate from infection in the teeth, upper respiratory tract, genitourinary system, biliary tract, and through skin lesions. The usual findings of weakness, anemia, weight loss, and sweats are common to many conditions affecting the older adult and may be obscured if renal or central nervous system disease is present. Also, cardiac murmurs in the older adult often are attributed to arteriosclerotic changes. In older adults with bacterial endocarditis, other findings may include pericarditis, hepatomegaly, splenomegaly, positive blood cultures, intractable heart failure, and possible low-grade fever.

Hypothyroid Heart Disease

Hypothyroid heart disease, or myxedema, is common among women and older adults sensitive to iodides. Common findings associated with this condition include pericardial effusion, increased heart muscle bulk, sluggish contractions, muffled heart sounds, bradycardia, decreased oxygen consumption, slower basal metabolic rate, decreased cardiac output, increased venous pressure, and prolonged circulation time. Physical findings in persons with myxedema include obesity, hoarse voice, sluggish speech, puffy eyelids, coarse facial features, and slowed responses. This condition is difficult to diagnose because symptoms (such as psychotic behavior, constipation, arthritis, and leg ulcers) may be erroneously attributed to old age, rather than to a pathology affecting the thyroid.

Hyperthyroid Heart Disease

Common classical findings of hyperthyroid heart disease, also called thyrotoxicosis, include bilateral exophthalmos, tachycardia, warm extremities, and adenomatous neck goiter. This condition may be masked in some older adults, with only the cardiac manifestation present in the form of various rapid arrhythmias, including paroxysmal atrial fibrillation and/or sinus tachycardia.

Abdominal Aortic Aneurysm

A throbbing abdominal mass, a sense of abdominal fullness, and abdominal pain are the clinical findings associated with an abdominal aortic aneurysm. Ruptured aneurysm is a significant risk accompanying this problem and is manifested by sudden unexplained pain in the abdomen or back, unexplained fever, decreased hemoglobin, ecchymosis of lower abdomen or perineum, and loss of deep-tendon reflexes in lower extremities.

Idiopathic Hypertrophic Subaortic Stenosis (IHSS)

IHSS is characterized by abnormal hypertrophy and disorganization of septal fibers, resulting in a thick akinetic septum. While IHSS is believed to be of congenital origin, it commonly appears first in persons over 60 years of age. It is often misdiagnosed initially as coronary artery disease in the older adult.

The most common complaints indicating IHSS are palpitations plus angina-like chest pain of long duration and with poor response to nitroglycerin. Other complaints include exertional dyspnea, fatigue, syncope, and symptoms of heart failure. Atrial fibrillation and a classical variable ejection murmur are present. They are increased by standing, Valsalva maneuver, and after inhalation of amyl nitrate. ECG or echocardiography will reveal left ventricular hypertrophy (LVH). The presence of IHSS is highly suspected if a female patient over 60 years of age presents with (a) a variable ejection murmur that increases after amyl nitrite inhalation, (b) unexplained LVH, and (c) palpitations, dyspnea, chest pain, or heart failure.

Cardiac Arrhythmias

Tachyarrhythmias and extrasystoles increase with aging. Arrhythmias in the older adult may be associated with many conditions affecting the heart, including: congestive heart failure, arteriosclerotic cardiovascular disease, myocardial infarction, anemia, fluid and electrolyte disorders, mineral abnormalities (calcium), drug toxicity (digitalis, potassium iodide), other body system disorders (thyroid disorders), acute infections, and hemorrhage. Assessment for extracardiac causes as well as cardiac causes of arrhythmias is essential for a complete evaluation of the older adult.

Your assessment also must include an evaluation of the arrhythmia's effect on the client. Atrial fibrillation may, for example, be well tolerated by some individuals, but be poorly tolerated by others. As cardiac output is decreased by certain arrhythmias, the effect of the reduced output may produce symptoms in certain persons. Evaluation must include investigation for complaints of chest pain, fatigue, dizziness, forgetfulness, or other mental status changes, plus examination for worsening heart failure.

"Sick Sinus Syndrome"

Sinoatrial dysfunction or "sick sinus syndrome" has occurred after cardioversion of clients with atrial fibrillation of long duration, and occurs spontaneously in association with arteriosclerotic heart disease, rheumatic and hypertensive heart disease, and as an idiopathic condition.

Features of this disorder include: inappropriate sinus bradycardia that does not respond to drugs or exercise; episodes of sinus arrest with occasional junctional escape rhythm; premature atrial contractions; sinoatrial block; and episodic rapid rhythm with intermittent atrial flutter, fibrillation, and tachycardia, sometimes with a rapid ventricular response. Assessment of the client should include checking for this bradycardia–tachycardia syndrome. Use of holter monitoring detects bradycardia–tachycardia periods and helps correlate symptoms to such events. In older adults, sick sinus syndrome is an important cause of dizzy spells, light-headedness, fainting, and possibly seizures. Clients may also complain of angina, symptoms of heart failure, and palpitations.

Congestive Heart Failure (CHF)

The inability of cardiac output to meet metabolic needs affects approximately two to three million people over age 60 (Fleg and Lakatta 1986). CHF in the older adult may be a result of many conditions. Examples of etiologic disorders contributing to CHF in the older adult are as follows:

- Valve disease and malfunctioning, including stenosis and insufficiency with regurgitation involving mitral and aortic valves
- Arrhythmias
- Myocardial infarction
- Presence of multiple abnormalities affecting the heart

Pulmonary edema may occur secondary to CHF when left atrial pressure rises to levels where capillary pressure is greater than the oncotic pressure of plasma proteins. Fluid then exudes into the lung interstitium and alveoli and thereby interferes with oxygen uptake and transport.

Symptoms the older adult may present as manifestations of heart failure include: mental status changes (for example, confusion, agitation, night wandering), depression, insomnia, anorexia, nausea, weakness, fatigue, shortness of breath, orthopnea, and bilateral pedal/ankle edema.

Peripheral Vascular Disease (PVD)

Blood vessel disease affecting vessels external to the heart is referred to as peripheral vascular disease. Older adults may present a variety of signs and symptoms suggestive of PVD, including pain at rest or with activity, skin discoloration including pallor, skin temperature changes, changes in size of the affected body part, neuropathies, thick dry nails, thin dry scaling skin, edema, chills, cramping of legs or intermittent claudication, ulceration, and gangrene.

Specific peripheral vascular disorders affecting the older adult include the following:

- *Aneurysms* of the aorta and peripheral vessels, which may be visible, palpable, painful masses, and are common at femoral and popliteal sites. Aneurysms may be associated with atherosclerosis, arteriosclerosis, trauma, infection, syphilis, and other conditions.
- Arterial embolism, which occurs secondary to atrial fibrillation, myocardial infarction, atherosclerosis, and arteriosclerosis.
- *Venous thromboembolism*, which is often associated with bedrest, postsurgical procedures, and leg fractures. Edema, warmth, and pain may be manifested. Calf muscles are most commonly affected.
- *Arteriosclerosis obliterans*, which may be manifested by pain with intermittent claudication and neuropathy. Common occlusive sites are femoral arteries involving popliteal or tibial artery systems.
- *Varicose veins*, which occur in the older adult in association with decreased exercise, long periods of standing while working, and decreased elasticity associated with aging changes. Dilated, tortuous veins may be visible, especially affecting lower extremities.

PVD has a higher incidence in the older diabetic. Neuropathies and infections are common complications. Manifestations of insufficient circulation may include pain at rest, intermittent claudications, absent or diminished peripheral pulses, skin discoloration, ulcerated lesions, and gangrenous changes.

Acute Rheumatic Fever (RF)

RF is a troublesome problem for the older adult because it tends to be recurrent and has a high incidence in the 50- to 80-year-old population. In addition, the classical signs and symptoms of RF are not presented by the older adult who has this condition. Instead, the usual presentation includes slight fever, moderate joint symptoms, and a protracted course.

In the older adult, acute RF may be difficult to diagnose for a variety of reasons. Often, acute RF may be mistaken for rheumatoid arthritis because it runs a similar course. As with some other conditions in the older adult, including MI, active RF may be silent. In addition, the presence of hypertension and/or arteriosclerosis may obscure rheumatic carditis occurring with acute RF.

The older adult with rheumatic carditis will usually present with unexplained fever and signs and symptoms of persistent congestive heart failure. Complete heart block with Stokes–Adams episodes may also appear in the presence of rheumatic carditis. Older adults with rheumatic carditis who are receiving digitalis therapy may develop adverse side effects to the drug, such as nausea, vomiting, diarrhea, and cardiac arrhythmias.

In contrast to acute RF, older adults with *chronic rheumatic heart disease* (CRHD) present with frequent dyspnea and cyanosis secondary to emphysema, pulmonary arteriosclerosis, or anemic hypoxia. Other conditions common in the older adult with CRHD are pneumonia, pulmonary infarction, and congestive heart failure.

This chapter has dealt primarily with assessment of the cardiovascular system and its functioning. It is important to note, however, that thorough assessment of the older adult's cardiovascular status includes more than a direct assessment of the cardiovascular system. A complete evaluation of the client's cardiovascular status includes assessing the cardiovascular system activity and functioning as it is reflected in other body organs and structures, such as the brain, lungs, and kidneys. Keep in mind your intent to assess not only for structural abnormalities in the heart and blood vessels, but also for aberrations in functioning of the cardiovascular system and possible disturbances in other body organs as a result of cardiovascular disease or dysfunction. A complete assessment also includes evaluating the role of drugs and other treatment in producing cardiac symptoms. Examples include the overzealous treatment of hypertension in some clients, which results in hypotensive complications. It must be remembered that the older adult's increased sensitivity to various drugs may lead to exaggerated response to the drugs and potential side effects. For example, while digitalis is used to treat cardiovascular problems, increased sensitivity and digitalis toxicity may produce other cardiac disorders such as bigeminy and other arrhythmias.

An important consideration in assessing cardiovascular status is the impact of cardiovascular problems on the older adult's ability to fulfill daily living activities. Cardiovascular-related physical problems, such as pain and shortness of breath, and psychologic problems, such as fear of causing a "heart attack," can limit the older adult's ability to obtain and prepare nutritious meals, travel to and participate in social activities, and maintain a clean environment. A variety of interventions may be necessary to help the client cope with these problems. Interventions may include counseling as to the realities of his or her condition, instruction in pacing activities, and the arrangement of shopping, housekeeping, and meal delivery services.

Other chapters in this book deal with selected manifestations of cardiovascular system disease and dysfunction. You are encouraged to consult other references for additional information on the manifestations and management of cardiovascular dysfunction in other body systems.

6 Chapter Summary

I. Age-related changes
   A. Cardiothorax ratio may increase due to decreased thorax width
   B. Valves become thick and rigid
   C. Endocardium thickens and scleroses
   D. Increased subpericardial fat
   E. Increased fibroelastic thickening in region of SA node
   F. Aorta and aortic branches dilate and become tortuous
   G. Carotid arteries become kinked
   H. More prominent and tortuous superficial vessels of forehead, neck, and extremities
   I. Difficult contraction and dilation of cardiac muscle due to decreased elasticity and increased rigidity
   J. Increased prevalence of arrhythmias
   K. Higher incidence of lower hemoglobin
   L. Slower heart rate
      1. Rate can range from 44 to 108 beats per minute
   M. Less efficient cardiovascular stress response
      1. Takes longer for elevated heart rate to return to normal
   N. Less efficient cardiac oxygen usage
   O. Higher systolic blood pressure due to loss of elasticity in peripheral vessels and increased peripheral resistance
   P. Increased vasopressor lability may raise both systolic and diastolic blood pressure
   Q. Decreased vasomotor tone
   R. Increased vagal tone
   S. Decreased baroreceptor sensitivity
   T. Heart more sensitive to carotid sinus stimulation; less sensitive to atropine
   U. EKG changes
      1. Possible decreased voltage of all waves
      2. Slight prolongation of all intervals
      3. Left axis deviation

II. Assessment
   A. Complaints related to cardiovascular disorder
      1. Confusion
      2. Dizziness
      3. Blackouts
      4. Syncope
      5. Ectopic beats: described as palpitations, butterflies, or skipped heart beats
      6. Murmurs
         a) Present in 60% or more older adult clients
         b) Most common: soft systolic ejection murmur heard at base of heart
      7. Coughs
      8. Wheezes
      9. Hemoptysis
      10. Shortness of breath, dyspnea, orthopnea
      11. Edema
      12. Chest pain
      13. Fatigue
   B. History of present illness
   C. Physical assessment
      1. Use a systematic approach
      2. Includes examination of arterial pulses and arterial blood pressure, venous pulses and pressure, and the heart
      3. Apical area
         a) Located at 5th LICS at or slightly medial to MCL
         b) Observe and palpate PMI

c) Record and describe
impulse location,
diameter, duration,
amplitude, and timing

4. Right ventricular area
   a) Located at lower, left
   sternal border
   b) Observe and palpate
   systolic impulse and
   thrills

5. Pulmonary area
   a) Located at 2nd LICS at
   base of heart
   b) Observe and palpate
   pulsation, thrill, and
   vibration of pulmonary
   valve closure

6. Aortic area
   a) Located at 2nd RICS
   b) Observe and palpate
   pulsation, thrill, and
   vibration of aortic valve
   closure

7. Epigastric area
   a) Observe and palpate
   pulsation of abdominal
   aorta

8. Heart size
   a) Percuss 3rd, 4th, and
   5th LICS for cardiac
   dullness; measure
   distance between
   midsternal line and
   border of dullness at
   each interspace
   b) Percussion should reveal
   no cardiac dullness
   beyond RSB

9. Auscultatory areas
   a) Apex (mitral area)
   b) LSB (tricuspid area)
   c) Erb's Point
   d) 2nd LICS (pulmonic
   area)
   e) 2nd RICS
   f) Listen for:
   S_1 intensity, variations,
   and effects of
   respiration
   S_2 intensity, variations,

and effects of
respiration
Systole: extra sounds
and murmurs
Diastole: extra sounds
and murmurs
   g) Note rhythm, extra
   sounds, and murmurs
   h) Describe murmurs in
   terms of timing,
   location, radiation to
   other areas, pitch,
   quality, grade

10. Jugular venous pressure
    a) Indirect assessment of
    central venous pressure
    using inspection
    b) Normal findings: when
    client is supine, full neck
    veins appear; at 45°
    angle elevation, venous
    pulse ascends a few
    millimeters above the
    clavicle

11. Hepatojugular reflux
    a) Used to check for
    right-sided heart failure
    b) Moderate firm pressure
    applied with palm of
    hand over right, upper
    quadrant of abdomen
    for $\frac{1}{2}$ to 1 minute
    c) Note jugular vein
    distention: increase
    greater than 1 cm is
    abnormal

12. Carotid arteries
    a) Inspect for large,
    bounding carotid
    arterial pulses
    b) Palpate both carotids
    and note rate, rhythm,
    equality, contour, and
    amplitude
    c) Auscultate to detect
    bruits
    d) Normal pulse
    characteristics: single
    positive wave, smooth
    and rapid upstroke,

dome-shaped summit, downstroke less steep than upstroke, dicrotic notch appears on downstroke and occurs nearly simultaneously with S_1

13. Blood pressure
   a) Arm positioned so that brachial artery is at heart level
   b) Measure bilaterally: normal variation up to 10 mm Hg between arms is acceptable
   c) Normal leg systolic pressure is 10 to 40 mm Hg higher than arm systolic
   d) Identify palpatory systolic pressure
   e) Note and record three auscultatory levels: level at which first beats are heard, level at which first sounds become muffled, level at which all sounds disappear
   f) Observe for auscultatory gap: silent period between systolic and diastolic blood pressure levels

III. Disorders
   A. Hypertension and hypertensive heart disease
      1. In older adults, blood pressure levels greater than 170/95 on repeated measurements for several weeks indicates high blood pressure
      2. Higher levels of blood pressure acceptable in the older adult
      3. Baseline tests to evaluate changes in other organs related to blood pressure include hematocrit, urinalysis, creatinine, blood urea nitrogen, serum potassium, and EKG
   B. Atherosclerosis
      1. Most common cause of heart disease in the older adult
      2. Manifestations: angina, myocardial infarction, arrhythmias, congestive heart failure, and sudden death
   C. Angina
      1. Presents with retrosternal pain or distress and radiating pain in neck, jaw, arms, and back
      2. May be precipitated by exertion, excitement, cold weather, or meals
      3. Nocturnal angina can indicate early left-sided heart failure
   D. Acute myocardial infarction
      1. May be manifested by dyspnea, congestive heart failure, moist pale skin, anginal symptoms, pressure of substernal distress, decreased blood pressure, arrhythmias, and low-grade fever
      2. Chest pain may not be present
      3. Many older adults experience silent MIs, which causes delay in seeking treatment
   E. Peripheral lesion
      1. Includes vascular ulcers and gangrenous lesions
   F. Mesenteric arteriosclerosis
      1. Can cause ischemic colitis, hemorrhagic enteropathy, and death
   G. Acute cor pulmonale
      1. Usually follows pulmonary infarction
      2. Other contributing factors: pulmonary embolus,

chronic congestive heart failure, and atrial fibrillation

H. Chronic cor pulmonale
  1. Usually associated with emphysema

I. Pulmonary embolus
  1. May be manifested by dyspnea, fever, pneumonitis, and changes in mental status
  2. Pain may or may not be present

J. Bacterial endocarditis
  1. High incidence in older adults
  2. Can originate in teeth, upper respiratory tract, genitourinary system, biliary tract, and through skin lesions
  3. Symptoms often confused with other geriatric disorders: weakness, anemia, weight loss, sweats, cardiac murmurs
  4. Pericarditis, hepatomegaly, splenomegaly, positive blood cultures, intractable heart failure, and low-grade fever may be present

K. Hypothyroid heart disease (myxedema)
  1. Findings: pericardial effusion, increased heart muscle bulk, sluggish contractions, muffled heart sounds, bradycardia, decreased oxygen consumption, slower basal metabolic rate, decreased cardiac output, increased venous pressure, and prolonged circulation time
  2. Signs include overweight, hoarse voice, sluggish speech, puffy eyelids, coarse facial features, and slowed response

L. Hyperthyroid heart disease (thyrotoxicosis)
  1. Findings: bilateral exophthalmos, tachycardia, warm extremities, adenomatous neck goiter
  2. Can be masked with various rapid arrhythmias, the only cardiac manifestations

M. Abdominal aortic aneurysm
  1. Findings: throbbing abdominal mass, sense of abdominal fullness, abdominal pain
  2. Ruptured aneurysm is a risk

N. Idiopathic hypertrophic subaortic stenosis (IHSS)
  1. Findings: palpitation, angina-like chest pain of long duration and with no response to nitroglycerin, exertional dyspnea, fatigue, syncope, atrial fibrillation, and symptoms of failure

O. Cardiac arrhythmias
  1. Can be associated with congestive heart failure, arteriosclerotic cardiovascular disease, myocardial infarction, anemia, fluid and electrolyte disorders, mineral abnormalities, drug toxicity, hemorrhage, acute infections, and other system disorders
  2. Client complaints may include chest pain, fatigue, dizziness, forgetfulness, mental status change, and symptoms related to heart failure

P. "Sick sinus syndrome" (Sinoatrial dysfunction)
  1. Can occur after cardioversion of clients with atrial fibrillation of long duration, as an

idiopathic condition, and in association with arteriosclerotic, rheumatic, and hypertensive heart disease

2. Findings include sinus bradycardia that does not respond to drugs or exercise, episodes of sinus arrest, pneumatic atrial contractions, sinoatrial block, and episodic rapid rhythm with intermittent atrial flutter, fibrillation, and tachycardia

3. Can cause dizzy spells, light-headedness, fainting, seizures, angina, palpitations, and heart failure

4. Holter monitoring useful in diagnosis

Q. Congestive heart failure (CHF)
   1. Contributing factors: valve disease and malfunctioning, arrhythmias, myocardial infarction, and multiple abnormalities affecting the heart
   2. Pulmonary edema may occur secondary to CHF
   3. Symptoms include mental status changes, depression, insomnia, anorexia, nausea, weakness, fatigue, shortness of breath, orthopnea, and bilateral pedal/ankle edema

R. Peripheral vascular disease (PVD)
   1. Blood vessel disease affecting vessels external to the heart
   2. Symptoms include pain at rest or with activity, skin discoloration, skin temperature changes, changes in size of affected part, neuropathies, thick dry nails, thin dry scaling skin, edema, chills, cramping of legs, intermittent claudication, ulceration, and gangrene
   3. Specific PVD affecting the older adult
      a) Aneurysms of aorta and peripheral vessels
      b) Arterial embolism
      c) Venous thromboembolism
      d) Arteriosclerosis obliterans
      e) Varicose veins
   4. PVD of high incidence among older diabetics

IV. Related nursing diagnoses
   A. Activity intolerance
   B. Decreased cardiac output
   C. Pain
   D. Diversional activity deficit
   E. Fear
   F. Fluid volume excess
   G. Impaired home maintenance management
   H. Potential for infection
   I. Potential for injury
   J. Knowledge deficit
   K. Impaired physical mobility
   L. Altered nutrition: more than body requirements
   M. Self-care deficit
   N. Personal identity disturbance
   O. Sexual dysfunction
   P. Impaired skin integrity
   Q. Sleep pattern disturbance
   R. Impaired social interaction
   S. Altered thought processes
   T. Altered tissue perfusion

READINGS AND REFERENCES

Andreoli KG et al. *Comprehensive Cardiac Care*, 6th ed. St. Louis: Mosby, 1987.

Bahr RT, Gress L. Blood pressure readings and selected parameter relationships on an elderly ambulatory population. *Journal of Gerontological Nursing* March 1982; 8(3):159–163.

Baldini J. Knowledge about hypertension in affected elderly persons. *Journal of Gerontological Nursing* September 1981; 7(9):542–551.

Bates B. *A Guide to Physical Examination*, 4th ed. Philadelphia: Lippincott, 1987.

Daniels L, Gifford RW. Therapy for older adults who are hypertensive. May/June 1980; 1:37–39.

Eliopoulos C. *Gerontological Nursing*, 2nd ed. New York: Lippincott, 1987, pp 169–182.

Fleg JL, Lakatta EG. Cardiovascular disease in old age. In: *Clinical Geriatrics*, 3rd ed. Rossman I (editor). Philadelphia: Lippincott, 1986, p 186.

Johnson J. Valvular heart disease in the elderly. *Journal of Cardiovascular Nursing* February 1987; 1(2):72–81.

Malasanos L et al. *Health Assessment*, 3rd ed. St. Louis: Mosby, 1986.

Moser M, Block H. Hypertension in the elderly. In: *Clinical Geriatrics*, 3rd ed. Rossman I (editor). Philadelphia: Lippincott, 1986, p 641.

Rossman I. Anatomy of aging. In: *Clinical Geriatrics*, 3rd ed. Rossman I (editor). Philadelphia: Lippincott, 1986, p 8.

Schroeder JS, Daily EK. *Techniques in Bedside Hemodynamic Monitoring*, 2nd ed. St. Louis: Mosby, 1980.

Steinberg FU (editor). *Cowdry's The Care of the Geriatric Patient*, 6th ed. St. Louis: Mosby, 1983.

7

Assessment of the Respiratory System

Hilary D. Sigmon, RN, MSN, CCRN

As with all body cells, death of respiratory cells begins at birth. The respiratory system's structure and function changes with normal growth and development. For example, the cartilagenous tracheal rings in the infant are extremely soft and pliable; to establish an airway, only slight hyperflexion of the neck is required. The 70-year-old person, however, has firm tracheal rings and would need the mandible firmly released with definite neck hyperflexion to create a comparable airway. The anatomy and physiology of the older adult must be understood to properly assess the respiratory system.

REVIEW OF THE RESPIRATORY SYSTEM

Air Exchange

Ventilation is initiated by movement of the thorax, which results in the flow of oxygen (O_2) into the lungs, and carbon dioxide (CO_2) out of the lungs. Cellular respiration is defined as cellular use of O_2 and production of CO_2. Random movement of O_2 and CO_2 results in a net flow of both gases from regions of abundance to regions of scarcity, a process known as diffusion. Diffusion is hindered between regions with distances of more than 20 microns in length or in thickness.

Structural Elements

The structure of the respiratory system begins with the *nasal turbinates*, which join to become one tube, the *trachea*. The trachea divides into two branches,

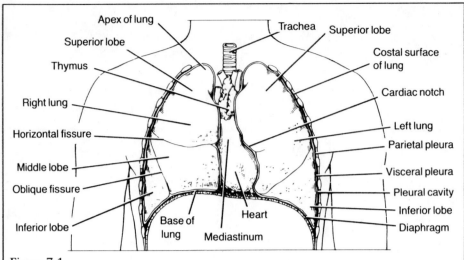

Figure 7-1
The respiratory system. Source: Spence AP, Mason EB. *Human Anatomy and Physiology*, 2nd ed. Redwood City, CA: Benjamin/Cummings, 1983.

the *right mainstem bronchus* and the *left mainstem bronchus*. Each bronchus divides into two subdivisions known as *bronchioles*, and these two into two more, and so on, completing approximately twenty-one bronchial subdivisions. These treelike projections end in terminal bronchioles. The part of the lung responsible for gas exchange is the alveolus, with 300 million grapelike *alveoli* in both lungs. The thin alveolar membrane (0.5 microns in thickness) is responsible for rapid diffusion of O_2 and CO_2 (Figure 7-1).

Ventilation of the alveoli is not enough to ensure adequate gas exchange. Movement of gas is dependent on an adequate blood supply and a pressure system supplied by expanding the volume of the thorax.

Muscular Activity

The *thorax* is a bony cage penetrated by an airway. The *diaphragm*, primarily responsible for enlarging the length of the thorax, is a dome-shaped muscle anchored around the circumference of the lower thorax that separates the thoracic cavity from the abdominal cavity. With inspiration, the diaphragm contracts (muscle shortening). This downward movement results in a longer, flatter, and wider thorax that increases its cross-sectional area for inspiration. This aids in drawing in air due to pressure differences. The lungs can easily expand because their covering (visceral pleura) is closely linked to the inner linking of the thorax (parietal pleura). Simultaneously, alveolar pressure drops below atmospheric pressure, creating a pressure difference that causes air to flow in through the nose, larynx, trachea, bronchi, bronchioles, and finally the alveoli of the lungs until the pressure is equalized. The amount of air inspired with a normal breath is called the *tidal volume* and measures 500 cc.

The diameter of the thorax also is changed by the *ribs*. The ribs are attached to the vertebral column posteriorly and to the sternum anteriorly. Skeletal muscle is arranged diagonally between the ribs. Muscle contraction on inspiration swings the ribs into a new position, upward and outward, increasing the anterior-posterior diameter of the thorax (Figure 7-2).

The descent of the diaphragm, and the activated movement and elevation of the ribs, expand the thorax for ventilation. The full expansion of the thorax is anatomically advantageous as it assures the maximum amount of air that

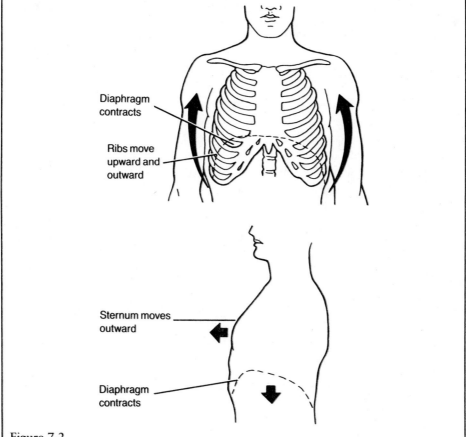

Figure 7-2
With inspiration, the diaphragm contracts and the ribs swing upward and out. Source: Kozier B, Erb G. *Techniques in Clinical Nursing: A Comprehensive Approach*. Menlo Park, CA: Addison-Wesley, 1982.

can be inhaled above and beyond the tidal volume, which is known as the *inspiratory reserve volume* (3000 cc).

The elastic tissue of the lungs is responsible for its *recoil properties* during expiration. This requires no active work for other organs, being analagous to a rubberband springing back into position after being stretched. The diaphragm regains its anatomic resting position with expiration. The recoil of its connective tissue and the release of stored energy (expended during inspiration) from thoracic skeletal muscle assist in the passive act of expiration. Active contraction of muscles during expiration occurs only with obstruction to the tracheobronchial tree or when ventilation is impaired due to loss of the lungs' elastic tissue. The maximum amount of air that can be exhaled is the *expiratory reserve volume* (2000 cc). The 5000 cc total volume of air that can be maximally exchanged in one breath is known as the *vital capacity*. This quantity of vital capacity is only possible with intact muscle activity of the thorax. In addition, there is approximately 1000 cc of reserve volume left in the lungs that is not expired.

AGE-RELATED CHANGES IN THE RESPIRATORY SYSTEM

The increased proportion of connective tissue distribution in the aging body affects all organ systems and accounts for regressive somatic changes. In older adults, all types of connective tissue required for respiration and ventilation are impaired, including skeletal muscle, connective tissue (such as elastin fibers), and smooth muscle. This change is particularly noted between the ages of 70 and 90, due to slower (and sometimes negligible) anabolic restoration of tissue, fibrosis, and atrophy of cells. The older adult can be assisted in adapting and modifying activities of daily living after understanding the expected normal growth and development changes in the pulmonary system.

Body Fluids

At birth, 80% of the body composition is water. Body water decreases to 60% total for those 30 to 40 years of age, and to approximately 50% for those 70 years old. This decline is a normal characteristic of aging, yet a drastic decline in body water (for example, dehydration from hyperthermia or heavy perspiration on hot summer days) adversely affects the respiratory system. Normally, moist mucous membrane lines the nose, larynx, trachea, bronchi, and bronchioles. The membrane's surface is covered with fingerlike hair projections called cilia. Mucus, a polysaccharide substance with a high water content, sits on top of the cilia, which constantly move to-and-fro. Potential upper airway and lung irritants, such as dust and dirt particles, stick to the thin mucus. Coughing or sneezing mobilizes the cilia-coated mucus, projecting the dirt- and dust-imbedded mucus out of the mouth or nose or down the esophagus into the stomach. A decrease in body fluid affects this process by causing the mucous membranes to be drier, thus impeding the removal of mucus. Thick plugs of mucus can obstruct the tracheobronchial tree, not only impairing the expectoration of mucus, but producing a breeding ground for bacteria that predisposes the client to bronchopneumonia.

Muscular Activity

Elastin and collagen, components of muscle within the lung, lose tensile strength and flexibility over the years. This loss impairs the normal elastic recoil of the lung during expiration. The client may develop anatomic emphysema, which differs from pathologic emphysema and is due to constant lung inflation from positive-end-expiratory pressure on the alveoli. Coupled with the loss of skeletal muscle strength in the thorax and diaphragm, the resilient force that normally holds the thorax in a slightly contracted position is lost, particularly in the lower chest. The result is the characteristic barrel chest seen in many older adults (Figure 7-3). Measurement of lung

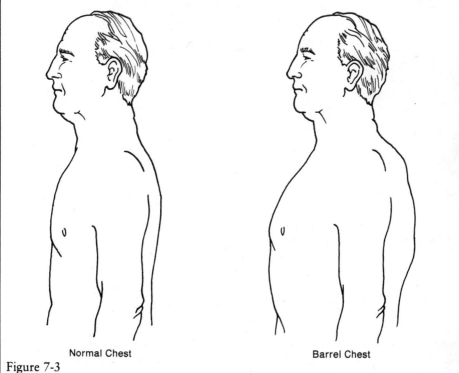

Normal Chest   Barrel Chest

Figure 7-3

Persons with pulmonary disease may have barrel chest, characterized by a rounded thorax resulting from an increased anteroposterior diameter.

volumes validate the significance of these physiologic and anatomic changes. Since inspiratory respiratory muscles become less powerful, some restriction in ventilation develops, and the inspiratory reserve volume is decreased. Expiration, no longer a totally passive activity, now requires the use of accessory muscles: intercostal, scalene, and diaphragmatic muscles. The expiratory reserve volume is substantially increased, due specifically to the increased amount of air remaining in the lungs at the end of a normal breath (residual volume).

Pulmonary Vasculature

There also are changes in the pulmonary vasculature with aging. Fine blood vessels, 0.5 micron in thickness, lie against the wall of each alveolus and enable quick diffusion for gas exchange. This capillary wall is composed of flat endothelial cells lying on its basement membrane. A small amount of interstitial fluid separates the membrane from the elastic tissue of the alveolus. With senescence, several changes occur to this membrane and its relationship to the alveolus. The elastic tissue of the alveolus loses its stretchability and morphologically changes to fibrous tissue. This thicker membrane curtails the amount of diffusion since the aging cross-sectional lung capillaries stunt pulmonary diffusion capacity. Arterial oxyhemoglobin saturation becomes slightly decreased and normal PaO_2 becomes 75 to 80 torr rather than 100 torr on room air. The $PaCO_2$ shows no appreciable change in the older adult, remaining at 35 to 46 torr as in the young individual. Blood pH remains between the parameters of 7.40 to 7.45.

Exertional capacity decreases in the older adult, since the diffusion capacity for oxygen cannot effectively meet the demands of an increase in basal metabolic rate.

ASSESSMENT OF THE RESPIRATORY SYSTEM

Inspection begins the instant you make contact with the client. As you visually examine the client, scrutinize the entire body, particularly the thorax and its accessory muscles. Compare and contrast findings with the client at rest and during activity.

As you introduce yourself, note the strength and quality of the client's verbal response. As mentioned in Chapter 1, extend your hand so that you can assess muscle grasp, skin color, and capillary refill of the nail beds. Observe posture in relation to body position and the impact of posture on respiration. At this time you should also assess the client's level of consciousness, especially in relation to time, place, and person. A change in mental status could be indicative of carbon dioxide retention.

Note the *color* of the face, trunk, and limbs. A ruddy, pink complexion is a deleterious rather than healthy sign. In fact, it can be a sign of hypoxia due to a high CO_2 level in the blood, which inhibits involuntary neurotransmission from the pons (part of the brain stem) to the diaphragm for inspiration. Persons with chronic obstructive lung disease are often referred to as "pink puffers" due to the presence of the sign. A blue or gray hue to the face and neck muscles is evident in persons with long-standing chronic bronchitis. Lack of oxygen binding to the hemoglobin muscle is the main cause of this cyanotic color. Persons with this sign are characteristically called "blue bloaters."

Listen to the client's *speech*. Assess his or her ability to communicate in sentences and phrases without shortness of breath. A nasal or bleating speech quality may signify congestion of nasal vessels and be a benign characteristic of a nose cold. On the other hand, hoarseness, stridor, or aphonia are cardinal signs of laryngeal cancer and edema to the laryngobronchiotrachial tree.

Assist the client or ask the client to remove his or her shirt so that *visualization of the anterior and posterior chest is possible*. Assess the chest for increased anterior–posterior diameter, kyphosis (curvature of the upper spine), scoliosis (curvature of the lower spine), or lordosis (curvature of the middle spine), all potentially decreasing inspiratory reserve volume. Inquire about the causes of any scars or bruises that may be present.

Watch the client breathe while he or she is in a sitting and lying position. Note any differences in rate, rhythm, type, depth, and length of respirations during the position change. Assess these characteristics during activity, such as eating, walking, and lifting. Observe for symmetrical expansion of the left and right chest. Unilateral expansion on inspiration can be caused by acute pleurisy, pleural fibrosis, or massive atelectasis. Decreased expansion of the left or right chest may be indicative of pulmonary emboli, pleural effusion, fractured ribs, or pain. If retractions and/or accessory muscles are used at rest or with activity note the location and degree. Determine the inspiration to expiration time, normally a one-to-one ratio. (Most older adults will reveal a ratio of one-to-three, and those with chronic pulmonary disease will have a longer expiration time.) Ask the client to inform you of any discomfort or pain during inspiration, expiration, coughing, or straining (for example, during a bowel movement). If pain is present, it should be characterized as to location, degree, mode of relief, and presence of radiation.

Question the client as to the frequency, effectiveness, productivity, and time (for example, upon awakening in smokers) of *coughing*. Sputum should be characterized as to color, odor, amount, and consistency.

Palpation

Prepare the client for palpation by explaining that you will be touching the front and back of his or her chest for further assessment of breathing ability.

While the client is in a sitting position, place your hands and outstretched fingers with thumbs close together on the base of the spinal cord. Ask the client to breathe in and out, slowly and deeply, inhaling through the nose and exhaling through pursed lips (the kissing position). Swiftly, but completely, move both hands after each complete breath, covering the entire lung field up the shoulders and axillae (Figure 7-4). Normally, as the fingers and thumbs move along the chest, palpation will elicit symmetry in distance and depth of respiration. During this activity, assess the temperature, moisture, and general turgor of the skin.

In addition to observing for edema, tenderness, and swelling, observe for *crepitus*. Crepitus is subcutaneous emphysema. It occurs when atmospheric

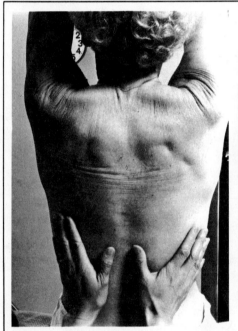
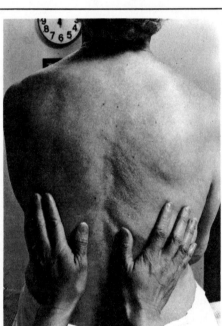
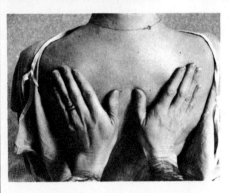

Figure 7-4
Positions of the hands to palpate the entire lung field.

air is trapped under the epidermis. The most likely cause would be a recent tracheostomy in which air has entered around the incision site and traveled to either the clavicle or nipple area. When crepitus is present, tactile stimulation creates a crunchy sensation described as a crackling sound.

Percussion

Percussion is the act of listening and feeling different qualities of air-filled spaces. Firmly place one hand on the chest wall with fingers slightly fanned. With the pad of the middle finger of your opposite hand, strike the middle finger of the hand that is on the chest wall. Begin at the apices of both lungs, and move towards the bases (Figure 7-5). The client's head should be flexed forward with his forearms at the waist to separate the scapulae. Compare both sides of the chest wall as you percuss. A resonant sound is a normal lung sound. It is clear and low-pitched due to the airways being appropriately filled with air. A hyperresonant sound is abnormal, characterized by a hollow, drumlike, high-pitched sound. It is characteristic of an overinflated organ found in emphysema (overinflation of the alveoli) or a pneumothorax (air in the thoracic space). A dull sound is caused by air spaces filled with solid

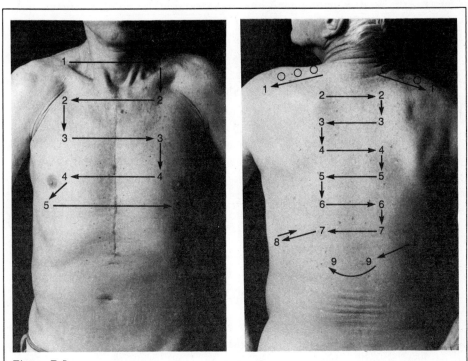

Figure 7-5
Percuss from the apices of the lungs to the bases.

material and is abnormal; pathologies such as consolidation, atalectasis, and a pleural effusion produce this sound. A flat sound is heard when bone is percussed; this is described as a dense sound.

Auscultation

Auscultation is the last phase of the physical examination and involves listening with a stethoscope to the pitch, intensity, quality, and duration of breath sounds. *Bronchial breathing* sounds are normally found at the trachea and are described by the duration of a short inspiration and a longer expiration. *Vesicular breathing* sounds are normal breath sounds heard over the entire lung, excepting the sternum and scapula. The duration of vesicular sounds are the opposite of the duration of bronchial sounds, having a long inspiration and a short expiration. *Bronchovesicular sounds* have an equal duration of inspiration and expiration and are normal when heard over the sternum and scapula.

Diminished or absent breath sounds occur with emphysema, shallow breathing, and impaired transmission of sound to the chest wall (for example, thickened pleura, and air or fluid in the pleural space). Increased breath sounds are abnormal transmissions of air originating in the larger airways and are found with extensively damaged lung (for example, tuberculosis, bronchiectasis, and types of chronic pulmonary fibrosis).

Rales are sounds indicative of an extra abundance of interstitial fluid. They are described as discontinuous and discrete clicking, popping, or bubbling sounds without a recognizable pitch or tone. These sounds usually are heard at the end of inspiration. Rales frequently exist in the presence of congestive heart failure, pulmonary edema, bronchitis, and pneumonia.

Rhonchi are sounds resulting from an abundance of mucus production, and usually can be differentiated from rales when they disappear after coughing or suctioning. Their sound is musical with a recognizable pitch and is heard on expiration. Rhonchi can indicate partial airway obstruction in the person with an asthma attack, severe bronchitis, or bronchiectasis.

Wheezes are abnormal sounds connoting airway narrowing. They are heard specifically in persons with asthma, pulmonary stenosis, and large amounts of tenacious mucus.

DISORDERS OF THE RESPIRATORY SYSTEM

Three molecular theories propose to account for the common respiratory diseases seen in the older adult (Comfort 1964, Strehler 1962). The commonly occurring diseases that could be explained by these theories are lung carcinoma (cancer), pulmonary tuberculosis, chronic bronchitis, emphysema, and pneumonia. One theory of aging states that at conception, each gene is assigned an age limit affecting every cell and causing cellular deaths as a natural part of the aging process. The second theory is the miscoding (replication errors) of RNA and DNA during protein synthesis, which causes genetic mutations and cellular aging due to a certain number of mitotic (cell division) accidents. The third theory is generally thought to reveal the culprit of the majority of diseases seen in the older adult. The hypothesis is that genetic miscodings are an insidious process throughout life. Nonetheless, immunologic processes of the body prevent disease *until* external, environmental variables produce additional internal assaults to mitosis. For example, changes in the mucous membrane of the lung occur with aging. Forty years of smoking combines the genetic changes with the environmental impact of tar and nicotine, possibly causing cancer.

Lung Cancer

Cancers (malignant tumors) of the lung are usually defined according to the anatomic area or cell type that has been invaded (for example, bronchogenic carcinoma invades the bronchus). Regardless of the type, lung cancers, like other malignant tumors, have the following characteristics:

1. Immature cell type
2. Anaplastic—less differentiated than the normal cell (parent cell) from which they are derived
3. Rapidly growing (usually)
4. Nonencapsulated
5. Metastatic growth capabilities—invades surrounding tissues in a wide area and forms secondary growths (sites) through both the lymph and bloodstream

Lung cancer is predominately a disease of late adult life, being relatively infrequent before the age of 40. There are several factors associated with lung cancer. Cigarette smokers have twice the incidence of lung cancer of nonsmokers. A history of exposure to such carcinogenic inhalants as asbestos, silicone, coal gas, radioactive dusts, chromates, and fiberglass particles predisposes persons to lung cancer. Persons over 40 years old, who have smoked 15 or more years, or who smoke more than a pack a day, and those who have had exposure to noxious inhalants, are "high risk" individuals for developing lung cancer. These individuals should receive yearly health exams with chest x-rays. Suspicious lesions should be further assessed with more elaborate studies such as tomograms, isotope scans, and open or closed lung biopsy.

Unfortunately, signs and symptoms of lung cancer occur long after its development, and present similarly to other lung diseases. Classic symptoms of lung cancer include shortness of breath (usually insidious in etiology) at rest or with activity, coughing (dry or productive), wheezing, numerous upper respiratory tract infections, chest pain during inspiration, and hemoptysis. Diagnosis is confirmed with roentgen studies, cytologic studies of sputum, bronchoscopy or mediastinoscopy, and lung biopsies.

Although the advantages of regular screening are controversial, screening has been shown to detect asymptomatic cancer, for which the five-year survival rate after resection is 70% or higher compared to a 8–10% survival rate in persons who were symptomatic (Flehinger et al 1984).

Pulmonary Tuberculosis

Tuberculosis is a granulomatous disease caused by the mycobacterium tubercle baccillus. When infecting the lung, the organism usurps healthy tissue (lung parenchyma, bronchi, bronchioles, mediastinal nodes, and/or lung pleura) with a mass of granules. Tuberculosis, commonly referred to as TB, is transmitted through water droplets from contaminated sputum emitted into the air by normal exhalation, coughing, or sneezing. These droplets lodge in susceptible tissues. Currently, the elderly constitute the largest group with active infection (Nagami and Yoshikawa 1983).

Exposure to TB does not always cause the disease. A history of poor nutrition and frequent illnesses, or an environment with little ventilation and lack of sunlight can lower immunity and predispose an individual to contacting TB. Though older adults may develop TB as a primary lung infection, they usually develop the disease from chronic endogenous reactivation. An age-related decline in cell-mediated immunity may influence the elderly's vulnerability to this condition. If immunity is successful, the TB organisms die, but the mass of granules (the tubercle) turn into fibrous tissue. Reinfection by a TB organism or (and most commonly) deterioration of the older adult's health state may cause erosion of the tubercle. Reactivation of the chronic endogenous tubercle results in active tuberculosis.

The older adult with TB presents symptoms of listlessness, fatigue, coughing with sputum production, anorexia, cachexia (a thin, pale, and weak stature), and fever with or without heavy perspiration. (Keep in mind, however that the hypothalamus, which regulates temperature control in the brain, is less sensitive to temperature control during senescence. Febrile states with compensatory sweating may not be observed.) The high prevalence of TB among the geriatric population suggests that skin testing for the disease be a routine part of the screening of patients entering institutional and other primarily geriatric settings.

Diagnosis is confirmed by chest x-ray, sputum cytology, gastric washings, and a positive Mantoux skin test. A tuberculin skin test can be negative in persons with *Mycobacterium tuberculosis* (Anderson et al 1986). Tuberculin sensitivity can be low in the aged and it may be necessary to repeat a negative test one week after the initial testing to detect the possibility of a waned response. While the diagnosis is pending, teach the client to cover his nose and mouth with tissue during coughing and to dispose of this material immediately. In an institutional setting, the contagious client should wear a face mask when he leaves his room, and those entering his room should wear one when approaching him. Gloves, head coverings, and gowns need only be worn by persons when contact with sputum is anticipated.

Chronic Bronchitis

Chronic bronchitis is classified as a chronic obstructive pulmonary disease (COPD). Chronic bronchitis is defined as a cough with mucus production that lasts a minimum of two months (not necessarily consecutive) and recurs for at least two years. This disease has an insidious onset. Contributing factors include years of exposure to lung irritants such as cigarette smoke, upper respiratory tract pathogens, and noxious fumes.

In chronic bronchitis, the mucous membrane of the bronchus and the bronchioles become inflamed and irritated, and often are hypertrophied. Hypersecretion of mucus coupled with the narrowed airways make the excessive amount of mucus difficult to expectorate. Symptoms of coughing with mucus production and shortness of breath with activity (and sometimes even at rest) ensue. Diagnosis is made by x-ray (large anterior–posterior diameter of the chest), physical examination (the diaphragm can be palpated lower than usual), and bronchoscopy.

Emphysema

Emphysema, another COPD, is defined as the permanent destruction of alveoli (air sacs). Thousands of healthy, grapelike clusters of alveoli lose their elasticity and become stiff and overfilled with air. These alveoli burst from the constant distention of air, and potentially one-hundred clusters of alveoli become one large alveolus. These damaged alveoli no longer have resiliency and more CO_2 becomes trapped in the lungs. The severe shortness of breath, wheezing, rhonchi, and coughing with sputum production in the emphysematous client are caused by three ventilation problems:

1. Hypoxia, caused by insufficient O_2 diffusing from the alveoli into the pulmonary capillaries
2. Hypercapnia (high $PaCO_2$ levels of 50 to 70 torr) resulting from air trapped during exhalation
3. Further airway narrowing caused by overinflation of the alveoli, which produces pressure on the bronchioles and bronchi during a forceful cough (Sigmon 1979)

The client with emphysema often has chronic bronchitis as well, further compromising ventilation.

Emphysema is diagnosed by the same methods as chronic bronchitis, and includes arterial blood gas determinations and blood pH (PaO_2: 60 torr, $PaCO_2$: 50 to 70 torr, pH: 7.30).

Pneumonia

Pneumonia is defined as partial consolidation of the lung with an inflammatory exudate in response to bacterium, lipid, a virus, or a chemical. The most common type of pneumonia seen in the older adult is bacterial pneumonia caused by pneumococcus, *staphylococcus aureus, Klebsiella pneumoniae*, hemolytic streptococcus, or *hemophilus influenzae*. Bacterial pneumonia is rampant during influenza season, when upper respiratory tract infections are common. The eradication of the invading organism is essential to prevent serious illness or death in immunologically compromised and debilitated persons.

Several normal physiologic changes in older adults contribute to their high incidence of pneumonia. Loss of skeletal muscle at the posterior pharynx reduces the gag reflex, predisposing the older adult to aspiration pneumonia. Less activity and mobility decreases deep expansion of the lungs. Decreased body fluids alter the effectiveness of the mucous membrane and cilia in removing foreign substances. There also is an age-related decline in the immunologic defense system.

Diagnosis of pneumonia can be difficult due to age-related changes that may alter symptoms. The typical presentation of fever may not exist due to the subnormal body temperatures found among many older adults. Altered pain sensations may mask the inspiratory pleuritic pain often accompanying pneumonia. Decreased respiratory activity may reduce coughing along with mucus production. General malaise and joint pain may be attributed to other geriatric conditions and not to pneumonia. Thus, early diagnosis often is difficult. Any suspicion of pneumonia should warrant evaluation. Diagnosis is confirmed with x-ray and sputum cultures.

Clients should be questioned as to if and when they have received influenza and pneumococcal pneumonia vaccines. These vaccinations are recommended for older adults.

7 Chapter Summary

I. Age-related changes
  A. Various connective tissues responsible for respiration and ventilation are weaker
  B. Decreased body fluid and drier mucous membranes impede removal of mucus and create greater risk of infection
  C. Elastic recoil of lung during expiration is impaired by weaker, less elastic collagen and elastin

D. Loss of resilient force, which holds thorax in a lightly contracted position, and decreased muscle strength in thorax and diaphragm, both promoting barrel chest

E. Decreased inspiratory reserve volume

F. Increased respiratory reserve volume

G. Expiration requires active use of accessory muscles

H. Alveoli are less elastic and contain fewer functional capillaries

   1. Arterial oxyhemoglobin saturation reduced to 93% to 94%

   2. PaO_2 becomes 75 to 80 torr

   3. $PaCO_2$ does not significantly change: 35 to 46 torr

   4. Blood pH remains 7.40 to 7.45

II. Assessment

A. Inspection

   1. Verbal response

   2. Muscle grasp

   3. Capillary refill of nail beds

   4. Posture

   5. Level of consciousness

   6. Color

     a) "Pink puffer": chronic obstructive lung disease; hypoxia

     b) "Blue bloater": chronic bronchitis; lack of oxygen binding to hemoglobin molecule

   7. Speech

     a) Nasal quality: congestion of nasal vessels

     b) Hoarseness, stridor, aphonia: laryngeal cancer; edema of laryngobronchial tree

   8. Anterior and posterior chest

   9. Respiratory rate, rhythm, depth, and length

   10. Symmetry of chest expansion

   11. Ratio of inspiration to expiration

     a) Usual ratio 1:3

     b) Longer expiratory time with chronic pulmonary disease

   12. Pain

   13. Coughing: frequency, effectiveness, productivity, time

   14. Sputum: color, odor, amount, consistency

B. Palpation

   1. Touching front and back of chest to assess breathing ability

   2. Note skin temperature, moisture, and turgor

   3. Hyperresonant sound (hollow, drumlike) is abnormal and indicates overinflated lung or pneumothorax

   4. Dull sound indicates air spaces are filled with material; can be caused by consolidation atelectasis, pleural effusion

   5. Flat, dense sound is heard over bone

C.. Percussion

   1. Act of listening and feeling different qualities of air-filled spaces

   2. Strike pad of middle finger on middle finger of other hand that is placed on chest wall

   3. Compare both sides of chest wall

   4. Normal lung sound

     a) resonant

     b) clear and low-pitched

   5. Abnormal lung sounds

     a) hyperresonant: hollow, drumlike, high-pitched, overinflated organ

b) dull sound: air spaces filled with solid material

6. Flat sound heard over bone

D. Auscultation
1. Use of stethoscope to assess pitch, intensity, quality, and duration of breath sounds
2. Bronchial breathing
   a) Short inspiration; long expiration
   b) Normally heard at trachea
3. Vesicular breathing
   a) Long inspiration; short expiration
   b) Normally heard over entire lung area
4. Bronchovesicular sound
   a) Equal expiration and inspiration
   b) Normally heard over sternum and scapula
5. Diminished or absent breath sounds: shallow breathing, thickened pleura, air or fluid in pleural space
6. Increased breath sounds: extensively damaged lungs
7. Rales: discontinuous, bubbling, or popping sound usually heard after inspiration:
   a) Extra interstitial fluid
   b) Indicates congestive heart failure, pulmonary edema, bronchitis, pneumonia
8. Rhonchi: musical sounds usually heard at expiration
   a) Increased mucus production
   b) Disappear after coughing or suctioning
   c) Indicates partial airway obstruction, as occurs with severe bronchitis or bronchiectasis

9. Wheezes
   a) Indicates airway narrowing or presence of large amounts of tenacious mucus
   b) Occurs with asthma and pulmonary stenosis

III. Pathologies
A. Lung cancer
1. Defined according to invaded anatomic area or cell type
2. Incidence higher with advanced age and among those who have smoked or have been exposed to asbestos, silicone, coal gas, radioactive dusts, chromates, fiberglass particles, and other carcinogenic inhalants
3. Symptoms often appear long after the disease develops and can resemble other lung diseases
   a) Shortness of breath
   b) Coughing
   c) Wheezing
   d) Recurrent upper respiratory tract infection
   e) Chest pain or inspiration
   f) Diagnosis confirmed through x-ray, sputum cytology, bronchoscopy, and lung biopsy
B. Pulmonary tuberculosis
1. Of high incidence in the geriatric population
2. Older adults usually develop TB from chronic endogenous reactivation
3. Symptoms
   a) Listlessness
   b) Fatigue
   c) Productive cough
   d) Anorexia
   e) Cachexia

f) Hemoptysis
g) Fever with or without heavy perspiration
4. Diagnosis confirmed by chest x-ray, sputum cytology, gastric washings, and tuberculin skin testing
C. Chronic bronchitis
1. A cough with mucus production lasting at least two months and recurring for at least two years
2. Contributing factors: chronic exposure to lung irritants and noxious fumes and upper respiratory tract infection
3. Symptoms
a) Productive cough
b) Shortness of breath
4. Diagnosis confirmed by x-ray and bronchoscopy
D. Emphysema
1. Permanent destruction of alveoli leading to CO_2 being trapped in lungs
2. Symptoms
a) Productive cough
b) Shortness of breath
c) Wheezing
d) Rhonchi
3. Diagnosis confirmed by x-ray, bronchoscopy, arterial blood gases, and blood pH
E. Pneumonia
1. Partial consolidation of lung with inflammatory exudate
2. In older adults, primarily caused by pneumococcus, staphylococcus, *Staphylococcus aureus, Klebsiella pneumoniae,* hemolytic streptococcus, or *Hemophilus influenzae*
3. Aging-related changes increase risk of pneumonia in old age

4. Symptoms
a) Pleuritic pain during inspiration
b) Fever
c) Malaise
d) Joint pain
e) Productive cough
5. Diagnosis confirmed by x-ray and sputum culture
IV. Related nursing diagnoses
A. Activity intolerance
B. Pain
C. Impaired verbal communication
D. Ineffective individual coping
E. Diversional activity deficit
F. Fear
G. Fluid volume deficit
H. Fluid volume excess
I. Altered health maintenance
J. Impaired home maintenance management
K. Potential for infection
L. Potential for injury
M. Knowledge deficit
N. Impaired physical mobility
O. Noncompliance
P. Altered nutrition: less than body requirements
Q. Altered oral mucous membrane
R. Ineffective airway clearance
S. Ineffective breathing pattern
T. Impaired gas exchange
U. Self-care deficit
V. Personal identity disturbance
W. Sexual dysfunction
X. Impaired skin integrity
Y. Sleep pattern disturbance
Z. Impaired social interaction
AA. Altered thought processes
BB. Altered tissue perfusion

READINGS AND REFERENCES

Anderson WM, Ryerson GG, Wynne JW. Pulmonary disease in the elderly. In: *Clinical Geriatrics*, 3rd ed. Rossman I (editor). Philadelphia: Lippincott, 1986, p 245.

Bates B. *A Guide to Physical Examination*, 4th ed. Philadelphia: Lippincott, 1987.

Battershill JH. Cutaneous testing in the elderly with tuberculosis. *Chest* February 1980; 77:180–189.

Comfort A. *Aging: the biology of senescence.* New York: Holt, Rinehart, & Winston, Inc., 1964.

Flehinger BJ et al. Screening for early lung cancer: Results of the Memorial Sloan-Kettering study in New York. *Chest* 1984; 86:44.

Nagami PH, Yoshikawa TT. Tuberculosis in the geriatric population. *Journal of the American Geriatrics Society* 1983; 31:356.

Reichel J. Pulmonary problems in the elderly. In: *Clinical Aspects of Aging*, 2nd ed. Reichel W (editor). Baltimore: Williams and Wilkens, 1983.

Sigmon H. *Chronic Lung Disease.* Bowie, MD: Brady, 1979.

Strehler BL. *Time, Cells, and Aging.* New York: Academic Press, 1962.

Wade JF. *Comprehensive Respiratory Care. Physiology and Technique*, 3rd ed. St. Louis: Mosby, 1982.

8

Assessment of the Gastrointestinal System

Charlotte Eliopoulos, RNC, MPH

Those working with older adults know that the gastrointestinal system is the source of much concern as well as the root of multiple health problems for them. Decreased interest in daily activities, mental status alterations, poor body image, weakness, and pain are among the problems emerging from gastrointestinal disorders. In turn, a variety of physical, emotional, and socioeconomic factors can influence the status of this system. Discrete assessment and problem identification of the gastrointestinal tract, therefore, are significant parts of the total assessment.

REVIEW OF THE GASTROINTESTINAL SYSTEM

The gastrointestinal system extends from the lips to the anus and functions to prepare food for absorption and to excrete waste materials (Figure 8-1).

Mouth

The mouth forms the entrance to the gastrointestinal system. This entranceway is bounded by the cheeks and lips. Capillary-rich skin covers the outer surface of the lips; mucous membrane lines the inner surface. A hard palate forms the anterior roof of the mouth. Posteriorly, a soft palate covers the roof

133

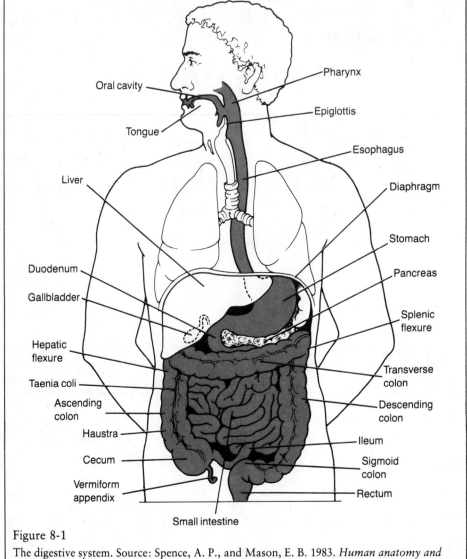

Figure 8-1

The digestive system. Source: Spence, A. P., and Mason, E. B. 1983. *Human anatomy and physiology.* 2nd ed. Redwood City, CA: The Benjamin/Cummings Publishing Company, Inc.

of the mouth and moves upward during the act of swallowing to block the nasopharynx.

Masticating and swallowing food, as well as speaking, are dependent on the action of an important accessory organ in the mouth: the tongue. Approximately two thirds of the anterior portion of the tongue is covered with papillae in which taste buds are located (Figure 8-2). Mastication is also dependent on the teeth, another set of accessory organs. The adult has 32 teeth

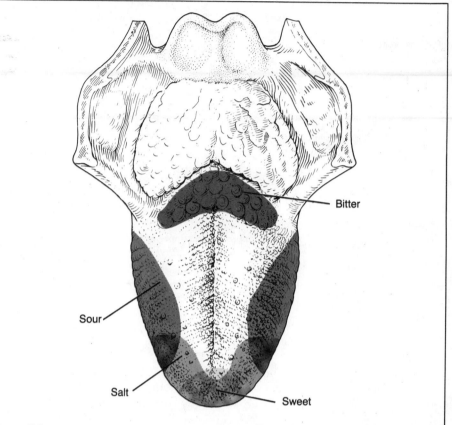

Figure 8-2

Various regions of the tongue have taste buds receptive to specific tastes. Source: Spence, A. P., and Mason, E. B. 1983. *Human anatomy and physiology.* 2nd ed. Redwood City, CA: The Benjamin/Cummings Publishing Company, Inc.

in his or her permanent set (Figure 8-3). Also in the mouth are salivary glands. These accessory organs produce saliva. Three sets of glands form the salivary glands: the parotid, submaxillary, and sublingual glands. Saliva keeps the mucous membrane moist, lubricates food, and assists with speech. It also starts the digestive process by breaking down complex starch molecules into dextrins and maltose. After food is chewed and mixed, the tongue elevates and throws the food into the pharynx.

Pharynx

The pharynx contains constrictor muscles that aid in swallowing and moving food to the esophagus. It also has another series of muscles that elevate the soft palate (closing the nasopharynx) and raise the pharynx during swallowing, thereby preventing respiration and potential aspiration of food into the lungs.

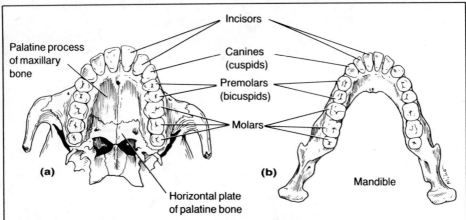

Figure 8-3
The normal adult has 32 permanent teeth in (A) the upper jaw, and (B) the lower jaw.
Source: Spence AP, Mason EB. *Human Anatomy and Physiology*, 2nd ed. Redwood City, CA: Benjamin/Cummings, 1983.

Esophagus

Behind the trachea, or windpipe, is a tube, the esophagus, which transports food from the laryngopharynx to the stomach, passing through the mediastinum and diaphragm en route. Its peristaltic muscular activity is responsible for the movement of food down this tube.

Stomach

Below the diaphragm is the stomach, which is a pouchlike structure that holds food during the early stages of digestion. Food usually remains in the stomach for five to seven hours following a meal. Fats remain in the stomach longer than other food substances. During this time, gastric juices break down food (primarily proteins to proteoses and peptones).

Food is prevented from backflowing from the stomach to the esophagus by the action of the cardiac sphincter. The pyloric sphincter serves a similar function between the stomach and the small intestine.

Small Intestine

The small intestine, which extends from the stomach to the large intestine, is divided into the duodenum, the jejunum, and the ileum. The duodenum is the shortest and widest portion and is curved somewhat in the shape of a "C." Within the concave portion of the duodenum lies the head of the pancreas. The jejunum and ileum form the largest portion of the small intestine. A sphincter, the ileocecal valve, is located between the ileum and large intestine.

Within the small intestine, muscular activity mixes the contents with the secretions present: pancreatic juice, bile, and intestinal juice. The stimulation of the taste receptors causes pancreatic juice to be secreted, by reflex, within one to two minutes after food enters the mouth. Pancreatic amylase digests uncooked starch, glycogen, and dextrin to maltose; proteins, proteoses, and peptones are turned to protease; and pancreatic lipase converts emulsified fats to fatty acids and glycerol.

Bile is produced in the liver and is temporarily stored in the gallbladder. It is released into the small intestine when the gastric contents are emptied into the duodenum. A major component of bile, bile salt, emulsifies fats and prepares them for action by pancreatic lipase.

Glands of the small intestine produce intestinal enzymes when the contents enter the duodenum. Several enzymes are present in intestinal secretions: proteases, which break protein to amino acids; enterokinase, which activates trypsinogen; sucrase, which breaks sucrose to glucose; maltose, which divides maltose to two molecules of glucose; and lactose, which reduces lactose to glucose and galactose.

Large Intestine

The large intestine is divided into four portions: the cecum, colon, rectum, and anal canal. The cecum is a blind pouch hanging at the area where the ileum meets the cecum. Approximately one inch from the ileocecal valve is the appendix, which stems from the cecum.

There are four portions of the colon: the ascending colon, transverse colon, descending colon, and sigmoid colon. Extending from the sigmoid colon is a 5- to 6-inch tube, the rectum, which connects with the anal canal. Two sphincters control the emptying of feces: the internal anal sphincter and the external anal sphincter. The anus is the terminal end of the gastrointestinal system.

Peristaltic activity moves the intestinal contents along to the sigmoid colon. Here, the contents remain until just before defecation, when the feces enter the rectum. The stretching of the nerve endings in the rectum arouses the sensation of the urge to defecate.

Other Accessory Organs

The liver, located in the upper portion of the abdominal cavity under the dome of the diaphragm, is the largest organ in the body and performs several important functions. As mentioned, bile is formed in the liver. The liver helps to regulate the blood glucose level by converting glucose to glycogen and storing it until a lowered blood glucose level demands it to be released. The liver metabolizes lipids and temporarily stores fat. The first step in urea formation occurs in the liver. The liver produces plasma proteins and temporarily stores amino acids. Vitamin A is formed and stored in the liver.

Vitamins D and B_{12} and a small amount of iron and copper are also stored in the liver. Phagocytic cells line the liver, providing protection to the body. The liver also produces heparin and detoxifies the blood.

Capillaries from the liver drain into small ducts that then join to form one large duct in each of the four lobes of the liver. Bile ducts from the right and left lobes form the hepatic duct, which joins with the cystic duct to form the common bile duct. The gallbladder, an organ shaped like a small pear, stores bile until it is ready to be secreted.

The pancreas is another important accessory organ. The head of the pancreas rests in the concavity of the duodenum and the tail extends towards the spleen. In addition to the secretion of pancreatic juices, the pancreas secretes insulin.

AGE-RELATED CHANGES IN THE GASTROINTESTINAL SYSTEM

The aging process affects virtually all parts of the gastrointestinal system, from entrance to exit. There is less salivary gland activity and the mucous membrane of the oral cavity is much drier. Wear and tear of the taste buds results in the loss of some taste sensations in old age, particularly those receptors for sweet and salty flavors. Smokers tend to suffer a greater loss of taste sensation than nonsmokers.

Teeth

Although tooth loss is not a normal outcome of aging, today's older population includes few individuals with a full set of natural teeth. Teeth often are missing, and if present, they tend to be in extremely poor condition. The enamel is thinner and the teeth may be extremely brittle. Caries are highly prevalent, resulting from poor dental care, a high carbohydrate diet, and insufficient intake of calcium. Periodontal disease becomes the major cause of tooth loss.

Gag Reflex

The gag reflex is weaker in old age. The esophagus becomes slightly dilated and esophageal motility is reduced. There is some relaxation of the cardiac sphincter. These factors predispose the older adult to aspiration problems.

Gastric Acids

Gastric acids are secreted in lesser amounts due to atrophic changes with age. Weaker musculature delays movement of material out of the stomach. These factors contribute to the difficulties older adults have in managing large quantities of food.

Small Intestine and Large Intestine

In the elderly there are fewer cells on the absorbing surface of the small intestine, along with a reduced functional capacity and decreased absorption of carbohydrates and fats (Brandt 1986a). There is also weakened intestinal musculature and decreased peristalsis in the large intestine. In addition to decreased peristaltic activity, there is a tendency for incomplete emptying of the bowel at one time and duller nerve sensations to the lower bowel that can cause a missed signal for defecation. Combine these changes with the altered dietary and activity patterns common among older adults, and it is understandable that constipation is a highly prevalent problem.

Liver

After the seventh decade, the liver decreases in size. Consequently the liver's storage capacity is reduced, as is its ability to synthesize protein. For the most part, the liver's functional capacity falls within a normal range with advanced age.

Gallbladder

Gallbladder function is affected by age, evidenced by more difficulty with emptying of the organ. Bile is present in lesser amounts and is thicker. Additionally, greater amounts of cholesterol are present in the bile of older adults.

Pancreas

Fewer digestive enzymes are produced by the aging pancreas. Insulin release also is altered with age. Studies have shown older persons to have normal rates of insulin released with high glucose levels (250 to 300 mg%) but diminished rates with moderately elevated levels (120 to 200 mg%) (Williams 1983).

ASSESSMENT OF THE GASTROINTESTINAL SYSTEM

Assessment of the gastrointestinal system includes the techniques of interview, inspection, auscultation, percussion, and palpation. An organized approach is to work from the entrance of this system to its end, combining the various techniques as you go along.

Lips

Inspect the client's lips for symmetry, color, and moisture. Because the lips are rich in capillaries, they can readily reflect insufficient oxygen through pale bluish discoloration and dehydration through dryness. Note any lesions or sores, and question the client as to the length of time they have been present and their related characteristics, for example, pain, bleeding, or crusting. Lesions and sores that do not heal within several weeks may be cancerous. Cracks and fissures at the mouth's angles can result from riboflavin deficiencies or overclosure of the mouth resulting from the lack of teeth or poorly fitting dentures. If cracks or fissures are present, it can be useful to ask the client to bite down (with dentures in if available) and observe if a tight bite causes a folding of skin at the angle of the mouth.

Mouth

Specifically note which teeth are missing and the condition of existing ones. Ask the client to describe his or her routine pattern of dental care and the date of his or her last visit to a dentist. If the client is wearing dentures, evaluate their fit and ask the client if the dentures produce any discomfort, if they can be worn throughout the entire day (especially at mealtime), and if they are loose or tight in any place. Observe if the dentures rub against the buccal mucosa. Request that dentures be removed for adequate examination of the mouth. You can use this opportunity to inspect the condition of the dentures, for example, broken parts or cleanliness.

Use a bright flashlight or other source of good light to inspect the oral cavity. A tongue depressor can assist you in moving the tongue, lips, and cheeks during the examination.

The mucous membrane is normally moist and of a light pink color. Black persons may have pigmented oral mucosa as a normal characteristic. Older adults may have a drier oral mucosa than younger persons due to decreased salivary gland activity. Extreme dryness can be associated with inadequate hydration.

Observe the lesions, discolorations and irritations of the mucous membrane. The client should be questioned as to how long sores or ulcers have been present, associated pain, and possible known factors that could have precipitated them, such as accidentally biting the membrane. Areas of irritation may be a result of friction from poorly fitting dentures or jagged teeth.

Moniliasis (thrush) infections can be present, evidenced by white patches resembling small beads of white milk. It must not be thought that because these patches can be scraped off with a tongue depressor that they are actually dried milk: moniliasis patches are able to be removed in such a manner. Only a culture can determine whether or not the patches are moniliasis. Occasionally, this problem is associated with diabetes and leukemia.

Discoloration, inflammation, and bleeding of the gums should be assessed. Some receding of the gums occurs with age. There also may be a brownish pigmentation to the gums, which is normal, especially in black persons. Periodontal disease, the primary cause of tooth loss in older adults, is characterized by swelling, redness, and bleeding of the gums. Dilantin therapy and leukemia can cause the gums to swell and partially cover the teeth. Although often associated with children, older adults can experience lead poisoning as a result of contact in their occupational experiences or in their home environment. A bluish-black line close to the edge of gums where teeth are present can indicate lead poisoning. This sign is not present in areas where teeth are missing; therefore, blood tests for lead screening may be indicated in the edentulous individual who is suspected of lead ingestion.

Ask the client to extend his or her tongue; observe the tongue's color, papillae, symmetry, and movement. Impaired function of certain cranial nerves can influence the tongue: the hypoglossal nerve affects movement, the trigeminal nerve affects touch, temperature, and pain; and the facial and glossopharyngeal nerves affect taste sensations.

Taste sensations may be anticipated to be duller in the older adult. It can be revealing to ask the client how much salt and sugar he or she adds to food, and if food tastes different than it did when he or she was younger.

A coated tongue does not indicate pathology. Wiping the tongue with dry gauze or brushing it with a toothbrush can remove accumulated materials and coatings from the tongue. Heavy coatings can be caused by poor oral hygiene and low fluid intake.

A smooth, red tongue can indicate a deficiency of iron, vitamin B_{12}, or niacin. Leukoplakia is characterized by a thick, white patch anywhere on the tongue, and can be precancerous; any lesion on the tongue that has existed for more than three weeks should give rise to suspicion of carcinoma.

The bottom surface and base of the tongue must not be overlooked. Varicosities may be seen on the tongue's undersurface: the tiny purple or bluish-black swollen areas under the tongue are not uncommon among older adults. Cancerous lesions occur more frequently on the bottom surface and base of the tongue than on the top of the tongue.

While examining the mouth, be alert to unusual odors. These odors can indicate poor oral hygiene, oral cavity disease, lung abscesses, and several systemic conditions.

Pharynx

To test the function of the vagus nerve (which causes the soft palate to rise and block the nasopharynx during swallowing), press a tongue blade on the middle portion of the tongue and ask the client to say "ah." The tongue depressor should not be far enough in the mouth to cause gagging. Under normal circumstances, the soft palate will rise when the client says "ah." If it fails to rise properly, aspiration of food is a threat. Some older persons will demonstrate a weakening of pharyngeal muscles.

Ask questions regarding swallowing problems. Complaints of "food sticking in the throat" may indicate cardiospasm, a condition in which the cardiac sphincter fails to relax properly while swallowing.

Soreness, redness, and white patches in the throat are associated with pharyngitis. Throat cultures are essential to identify the exact cause.

Esophagus

The client may complain of feeling uncomfortable and full in his or her chest after meals. These symptoms are related to esophageal changes associated with the aging process.

Since they communicate with the gastric veins of the portal system, esophageal veins can become dilated and tortuous if related problems exist. Bleeding and irritation of the esophagus are indicative of esophageal varicosities.

Esophageal diverticulum can cause gagging, dysphagia, regurgitation of undigested food, and foul breath odor resulting from food materials accumulated in the diverticulum. A barium swallow is necessary to confirm the diagnoses.

Excessive salivation, hiccups, dysphagia, anemia, thirst, and chronic bleeding can indicate cancer of the esophagus. A high incidence of esophageal cancer occurs in males, blacks, and alcoholics. A barium swallow, esophagoscopy, and biopsy are usually performed when esophageal cancer is suspected.

Stomach

Indigestion and intolerance to certain foods are common problems of the older adult due to decreased gastric acid secretion and delayed emptying time of the stomach. Question the client as to the presence and management of indigestion, as well as to the quantity and quality of meals.

Complaints of nausea can result from gastrointestinal disturbances, medications, and inner ear problems. In addition to gastrointestinal disturbances, vomiting can be associated with medications, poisoning, and brain tumors. The frequency, precipitating factors, management, and characteristics of nausea and vomiting should be explored. Question the client for symptoms of gastric problems. Specifically investigate complaints of heartburn, belching, dysphagia, regurgitation, gastric irritation, and pain.

Small Intestine

Indications of small intestinal problems can be obtained during physical assessment of the abdomen, and through symptoms such as pain, vomiting, constipation, distension, and flatus.

Intestinal obstruction can occur among older adults. Strictures from an ulcer, peritonitis, adhesions, parasites, diverticulitis, gallstones, hernias, and tumors can result in a mechanical obstruction of the intestine. Paralytic ileus, an obstruction associated with a paralyzed bowel, can be caused by a low potassium level, a myocardial infarction, and infections such as pneumonia, septicemia, peritonitis, and pancreatitis; it also can be a complication following abdominal or pelvic surgery. Vomiting, distension, and constipation can indicate an intestinal obstruction. Bowel sounds can be present with a mechanical obstruction, whereas they are absent with paralytic ileus. Pain tends to be more severe with mechanical obstructions.

Small intestine diverticuli occur less frequently than large intestine diverticuli. Symptoms associated with osteomalacia, and iron and vitamin B_{12} deficiencies can be clues to this problem.

If the client has an ileostomy, note when and why it was performed, the general condition, the method in which the client cares for it, and other significant data.

Large Intestine

A careful history of bowel habits should be obtained from the older adult. Do not rely on the client's assessment of constipation.

Many older persons erroneously believe that the absence of a daily bowel movement means constipation. Diet, activity, medications, frequency of elimination, characteristics of the feces, and ease of passage of the bowel movement all must be considered in assessing for constipation. Question the client as to his or her frequency in the use of elimination aids (for example, laxatives, suppositories, or enemas) and the method in which they are administered. Note the impact of foods and other natural products on the client's elimination pattern.

Older adults have higher incidences of cancer at all sites along the large intestine, although the sigmoid colon and rectum are the most common sites. Indications of the problem include a change in bowel function, bloody feces, epigastric pain, jaundice, anorexia, and nausea. Digital rectal examination detects half of all large bowel and rectal carcinomas.

If the client has a colostomy, note when and why it was performed, the pattern of elimination, its condition, how it is cared for, and other significant data.

Accessory Organs

Examination of the abdomen contributes a great deal of information about the accessory organs, but much can be learned through taking the patient's history.

Jaundice is often a sign of liver disease. Hepatitis occurs in older adults, although less frequently than in younger people. The US National Center for Health Statistics states that cirrhosis is among the ten leading causes of death in the older population. This problem is commonly associated with alcoholism and chronic nutritional deficiencies. Drug detoxification is a problem for individuals with liver damage. The icterus index gives an indication of bilirubin concentration and general liver function.

Disorders of the pancreas are difficult to detect due to altered or vague symptoms. Pancreatitis can be confused with liver or gallbladder diseases. Pancreatitis symptoms include anorexia, weight loss, malaise, nausea, vomiting, and epigastric pain radiating to the back and abdomen. Chronic pancreatitis can have similar symptoms to acute pancreatitis, as well as symptoms of jaundice and constipation. Cancer of the pancreas mimics chronic pancreatitis in symptoms, and, unfortunately, it is usually in an advanced state before these symptoms occur. Characteristic of pancreatic cancer is pain in the recumbent position that is relieved when the affected person leans forward.

Biliary tract disease increases in incidence with age, and cholecystectomy (removal of the gallbladder) is the most common type of abdominal surgery in the aged (Brandt 1986b). Gallstones, which affect women more frequently than men, can be asymptomatic or can be present with symptoms of nausea, vomiting, indigestion, obstructive jaundice, and pain in the upper right quadrant of the abdomen or in the right shoulder. Gallstones can obstruct the common or cystic ducts and lead to inflammation and infection. Cancer of the gallbladder, although rare, affects older adults more than younger adults. Because its symptoms can be confused with those of gallstones or liver disorders, detection is often delayed.

Examination of the Abdomen

Crucial to a complete assessment of the gastrointestinal system is examination of the abdomen. All four methods of examination—inspection, auscultation, palpation, and percussion—are used to examine the abdomen. Because touch stimulates movement in the bowel, which in turn alters sounds, inspection and auscultation are performed prior to palpation and percussion.

To prepare for examination of the abdomen, have the client:

1. Void
2. Lie supine on a firm surface with hands at side or folded across the chest
3. Relax abdominal muscles (Relaxation can be aided by creating a comfortable atmosphere, providing a warm environment to prevent shivering, and placing a pillow under the client's knees)

For the purpose of examination, the abdomen is divided into four quadrants with the umbilicus at the center. See Figure 8-4.

To inspect the abdomen, fully expose the abdominal region. General *skin condition* should be noted. Scars can indicate prior surgery that the client failed to mention during the interview, perhaps because of a memory deficit or

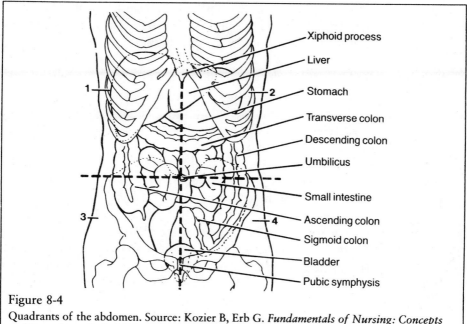

Figure 8-4
Quadrants of the abdomen. Source: Kozier B, Erb G. *Fundamentals of Nursing: Concepts and Procedures*, 2nd ed. Menlo Park, CA: Addison-Wesley, 1983.

the blocking of information associated with the stress of being examined. Reduced touch and pressure sensations can result in skin injuries, indicated by scars, that the individual is unaware of. Deep irregular scars are usually associated with burns. When scars exist, describe the shape, size, and location (for example, scar, straight line, 7 cm, RLQ).

Striae, "stretch marks" resulting from disruption to the elastic fibers of the reticular layer of the cutis, should be noted. These marks are pink or blue if recently developed and become silvery white with time. Striae can occur with an abdominal tumor, ascites, and obesity. Purple striae are associated with Cushing's syndrome.

Abdominal skin color is a good indication of the individual's normal skin color because it tends to be protected and untanned. Jaundice can be detected by abdominal skin discoloration. A glistening abdomen can occur with ascites.

Rashes may appear on the abdomen, resulting from drug reactions, irritation from soap or clothing, or nervous itching. Small, hard, painless nodules can be carcinoma of the skin.

The *contour* of the abdomen is another factor to be noted during the inspection of this region. The right and left quadrants should be symmetrical. A method to assess contour is to sit beside the client while he or she is lying down and observe the abdomen. The greatest height of convexity will be at the umbilicus when the client is lying down. When the client stands, the greatest height of convexity drops between the umbilicus and symphysis pubis because of the pull of gravity. Many older adults have rounded abdomens due to weaker muscles and greater amounts of adipose tissue.

The abdominal surface should be smooth, without dilated vessels or bulging areas. By having the client raise his head while lying, umbilical and incisional hernias may be made apparent.

Distention is an abnormal finding and indicates an unusual stretching of the abdominal wall (Figure 8-5). Generalized symmetrical distention can be caused by obesity, tumors, or ascites. A symmetrical distention can be due to tumors, hernias, or bowel obstruction. Central, lower-quadrant distention can result from bladder enlargement, ovarian tumors, or uterine tumors. Central, upper-quadrant distention can be an outcome of gastric dilatation or pancreatic tumors or cysts.

Activity is also noted during inspection of the abdomen. The abdomen may move in relation to respirations; this is less common in females because they have more costal movement with respiration. Limited respiratory movement may be associated with peritonitis or abdominal infection.

Peristaltic activity can be observed by sitting by the client's side and looking across the abdomen. Peristalsis is easier to detect in thin persons.

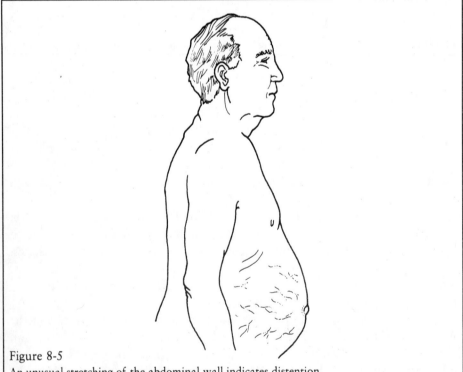

Figure 8-5
An unusual stretching of the abdominal wall indicates distention.

Touching the abdomen is a means of stimulating peristalsis. Strong, visible contractions can be noted when there is bowel obstruction.

Abdominal-intestinal sounds are primarily high-pitched sounds and are best heard using the diaphragm of the stethoscope. The bell portion is used in assessing vascular sounds. Auscultation should be performed for all four quadrants.

Peristaltic Sounds

Listen to the *peristaltic sounds* using the diaphragm of the stethoscope. Normal bowel sounds occur once every 5 to 15 seconds, and can last from 1 to several seconds. There is no regular pattern to bowel sounds, thus several minutes of listening may be necessary to assess peristaltic activity accurately.

The lack of bowel sounds indicates no intestinal motility. Due to the irregularity of bowel sounds, it is advisable to listen for at least five minutes before determining that bowel sounds are absent. Often, flecking your finger on the abdominal wall can trigger bowel sounds. Reduced bowel sounds can result from peritonitis, electrolyte imbalances, handling of the bowel during surgery, late bowel obstruction, and pneumonia.

Loud, gurgling, and frequent bowel sounds indicate increased peristaltic activity. This can be due to gastroenteritis, diarrhea, laxative use, and early obstruction of the bowel. Continuous sounds may be heard if there has been food intake four to eight hours prior to auscultation.

Vascular Sounds

To hear *vascular sounds*, hold the bell portion of the stethoscope lightly against the abdomen.

Bruits, associated with dilated or constricted vessels, can be heard as murmurs over the areas of major arteries. A loud murmur over the abdominal aorta can indicate an aneurysm. Low pitches to medium murmurs over a renal artery can be due to renal arterial stenosis. Cardiac murmurs can radiate sounds to the abdomen. Thus it is useful to have knowledge of cardiac murmurs if murmur sounds are present.

A continuous, medium-pitched hum is heard over the inferior vena cava and its large tributaries. A venous hum in the right upper quadrant is an abnormal finding and is associated with increased collateral circulation resulting from obstructed portal circulation; this occurs with hepatic cirrhosis. Exerting too much pressure on the stethoscope can cause the hum to be missed.

Friction Rub

A rough, grating sound over the spleen or liver similar to shoes rubbing on a cement surface can indicate a *friction rub*. Friction rubs are created by these

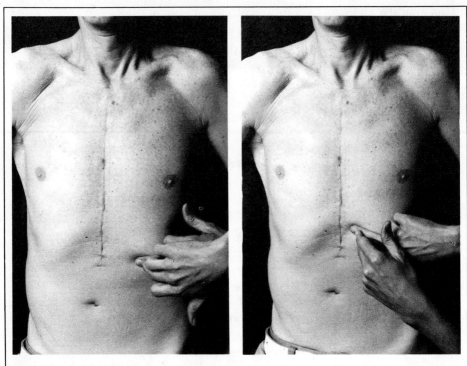

Figure 8-6
To assess tympany of the stomach, percuss (A) in the left anterior rib cage, and (B) in the left epigastric region.

organs, which have large surfaces, coming in contact with the peritoneum. Infections, abscesses, or tumors of the liver or spleen can cause this problem.

Percussion determines the presence of fluid, gas, and masses. The entire abdomen is percussed for areas of tympany and dullness. Dullness indicates solid masses; tympany indicates the presence of gas and will predominate in the small and large intestines. (Refer to technique for percussion in Chapter 1.) To ascertain the distribution of tympany and dullness, gently percuss the abdomen in all four quadrants.

To assess the tympany of the *stomach*, percuss in the left lower anterior rib cage and the left epigastric region (Figure 8-6). The tympany of the stomach is of a lower pitch than that of the intestines. Tympany of the gastric air bubble will vary: increase in the gastric air bubble size within an individual who also demonstrates a distended abdomen can be due to gastric dilatation.

Ascites

Ascites should be differentiated from other causes of abdominal distention. To do so, percuss the abdomen as the client lies supine. Fluid causes dullness laterally in the flank and tympany at the midpoint of the abdomen. Carefully identify the point between the dull and tympanic sounds, and mark that area. Turn the client to his or her side and percuss the abdomen. Mark that area and turn the client to the other side, repeating the same procedure. If ascites is present, the area of dullness will be closer to the umbilicus due to free fluid shifting as the client turns. This procedure can be done on a daily basis to estimate changes in fluid volume for individuals with ascites.

Liver Span

To obtain a gross estimate of the *liver span*, follow the midclavicular line below the umbilicus and percuss in an area of tympany. Continue percussing from this area upward along the midclavicular line until the tympanic sounds change to dull ones, which denotes the lower border of the liver. Mark this area (Figure 8-7). To identify the upper portion of the liver, percuss from the

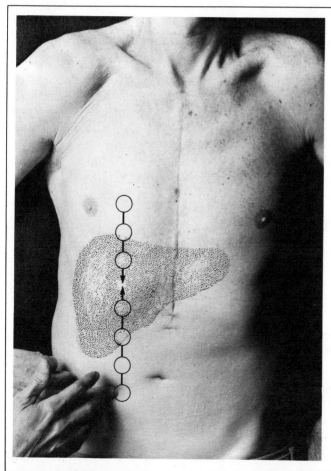

Figure 8-7
Determine liver span by locating the lower and upper borders of the liver.

midclavicular line downward until dullness is noted (usually between the 5th to 7th interspace) and mark the area. Liver span is related to body height; for example, taller persons will have a longer liver span. Men tend to have a greater liver span than women. Spans ranging between 6 and 12 cm at the midclavicular line are considered normal. If the liver is suspected of being enlarged, percussion may be done along the midsternal line in the same method that was used along the midclavicular line. The normal span in the midsternal line ranges between 4 and 8 cm.

Each border of dullness may occasionally be obscured. Gas in the colon can obscure the lower border, and the upper border can be obscured if there is pleural effusion or lung consolidation. Caudal displacement of the liver can occur with pulmonary edema, and upward displacement can indicate ascites or tumors.

Spleen

The *spleen* is somewhat easier to assess than the liver. Splenic dullness can be percussed in a small area posterior to the midaxillary line, between the 6th and 10th ribs (Figure 8-8). Gas in the stomach or colon can obscure the splenic dullness. Increased areas of dullness are associated with enlargement of the spleen. Palpation is more reliable in assessing splenic enlargement since the spleen is normally not palpable in the adult.

The most beneficial method to identify abdominal abnormalities is palpation. Help the client to relax prior to beginning palpation. If the client does not voluntarily relax his abdominal muscles, apply gentle pressure on the lower sternum with one hand as you palpate with the other. This maneuver forces a deeper respiration and inhibits abdominal muscle contraction. It is generally useful to position yourself on the side of the examining table so that your dominant hand is closest to the client.

Light palpation is performed first to determine the presence of slight tenderness, muscle resistance, and large masses. The pads of the fingers, not the tips, are depressed in the abdominal wall approximately 1 cm. With a gentle, smooth motion, palpate all quadrants. Note areas of sensitivity, spasm or rigidity, and avoid aggressive manipulation of these areas.

Involuntary muscle contraction (rigidity) is associated with peritoneal irritation. Carefully palpate to determine if this finding is unilateral or bilateral. To identify specific problem areas, ask the client to raise his head without using his arms. The client will feel unilateral pain if problems are present. Rigidity in the right upper quadrant can be associated with acute cholecystitis. Boardlike rigidity of the abdominal wall is a sign of peritonitis. It is important to remember that peritoneal irritation can be present, but because of altered pain sensations in the older adult, the client may not give the customary description of severe pain.

After light palpation, moderately palpate all four quadrants using the side of the hand. This technique is most useful in assessing the liver and spleen,

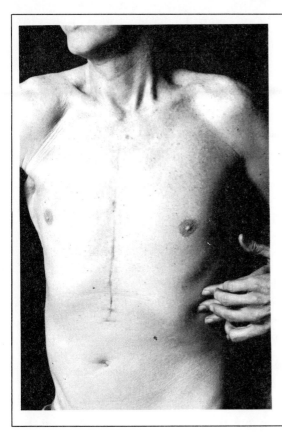

Figure 8-8
Percuss splenic dullness posterior
to the midaxillary line, between
the 6th and 10th rib. Increased
areas of dullness are associated
with splenic enlargement.

which move in relation to respirations. Normally, on inspiration, an abdominal organ is pushed downward against the examining hand. The presence of pain is an abnormal finding.

Deeper palpation is necessary to detect organ tenderness and masses missed during light and moderate palpation. All quadrants are palpated by indenting the distal half of the palmar surfaces of the fingers into the abdominal wall. In the presence of obesity or muscle resistance, two hands may be needed to palpate: one to feel the organs and the other to exert pressure on the examining hand.

Rebound Tenderness

Masses should be thoroughly described as to their location, size, shape, tenderness, pulsations, and relation to activity (such as respiration and coughing). Note areas of tenderness and obtain information from the client as to prior awareness of the problem, length of time present, and relationship to other factors (such as trauma or onset of specific symptoms). Some tenderness over the cecum, sigmoid colon, and aorta is normal. Tenderness can be associated with peritoneal irritation. When tenderness is present, test for *rebound tenderness*. This testing is done by pushing the pads of the fingers deeply into the tender area and rapidly withdrawing them. Stabbing pain will result at the source of inflammation.

The spleen, pancreas, and gallbladder are not palpable unless enlarged. Although normally not palpable, the liver sometimes may be felt in thin persons.

Rectal Examination

The many problems affecting the older adult's rectosigmoid area make rectal examination an essential component of the gastrointestinal system's assessment. As you prepare the client for the procedure, elicit information regarding bowel patterns, stool characteristics, incontinence, hemorrhoidal problems, the presence of rectal bleeding, and other data pertaining to this region.

Rectal examination can produce anxiety in many persons. Some are embarrassed by the procedure and are fearful that they may involuntarily have a bowel movement while being examined. Others find the examination uncomfortable. Concern about possible findings can be a cause for anxiety also. Reassurance, explanations, and adequate draping can help relax clients.

Among the many positions that can be used for rectal examination, the left lateral and standing positions are the most popular. In the left lateral position, the client rests on the left side, slightly flexing the right hip and knee. The standing position allows better palpation of the prostate and requires that the client stand and flex the hips to allow his upper extremity to rest across the examining table or bed.

Begin the examination by spreading the buttocks and inspecting the perianal region. Note the presence of external hemorrhoids (painful or painless flaccid skin sacs around the anus), rashes, lesions, tumors, fissures, inflammation, and other unusual observations. Drier membrane predisposes the older adult to a greater risk of skin cracking and irritation. Indications of hygienic practices may also be present: for example, irritation from harsh wiping or evidence that fecal material is being wiped toward the vaginal opening.

Ask the client to strain and bear down as if trying to have a bowel movement. Hemorrhoids and rectal prolapse can be revealed by this maneuver. As the client continues to bear down, gently insert a lubricated, gloved finger into the anal canal toward the direction of the umbilicus. You can reassure the client that it is normal to feel as if a bowel movement is occurring. The strength of the sphincter can be assessed by asking the client to tighten the muscles around your finger.

Palpate the rectal wall and canal by rotating your finger. Be alert to masses and other irregularities. Fecal impactions should not be confused with masses.

A fecal impaction can be detected as a hard mass that blocks your palpation of the rectum. It may or may not be moveable. You will notice fecal material, as well as some oozing of diarrhealike discharge, on your withdrawn finger if an impaction is present.

Prostate Gland

The prostate gland can be palpated along the anterior wall of the rectum. Normally, the prostate is a firm, smooth structure consisting of two lobes joining in somewhat of a heart shape. It is approximately 4 cm in diameter and 2.5 cm in length. Masses may be more evident by asking the client to bear down. Any irregularity in size, consistency, and tenderness should be noted. Benign prostatic enlargement is present in most older males. With this condition, the gland is symmetrically enlarged and smooth.

The cervix can be palpated through the anterior wall of the female's rectum. The cervix feels like a small round mass. Be alert to tenderness and masses.

Stool Examination

After completing the palpation and withdrawing your examining finger, examine the fecal material that has adhered to the glove's surface for unusual color or content characteristics. Tarry, *black stool* can be associated with upper gastrointestinal bleeding or the ingestion of iron substances; *bright red blood* can be due to lower bowel problems, for example, hemorrhoids. It is beneficial to perform a guaiac test for occult blood as a routine measure. Obstructive jaundice can cause the stool to *lack pigmentation* and *appear gray or tan. Pale stool*, which is also of a fatty nature, is associated with absorption problems. *Mucous particles* present in stool can indicate an inflammatory process. The existence of any parasites, such as pinworms, should be noted also.

DISORDERS OF THE GASTROINTESTINAL SYSTEM

Hiatus Hernia

Displacement of the stomach above the diaphragm is known as a hiatus hernia. The incidence of hiatus hernia increases with age to the extent that it is believed that more than 50% of all older adults experience this condition. Heartburn, dysphagia, belching, vomiting, and regurgitation characterize this disorder. Bleeding and pain, often mistaken for cardiac disorder, also may accompany a hiatus hernia. Symptoms are more pronounced when the affected individual is in a recumbent position. A barium swallow and esophagoscopy will confirm the presence of the condition.

Ulcers

Ulcers can be present in older adults as a new problem or as an outgrowth of a chronic ulcer problem throughout their lifespans. Older women develop ulcers more often than older men. Duodenal ulcers occur two to three times more frequently than gastric ulcers, although more deaths are related to gastric ulcer (Brandt 1986c). A predisposition to ulcers may exist among persons with a family history of ulcers, a stressful life-style, and who ingest a diet known to contribute to gastric irritation and ulcer formation. Persons with chronic obstructive pulmonary disease often experience ulcers as a complication. Also, many drugs prescribed for older individuals carry the risk of increasing gastric secretions and reducing the resistance of the gastric mucosa. Examples of such drugs include aspirin, reserpine, phenylbutazone, phenobarbital, tolbutamide, and adrenal corticosteroids.

Symptoms of ulcers may be atypical among older adults. Gastric pain may be less severe than expected, or it may be absent. Weight loss, painless vomiting, and anemias may be among the first indicators of this disorder. In addition to the client's history, a barium swallow and gastroscopy will aid in the diagnosis.

Stomach Cancer

Although stomach cancer decreases in incidence with age, it is far from an uncommon problem affecting older adults. Those persons who have a higher incidence of stomach cancer are males, those having pernicious anemia or atrophy of the gastric mucosa, or those in the 75- to 85-year-old group (Berman and Kersner 1983). Symptoms of this disorder often mimic those associated with gastric ulcers and include anorexia, weight loss, anemia, and epigastric pain. If the client chronically uses antacids, gastric symptoms may be masked; weight loss and bloody vomit or feces may be the primary clues. A barium swallow and gastroscopy with biopsy confirm this diagnosis.

Diverticulosis and Diverticulitis

Atrophy of the intestinal wall muscles with age, obesity, chronic constipation, and hiatus hernia contribute to the formation of multiple pouches of intestinal mucosa in the weakened muscular wall of the large intestine. This condition, diverticulosis, is common among older adults.

Although medical management usually is sufficient in controlling diverticulosis, situations can occur when bowel contents accumulate in the diverticuli, decompose, and cause inflammation and infection. This condition is known as diverticulitis and can be triggered by overeating, straining during a bowel movement, and the ingestion of irritating foods and alcohol. Symptoms of diverticulitis include nausea, vomiting, constipation, diarrhea, low-grade fever, blood or mucus in the feces, and pain in the left lower quadrant.

Colorectal Cancer

Cancers of the large intestines, rectosigmoid, and rectum occur primarily in persons age 50 or older and rank second to lung cancer in men and breast cancer in women as the major cause of cancer death in late life. Colorectal cancer is closely related to the consumption of a high meat and fat, low fiber diet; a history of ulcerative colitis is also a related factor.

Often, symptoms related to anemia from the blood loss associated with the disease are the first indication of the problem. Later signs include narrow ribbonlike stools, rectal bleeding, alteration in bowel habits, weight loss, fatigue, and the complaint of vague abdominal pain. A mass may be palpable on rectal examination.

To facilitate early detection of this highly prevalent condition it is recommended that persons over age 40 receive regular digital examination or sigmoidoscopy and a guaiac test of stool.

Appendicitis

Six to eight percent of all appendectomies are performed in persons aged 60 and over (Fenyo 1982). Although its incidence is not high, morbidity and mortality associated with appendicitis are due to the difficulty in identifying this problem early and the speed with which this condition progresses in older adults.

Fever may not be present with appendicitis in the elderly. Pain over the appendix may not be present or may be referred to another area. Rebound tenderness is usually present. Abdominal distention, constipation, nausea, vomiting, tachycardia, and leukocytosis are findings consistent with the diagnosis.

Regular assessment of the client postoperatively is important because peritonitis develops more commonly and perforation occurs two to three times more often in older persons (Fenyo 1982).

8 Chapter Summary

I. Age-related changes
- A. Teeth not normally lost with age but high prevalence of denture use among older adults
- B. Decreased salivary gland activity; dried oral mucosa
- C. Loss of taste buds, especially for sweet and salty flavors
- D. Weakening of pharyngeal muscles in some older adults
- E. Esophagus becomes slightly dilated; esophageal mobility decreased
- F. Delayed emptying time of stomach; decreased gastric acid secretion

G. Weaker intestinal musculature

H. Decreased peristalsis

I. Liver smaller in size and reduced in storage capacity

J. Less digestive enzymes produced by pancreas

K. Altered rates of insulin release

II. Assessment

  A. Inspection and general review

    1. Lips

      a) Symmetry

      b) Color

      c) Moisture

      d) Lesions, sores, cracks

    2. Teeth and Dentures

      a) Presence

      b) Condition

    3. Mucous membrane of mouth

      a) Color

      b) Lesions

      c) Irritations caused by friction from teeth or dentures

    4. Gums

      a) Color

      b) Condition

      c) Swelling, irritation, bleeding

    5. Tongue

      a) Color

      b) Papillae

      c) Symmetry

      d) Movement

      e) Taste sensation

    6. Pharynx

      a) Vagus nerve function

      b) Swallowing

      c) Soreness, redness, white patches

    7. Esophagus

      a) Mobility: ease of digestion

      b) Bleeding, gagging, dysphagia, regurgitation of undigested food, breath odor

    8. Stomach

      a) Digestion

      b) Quality and quantity of meals

      c) Dysphagia, indigestion, belching, nausea, vomiting, regurgitation, indications of bleeding

    9. Small intestine

      a) Indications of vitamin or mineral deficiencies

      b) Pain, vomiting, constipation, distention, flatus

      c) Presence of ileostomy

  B. Examination of the abdomen

    1. Prepare client for examination

    2. Inspect abdomen

      a) Skin condition

      b) Contour

      c) Activity

    3. Auscultation

      a) Diaphragm of stethoscope used for high-pitched, abdominal-intestinal sounds, bell portion used for vascular sounds

      b) Peristaltic sounds: heard irregularly every 5 to 15 seconds

      c) Vascular sounds: murmurs, hums

      d) Friction rub: organ coming in contact with peritoneum

    4. Percussion

      a) Determines presence of fluid, gas, and masses

      b) Dullness indicates solid masses; tympany indicates gas

      c) Percuss: tympany in stomach and small and large intestine; liver span; splenic size; and ascites

    5. Palpation

      a) Light palpation, using pads of fingers, performed to detect slight tenderness, muscle resistance, and large masses

      b) Moderate palpation, using side of hand,

performed to assess liver and spleen

   c) Deeper palpation, using distal half of palmar surfaces of fingers, performed to detect organ tenderness and masses

   d) Spleen, pancreas, gallbladder, and liver not palpable normally, although liver may be palpated in a thin client

   e) Note masses and tenderness

C. Rectal examination
1. Preparation and positioning of client
2. Inspection of perianal region
   a) Note hemorrhoids, rashes, lesions, rectal prolapse, tumors, fissures, inflammation, hygienic practices
3. Palpation of rectal wall and canal
   a) Note masses, fecal impactions, irregularities
4. Examination of fecal material

III. Pathologies
A. Oral cavity
1. Insufficient oxygen or dehydration
   a) Lips dry, pale blue
   b) Coated tongue
2. Cancer of the lips
   a) Lesions and sores that do not heal
3. Riboflavin deficiencies
   a) Cracks and fissures at angle of mouth
4. Moniliasis infection
   a) White patches resembling small beads of dried milk
   b) Can be associated with diabetes or leukemia
5. Periodontal disease
   a) Primary cause of tooth loss in aging adults
   b) Swelling, redness, bleeding gums

6. Iron, vitamin B_{12}, or niacin deficiencies
   a) Smooth red tongue
7. Cancer of tongue
   a) Leukoplakia lasting more than three weeks is strong indication

B. Pharynx
1. Weak pharyngeal muscles
   a) Soft palate fails to rise properly when client says "ah" while tongue depressor is pressed on middle portion of tongue
   b) Risk of aspiration
2. Cardiospasm
   a) Cardiac sphincter fails to relax properly during swallowing
   b) Client complains of "food sticking in throat"
3. Pharyngitis
   a) Soreness, redness, white patches in throat
   b) Confirmed through throat culture

C. Esophagus
1. Esophageal varicosities
   a) Dilated and tortuous esophageal veins
   b) Bleeding, irritation of esophagus
2. Esophageal diverticulum
   a) Accumulation of food in pouches along esophagus
   b) Gagging, dysphagia, regurgitation of undigested food, foul breath odor
   c) Confirmed through barium swallow
3. Cancer of the esophagus
   a) Higher incidence among blacks, males, and alcoholics
   b) Excessive salivation, hiccups, dysphagia, anemia, thirst, chronic bleeding
   c) Confirmed by barium swallow, esophagoscopy, and biopsy

D. Stomach
  1. Hiatus hernia
     a) Squeezing of stomach above diaphragm
     b) Heartburn, dysphagia, belching, vomiting, regurgitation, pain, bleeding
     c) Symptoms more pronounced when in recumbent position
  2. Ulcers
     a) Symptoms may be atypical: less severe gastric pain, weight loss, painless vomiting, anemia
  3. Stomach cancer
     a) Symptoms can mimic gastric ulcer and can be masked by chronic antacid use
     b) Primary clues: weight loss, bloody vomit or feces
     c) Confirmed by barium swallow, gastroscopy, biopsy

E. Small intestines
  1. Intestinal obstruction
     a) Mechanical causes: ulcer, peritonitis, adhesions, parasites, diverticulitis, gallstones, hernias, tumors
     b) Neurologic causes: low potassium level, myocardial infarction, infection, surgery
     c) Vomiting, distention, constipation, pain (more severe with mechanical obstruction)
     d) Bowel sounds can be present with mechanical obstruction
  2. Diverticuli
     a) Less common than large intestine diverticuli
     b) Symptoms associated with osteomalacia, and deficiencies of iron and vitamin B_{12}

F. Large intestine
  1. Constipation
     a) Irregular and difficult passage of hard feces: lack of daily bowel movement alone not indicative of constipation
     b) Common among older adults due to multiple predisposing factors
     c) Assess frequency of elimination, characteristics of feces, ease of stool passage, diet, activity, and medications
  2. Diverticulitis
     a) Pouches on weakened intestinal wall that have accumulated bowel contents leading to inflammation and infection
     b) Pain over sigmoid area, nausea, vomiting, constipation, diarrhea, low-grade fever, blood or mucus in feces
  3. Cancer of the large intestine
     a) One half of all bowel and rectal carcinomas detectable through rectal examination
     b) Sigmoid colon and rectum most common sites, although higher incidence of cancer all along large intestines in older adults
     c) Change in bowel function, bloody feces, epigastric pain, jaundice, anorexia, nausea

G. Accessory organs
  1. Cirrhosis of the liver
     a) One of the major causes of death among older adults
     b) Commonly associated with alcoholism and chronic nutritional deficiencies

c) Icterus index helpful in diagnosis
2. Pancreatitis
   a) Anorexia, weight loss, malaise, nausea, vomiting, epigastric pain radiating to back and abdomen, jaundice, constipation
3. Gallstones
   a) Increased incidence with age; affects women more often than men
   b) Nausea, vomiting, indigestion, obstructive jaundice, pain in upper right quadrant of abdomen or in the right shoulder; can be asymptomatic
4. Appendicitis
   a) Higher morbidity and mortality among aged
   b) Early detection difficult; fever and pain may not be present

IV. Related nursing diagnoses
   A. Constipation
   B. Diarrhea
   C. Pain
   D. Fluid volume deficit
   E. Potential for infection
   F. Knowledge deficit
   G. Noncompliance
   H. Altered nutrition: more than body requirements
   I. Altered nutrition: less than body requirements
   J. Altered oral mucous membrane
   K. Self-care deficit
   L. Altered thought processes

READINGS AND REFERENCES

Bates B. *A Guide to Physical Examination*, 4th ed. Philadelphia: Lippincott, 1987.

Berman PM, Kersner JB. Gastrointestinal problems. In: *Cowdry's The Care of the Geriatric Patient*, 6th ed. Steinberg FU (editor). St. Louis: Mosby, 1983.

Brandt LJ. Gastrointestinal disorders in the elderly. In: *Clinical Geriatrics*, 3rd ed. Rossman I (editor). Philadelphia: Lippincott, 1986, a) p 271, b) p 318, c) p 266.

Cowman SC. The elderly patient: A dental thought. *Age and Aging* May 1978; 7(2):65–67.

Fenyo G. Acute abdominal disease in the elderly. Experiences in two series in Stockholm. *American Journal of Surgery* 1982; 143:751–754.

Hudis MM. Dentistry for the elderly in health and illness. In: *Clinical Aspects of Aging*, 2nd ed. Reichel W (editor). Baltimore: Williams and Wilkens, 1983, pp 498–509.

Kravitz S. Anemia in the elderly. In: *Clinical Aspects of Aging*, 2nd ed. Reichel W (editor). Baltimore: Williams and Wilkens, 1983.

Malasanos L et al. *Health Assessment*, 3rd ed. St. Louis: Mosby, 1986.

Williams FT. Diabetes mellitus in older people. In: *Clinical Aspects of Aging*, 2nd ed. Reichel W (editor). Baltimore: Williams and Wilkens, 1983.

9

Assessment of Nutritional Status

Peggy Yen, RD, MPH

Among the many influences on the health and well-being of people as they age is nutrition. A good nutritional status significantly helps maximize the functional capacity and independence of the older adult. Illness can be avoided or better managed by individuals who have a proper dietary intake. Proper diet can improve surgical and medical outcomes, and rehabilitation as well.

Certain nutrients are essential to life, yet harmful effects can develop from excessive or deficient intake of these nutrients. However, determining a diet that will guarantee optimum functioning but not result in over- or undernutrition is difficult. Since information on the older adult's nutritional needs is limited, we can only assume that they need about the same amount of nutrients as other adults. The recommended dietary allowance (RDA) for thiamin, riboflavin and niacin is related to caloric intake. When the RDA for energy declines, the RDA for these nutrients also declines. The RDA for iron decreases for females 51 and over due to menopause.

As the body ages, some cells die and are not replaced. The cellular loss leads to a decrease in lean body mass and a relative increase in adipose tissue. Adipose tissue has a lower metabolic rate than lean tissue. Because activity also tends to decrease with age, an overall decline occurs in the older adult's caloric need. The lower an individual's caloric intake, the less room exists for foods that contain little else but calories.

Although the recommended dietary allowances of the Food and Nutrition Board suggest calorie levels for two age groups over fifty, caloric needs depend on personal characteristics such as body size, health status, and activity. The

RDA for energy (calories) is an amount that is estimated to meet the need of the *average* healthy person. It may overestimate or underestimate the individual's need.

The RDA for nutrients is an amount estimated to meet the needs of *most* healthy people, and therefore may overestimate an individual's need. Even so, a diet that meets the RDA for nutrients will probably be adequate for a healthy older adult. The diet may be inadequate for one who is ill or debilitated.

DIETARY INTAKE OF OLDER ADULTS

Dietary patterns of older adults, when compared to patterns of the general population, show that older adults eat less meat, fewer fruits and vegetables, proportionately larger amounts of breads and cereals, and about the same amounts of fats and sweets. These patterns have plausible reasons. For example, meats are usually the most expensive grocery item, require the most preparation, require careful storage, and are often inconveniently packaged. Fruits and vegetables also seem expensive per unit; some require preparation or are difficult to chew or digest. Breads and cereals are cheaper and easier to store, prepare, and eat.

The elimination of foods from a particular food group, as noted above, indicates that an older adult's diet may lack an adequate amount of one or more major nutrients. This practice can be complicated by other dietary habits. For example, greater consumption of breads combined with a habit of drinking tea can affect iron absorption. Breads, even when enriched, are not the best dietary source of iron. Chemical compounds in tea can inhibit even this iron absorption.

Many factors affect the dietary intake of older adults (Table 9-1). Although only a small percentage of older adults are institutionalized, they are the group most in need of nutritional assessment. This is because they are more likely to be inactive, to have dietary restrictions, and to have multiple medical problems and therefore multiple drug therapies.

In addition, many older people misjudge the adequacy of their own diets. Nutritional assessment provides information on which to base the education of older adults for improvements in diet.

NUTRITIONAL ASSESSMENT

Nutritional assessment of the individual requires dietary assessment as well as clinical, anthropometric, and biochemical data.

Table 9-1 Factors that Lead to Nutritional Problems in the Older Adult

FACTORS	ASSOCIATED CHARACTERISTICS	EFFECTS
Dental and oral		
Lack of good dental care	Chewing discomforts	Limits choice of foods to those easily chewed
Missing or decayed teeth; ill-fitting dentures	Chewing discomforts	Limits choice of foods to those easily chewed
Change in taste sensitivities	Decreases appetite or interest in food	Limits intake of foods
Bowel		
Constipation or diarrhea	Discomfort	May lead to elimination of certain foods in the mistaken belief that they cause bowel problems
	May overuse laxatives	Overuse of laxatives may affect nutrient absorption
Muscle		
Weakness	Interferes with food shopping and preparation	Limits choice of foods and preparation of nutritious meals
Lack of physical activity	Aggravates muscle weakness	Decreases interest in day-to-day activities, including eating
Chronic disease		
Diabetes mellitus, high blood pressure, cancer, and pulmonary, cardiac, renal, and gastrointestinal diseases are common	Need to modify normal diet due to disease process	Imposes further restrictions on food intake and appetite
	Physiologic status changes; drug, radiation, or surgical treatments may be required	Interferes with digestion, absorption, and use of nutrients
Drugs		
Self- or physician-prescribed		May cause some interference with nutrient absorption and use; alcohol may do likewise and may act as substitution for food calories
Mood		
Depression and/or loneliness	Decreases interest in food and proper diet	Limits intake of food
Institutionalization		
Inability to adapt to new situation; inactivity; no control over meal plans	Decreases interest in food and decreases incentive to follow dietary advice	Limits intake of foods and choice of foods

Table 9-2 Physical Signs Indicative or Suggestive of Malnutrition

BODY AREA	NORMAL APPEARANCE	SIGNS ASSOCIATED WITH MALNUTRITION
Hair	Shiny; firm; not easily plucked	Lack of natural shine; hair dull and dry; thin and sparse; hair fine, silky, and straight; color changes (flag sign); can be easily plucked
Face	Skin color uniform; smooth, pink, healthy appearance; not swollen	Skin color loss (depigmentation); skin dark over cheeks and under eyes (malar and supra-orbital pigmentation; lumpiness or flakiness of skin of nose and mouth; swollen face; enlarged parotid glands; scaling of skin around nostrils (nasolabial seborrhea)
Eyes	Bright, clear, shiny; no sores at corners of eyelids; membranes a healthy pink and are moist. No prominent blood vessels or mound of tissue on sclera	Eye membranes are pale (pale conjunctivae); redness of membranes (conjunctival injection); Bitot's spots; redness and fissuring of eyelid corners (angular palpebritis); dryness of eye membranes (conjunctival xerosis); cornea has dull appearance (corneal xerosts); cornea is soft (keratomalacia); scar on cornea; ring of fine blood vessels around corner (circumcorneal injection)
Lips	Smooth, not chapped or swollen	Redness and swelling of mouth or lips (cheilosis), especially at corners of mouth (angular fissures and scars)
Tongue	Deep red in appearance; not swollen or smooth	Swelling; scarlet and raw tongue; magenta (purplish) color of tongue; smooth tongue; swollen sores; hyperemic and hypertrophic papillae; and atrophic papillae
Teeth	No cavities; no pain; bright	May be missing or erupting abnormally; gray or black spots (fluorosis); cavities (caries)

	Normal	Abnormal
Gums	Healthy; red; do not bleed; not swollen	"Spongy" and bleed easily; recession of gums
Glands	Face not swollen	Thyroid enlargement (front of neck); parotid enlargement (cheeks become swollen)
Skin	No signs of rashes, swellings, dark or light spots	Dryness of skin (xerosis); sandpaper feel of skin (follicular hyperkeratosis); flakiness of skin; skin swollen and dark; red swollen pigmentation of exposed areas (pellagrous dermatosis); excessive lightness or darkness of skin (dyspigmentation); black and blue marks due to skin bleeding (petechiae); lack of fat under skin
Nails	Firm, pink	Nails are spoon-shape (koilonychia); brittle, ridged nails
Muscular and skeletal systems	Good muscle tone; some fat under skin; can walk or run without pain	Muscles have "wasted" appearance; bleeding into muscle (musculoskeletal hemorrhages); person cannot get up or walk properly
Internal systems: Cardiovascular	Normal heart rate and rhythm; no murmurs or abnormal rhythms; normal blood pressure for age	Rapid heart rate (above 100 tachycardia); enlarged heart; abnormal rhythm; elevated blood pressure
Gastrointestinal	No palpable organs or masses (in children, however, liver edge may be palpable)	Liver enlargement; enlargement of spleen (usually indicates other associated diseases)
Nervous	Psychologic stability; normal reflexes	Mental irritability and confusion; burning and tingling of hands and feet (paresthesia); loss of position and vibratory sense; weakness and tenderness of muscles (may result in inability to walk); decrease and loss of ankle and knee reflexes

Source: Christakis G. Nutritional assessment in health programs, Table 1. *American Journal of Public Health* November 1983; 63(2):19.

Clinical Assessment

Clinical assessment involves physical examination of the client for clinical signs of malnutrition (Table 9-2), and is best done by a trained examiner. These signs are not generally observed in the US population, although the older adult population is perhaps more likely to exhibit these signs than the general population. Most of the signs are not exclusive to nutritional deficiency; environmental or disease processes can be the cause. Untrained examiners can look for gross deviation from the norm and refer questionable signs to a clinical expert.

Anthropometric Assessment

Anthropometric assessment is the measurement and evaluation of physical parameters of body size such as height, weight, and triceps skinfold thickness.

Table 9-3 Comparison of the Weight-for-Height Tables from Actuarial Data (Build Study): Non-Age-Corrected Metropolitan Life Insurance Company and Age-Specific Gerontology Research Center Recommendations*

Height	Metropolitan 1983 Weights for Ages 25–29[†]		Gerontology Research Center Weight Range for Men and Women by Age (Years)[‡]				
	Men	Women	25	35	45	55	65
ft–in					lb		
4–10	· · ·	100–131	84–111	92–119	99–127	107–135	115–142
4–11	· · ·	101–134	87–115	95–123	103–131	111–139	119–147
5–0	· · ·	103–137	90–119	98–127	106–135	114–143	123–152
5–1	123–145	105–140	93–123	101–131	110–140	118–148	127–157
5–2	125–148	108–144	96–127	105–136	113–144	122–153	131–163
5–3	127–151	111–148	99–131	108–140	117–149	126–158	135–168
5–4	129–155	114–152	102–135	112–145	121–154	130–163	140–173
5–5	131–159	117–156	106–140	115–149	125–159	134–168	144–179
5–6	133–163	120–160	109–144	119–154	129–164	138–174	148–184
5–7	135–167	123–164	112–148	122–159	133–169	143–179	153–190
5–8	137–171	126–167	116–153	126–163	137–174	147–184	158–196
5–9	139–175	129–170	119–157	130–168	141–179	151–190	162–201
5–10	141–179	132–173	122–162	134–173	145–184	156–195	167–207
5–11	144–183	135–176	126–167	137–178	149–190	160–201	172–213
6–0	147–187	· · ·	129–171	141–183	153–195	165–207	177–219
6–1	150–192	· · ·	133–176	145–188	157–200	169–213	182–225
6–2	153–197	· · ·	137–181	149–194	162–206	174–219	187–232
6–3	157–202	· · ·	141–186	153–199	166–212	179–225	192–238
6–4	· · ·	· · ·	144–191	157–205	171–218	184–231	197–244

* Values in this table are for height without shoes and weight without clothes. To convert inches to centimeters, multiply by 2.54; to convert pounds to kilograms, multiply by 0.455.
† The weight range is the lower weight for small frame and the upper weight for large frame.
‡ Data from Andres (9).

In older adults, the most useful measurements include height, weight, skinfold, and arm circumference. A new reference chart (Table 9-3) that provides age-specific height–weight standards has replaced the previously used Metropolitan Life Insurance scales. The most reliable skinfold measurements are obtained from the right of the umbilicus and over the hip area in men, and in women from the umbilicus and upper arm (Rossman 1986). Of all the nutritional asssessment data available, weight and height are probably the most important. They are available in every setting; even the homebound can be weighed on a portable scale and have their height measured or at least estimated. Weight and height in older adults do not always accurately reflect nutritional status because of osteoporotic changes. This fact makes evaluating a single weight measurement difficult. It is important, therefore, to observe body weight over time as a measure of change in nutritional status.

Biochemical Assessment

Biochemical assessment is the measurement and evaluation of the levels of various substances in body fluids and tissues. In older adults, hemoglobin, hematocrit, total iron binding capacity (TIBC), and transferrin saturation are useful measurements for assessing iron nutriture, a common problem. Serum or urine vitamin levels may give evidence of dietary problems, but low levels generally will not occur in any but the most deficient individuals (Table 9-4). Some vitamin measurements reflect the intake of a vitamin, such as for vitamin C, immediately preceding the test. A low-blood vitamin or mineral level demands clinical attention.

Dietary Assessment

Dietary assessment involves interviewing or otherwise collecting information about food intake and habits as well as socioeconomic influences on these factors. Food intake is evaluated by comparing it to a standard such as the basic food groups or the RDAs. Factors to note that could increase an older adult's risk for poor dietary intake include living alone, isolation, and physical and mental disability.

FOOD INTAKE AND HABITS

Food intake data is obtained by a twenty-four-hour dietary recall, food record, or food frequency checklist.

Dietary Recall

A twenty-four-hour *dietary recall* is a recording of the client's recollection of his or her intake over the preceding twenty-four hours. Training, practice, and

Table 9-4 Current Guidelines for Criteria of Nutritional Status for Laboratory Evaluation

Nutrients and Units	Age of Subject (years)	Criteria of Status		
		Deficient	Marginal	Acceptable
*Hemoglobin	6–23 mos.	Up to 9.0	9.0– 9.9	10.0+
(g/100 mL)	2–5	Up to 10.0	10.0–10.9	11.0+
	6–12	Up to 10.0	10.0–11.4	11.5+
	13–16M	Up to 12.0	12.0–12.9	13.0+
	13–16F	Up to 10.0	10.0–11.4	11.5+
	16 + M	Up to 12.0	12.0–13.9	14.0+
	16 + F	Up to 10.0	10.0–11.9	12.0+
	Pregnant (after 6 + mos.)	Up to 9.5	9.5–10.9	11.0+
*Hematocrit	Up to 2	Up to 28	28 30	31+
(Packed cell volume	2–5	Up to 30	30–33	34+
in percent)	6–12	Up to 30	30–35	36+
	13–16M	Up to 37	37–39	40+
	13–16F	Up to 31	31–35	36+
	16 + M	Up to 37	37–43	44+
	16 + F	Up to 31	31–37	33+
	Pregnant	Up to 30	30–32	33+
*Serum Albumin	Up to 1	—	Up to 2.5	2.5+
(g/100 mL)	1–5	—	Up to 3.0	3.0+
	6–16	—	Up to 3.5	3.5+
	16+	Up to 2.8	2.8–3.4	3.5+
	Pregnant	Up to 3.0	3.0–3.4	3.5+
*Serum Protein	Up to 1	—	Up to 5.0	5.0+
(g/100 mL)	1–5	—	Up to 5.5	5.5+
	6–16	—	Up to 6.0	6.0+
	16+	Up to 6.0	6.0–6.4	6.5+
	Pregnant	Up to 5.5	5.5–5.9	6.0+
*Serum Ascorbic Acid (g/100 mL)	All ages	Up to 0.1	0.1–0.19	0.2+
*Plasma vitamin A (μg/100 mL)	All ages	Up to 10	10–19	20+
*Plasma Carotene	All ages	Up to 20	20–39	40+
(μg/100 mL)	Pregnant	—	40–79	80+
*Serum Iron	Up to 2	Up to 30	—	30+
(μg/100 mL)	2–5	Up to 40	—	40+
	6–12	Up to 50	—	50+
	12 + M	Up to 60	—	60+
	12 + F	Up to 40	—	40+
*Transferrin Saturation	Up to 2	Up to 15.0	—	15.0+
(percent)	2–12	Up to 20.0	—	20.0+
	12 + M	Up to 20.0		20.0 I
	12 + F	Up to 15.0	—	15.0+
**Serum Folacin (ng/mL)	All ages	Up to 2.0	2.1–5.9	6.0+

Table 9-4 (*Continued*)

Nutrients and Units	Age of Subject (years)	Criteria of Status		
		Deficient	Marginal	Acceptable
*Serum vitamin B$_{12}$ (pg/mL)	All ages	Up to 100	—	100+
*Thiamine in Urine (μg/g creatinine)	1–3	Up to 120	120–175	175+
	4–5	Up to 85	85–120	120+
	6–9	Up to 70	70–180	180+
	10–15	Up to 55	55–150	150+
	16+	Up to 27	27– 65	65+
	Pregnant	Up to 21	21– 49	50+
*Riboflavin in Urine (μg/g creatinine)	1–3	Up to 150	150–499	500+
	4–5	Up to 100	100–299	300+
	6–9	Up to 85	85–269	270+
	10–16	Up to 70	70–199	200+
	16+	Up to 27	27– 79	80+
	Pregnant	Up to 30	30– 89	90+
*RBC Transketolase-TPP effect (ratio)	All ages	25+	15– 25	Up to 15
*RBC Glutathione Reductase-FAD effect (ratio)	All ages	1.2+	—	Up to 1.2
*Tryptophan Load (mg Xanthurenic acid excreted)	Adults (Dose: 100 mg/kg body weight)	25 + (6 hrs) 75 + (24 hrs)	— —	Up to 25 Up to 75
*Urinary Pyridoxine (μg/g creatinine)	1–3	Up to 90	—	90+
	4–6	Up to 80	—	80+
	7–9	Up to 60	—	60+
	10–12	Up to 40	—	40+
	13–15	Up to 30	—	30+
	16+	Up to 20	—	20+
*Urinary N'methyl nicotinamide (mg/g creatinine)	All ages	Up to 0.2	0.2–5.59	0.6+
	Pregnant	Up to 0.8	0.8–2.49	2.5+
*Urinary Pantothenic Acid (μg)	All ages	Up to 200	—	200+
*Plasma vitamin E (mg/100 mL)	All ages	Up to 0.2	0.2–0.6	0.6+
*Transaminase Index (ratio)				
†EGOT	Adult	2.0+	—	Up to 2.0
‡EGPT	Adult	1.25+	—	Up to 1.25

Source: Adapted from the Ten State Nutrition Survey. In: Nutritional assessment in health programs. *American Journal of Public Health* November 1973; 63(2):34–35.
* Criteria may vary with different methodology.
† Erythrocyte Glutamic Oxalacetic Transaminase
‡ Erythrocyte Glutamic Pyruvic Transaminase

a knowledge of food composition and preparation will help you obtain reliable information. For example, an inexperienced interviewer may ask "What did you have for breakfast yesterday?" and receive the reply, "I didn't eat breakfast." In this case the client doesn't consider a glass of orange juice to be breakfast, but it is part of his or her intake. A good interviewer would ask, "What was the first thing you had to eat or drink yesterday?" and receive the reply, "Orange juice."

Poor memory can interfere with the use of this method. Another pitfall of the twenty-four-hour recall is that the twenty-four hours may not represent a "typical" day. That is, the client may have eaten quite a bit more or less than usual, or in an unusual way. To ascertain this fact, ask the client if his or her intake was typical and check for the frequency of ingestion of certain foods.

Food Frequency Checklist

A *food frequency checklist* is used to interview the client for the frequency with which he or she eats foods from the major food groups as well as extras such as sweets or alcohol. A sample from a frequency checklist for the meat group might look like Table 9-5.

Food Record

A *food record* is a written record of what the client ate for a one-day period or longer. The individual records this information when the food is consumed. Careful instructions must be given to record all foods and beverages as well as amounts and methods of preparation.

The data from either a twenty-four-hour recall, a food frequency checklist, or a food record can be compared to the RDAs after calculating

Table 9-5 Sample from Food Frequency Checklist

Type of Meat	Usual Portion	Times per Week
Beef, veal	Small hamburger (4 oz)	3
Pork, ham	2 large pork chops (6 oz)	2–3
Lamb	—	—
Chicken, turkey, other poultry	1 breast (4 oz)	2–3
Fish	Small piece (6 oz)	1
Shellfish	—	—
Egg	3 large eggs (fried)	Every morning
Dried beans, peas	1 cup	2
Peanut butter	—	—
Nuts	$\frac{1}{2}$ cup	5

nutrient content with a resource such as the USDA Handbook 8, *Composition of Foods*. This is a tedious process, best done by computer, and is not suited to most patient care situations. The alternative is to compare intake to the food groups in Table 9-6 to determine the likelihood that the client's diet contains adequate amounts of important nutrients. Pay particular attention to those foods that are sources of protein, carbohydrate, fat, calcium, iron, vitamins A and C, and the B vitamins thiamin, riboflavin, and niacin. While an adequate

Table 9-6 Recommended Dietary Intake and Significance of Insufficiencies

Group	Suggested Servings per Day for Older Persons	Size of Serving	Possible Significance of Eating Less than Suggested Amounts
Meat, fish, poultry, beans, and nuts	2	2–3 ounces meat, fish, poultry (cooked) 2 large eggs 1 cup cooked dry beans or peas 3 tablespoons peanut butter $\frac{1}{2}$ cup nuts	Insufficient protein or iron intake
Milk and milk products	2	1 cup milk, yogurt $\frac{1}{2}$ cup cottage cheese 1 ounce hard or processed cheese $\frac{1}{2}$ cup ice cream or custard	Insufficient calcium or riboflavin intake
Fruits and vegetables	4	$\frac{1}{2}$ cup raw, canned, or cooked fruit or vegetable 1 small, whole fruit or vegetable	Insufficient vitamin A or C
Breads, cereals, and grains	4	1 slice enriched or whole-grain bread 1 enriched or whole-grain biscuit, roll, muffin 1 ounce ready-to-eat cereal $\frac{1}{2}$ cup cooked cereal $\frac{1}{2}$ cup enriched rice, pasta	Insufficient protein and vitamin B intake if in combination with less than two servings from meat group
Fats, sweets, and alcohol	As calories permit		*Note*: Intake can be rounded out with additional servings from the above groups or with extras from this group as calories and preferences permit

intake of these ten nutrients does not guarantee an adequate diet for the older adult, it will usually provide other necessary nutrients in sufficient amounts for the healthy person. A determination of possible dietary inadequacy can be made by using the food group comparison. For example, the female older adult whose dietary assessment shows an intake of only two servings per week from the milk group may be at risk of calcium deficiency. Dietary evaluation does not *prove* nutrient deficiency, it only uncovers the possibility of it. Remember also that any method of collecting dietary information can be inaccurate due to deliberate false reporting, poor memory, and other problems. When assessing a client's diet using the food groups, use the following additional information:

Meat, Fish, Poultry, Beans, and Nuts Group

- Primarily a source of protein, iron, and B vitamins
- If beans and/or nuts are used exclusively, they must be combined with milk in the same meal or with selected vegetable protein sources to ensure the intake of high quality (complete) protein.
- Larger amounts of milk or cheese can supply protein needs if meat group servings are limited. One cup of milk or one ounce of cheese is equivalent in protein to one ounce of meat. Other groups provide incomplete proteins that can be supplemented to furnish complete proteins (Lappe 1971). Alternative protein sources such as milk, cheese, peanut butter, and nuts are not good iron sources.

Milk and Milk Products

- Primarily a source of protein and calcium.
- Calcium content varies widely. If milk or cheese is not eaten, consider the following calcium equivalents: 2 cups of ice cream or $1\frac{1}{2}$ cups of cottage cheese is equivalent to 1 cup of milk in calcium.

Fruits and Vegetables

- Primarily a source of vitamin A, vitamin C, and fiber.
- Vitamin C equivalents are:

6 ounces citrus juice	1 cup strawberries
16 ounces tomato juice	$\frac{3}{4}$ cup broccoli
1 whole orange	$\frac{1}{2}$ large canteloupe
$\frac{1}{2}$ grapefruit	$1\frac{1}{2}$ cups raw cabbage
2 medium tomatoes	

- Vitamin A equivalents are $\frac{1}{2}$ cup of any dark green or deep yellow fruit or vegetable such as peaches, cantaloupe, carrots, sweet potatoes, spinach, broccoli, kale, collards, pumpkin, and apricots. Check other sources of vitamin A such as liver if intake of fruits and vegetables is limited. A single serving of beef liver provides a two-week supply of vitamin A.

- Some iron is found in dark green, leafy vegetables. If protein sources of iron are limited, consider this group.
- Dark green, leafy vegetables (except spinach) provide some calcium. A 1-cup serving is equal in calcium to about $\frac{1}{2}$ cup of milk.

Breads, Cereals, and Grains

- Primarily a source of B vitamins, iron, and fiber.
- Enriched and whole-grain products provide B vitamins and iron, which are lacking in unenriched products.
- Calorie, fat, and cholesterol content varies.
- This group should not represent the client's major protein source unless carefully combined with other vegetable foods to supply complete protein.

Fats, Sweets, and Alcohol

- Primarily a source of calories.
- Butter and margarine supply vitamin A. Two teaspoons of either provides about $\frac{1}{9}$ the RDA for vitamin A.
- Cholesterol and saturated fat content varies.
- Exclusion of foods from the above four groups in favor of this group implies dietary inadequacy. Even if suggested amounts of the above foods are consumed, this group may be an important source of excess calories.

Miscellaneous

- The recommended number of servings as listed in the first four groups of Table 9-5 supplies about 1200 calories. Adequacy of caloric intake depends on the client's present weight and the desirability of that weight. Monitoring weight loss or gain is the best way to determine adequacy of caloric intake.
- A varied diet is most likely to provide the nutrients needed for health. A client who consumes the suggested amounts from the food groups, but chooses the same foods every day, may not be getting adequate amounts of some micronutrients.
- Fluids are important from the standpoint of their possible nutrient content as well as the older adult's need for adequate fluids. Six to eight cups of fluid per day is recommended.
- Ask about dietary supplements, including vitamin and mineral preparations and tonics as well as "health foods" such as brewer's yeast. Consider the content of the supplement and the regularity with which the client takes it. Reliance on supplements to the exclusion of necessary foods may cause deficiency of nutrients not provided by the supplement and may also waste money.

Food habits, the other half of dietary assessment, refers to the circumstances and factors that influence food consumption. Examples are financial means, living arrangements, work schedule, education, and culture. Aspects of food habits to keep in mind when assessing diet include:

Food budget
- May limit food choices or require supplementation such as food stamps.

Living arrangements
- May indicate barriers to good nutrition such as lack of food storage or preparation facilities, social pressures, or loneliness. Knowing who prepares the client's food means knowing who largely controls the client's dietary intake.

Cultural, religious, or regional influences
- Affect types of foods chosen and must be considered in developing intervention.

Previous dietary regimen
- Knowing history of previous dietary prescription helps avoid confusion with a new one.
- Self-prescribed diets may indicate a "fad" approach to diet or, conversely, a real interest in health.

Use of convenience foods
- May indicate lack of interest and/or knowledge of meal planning and cooking.
- May take up too much of the food dollar.

COMMON NUTRITIONAL PROBLEMS AND THEIR ASSESSMENT

Obesity

Table 9-3 shows desirable weights for healthy people according to height. Studies by the National Institute on Aging suggest that weight in a healthy older adult that is up to 10% over "desirable" weight is acceptable. Mortality for the slightly "overweight," by this definition, is less than for those under this weight. The term obesity technically refers to excess adipose tissue but is often defined as weight greater than 20% of desirable weight. Measurement of skinfold thickness using calipers is a more reliable way to assess body fatness, although the standards used are not based on measurements of older people

(Table 9-7). Proper technique with the calipers will assure dependable measurements (Figure 9-1).

The real value of weight assessment is what it reveals about change in status. Weight loss or gain of more than a few pounds should be investigated to ascertain the reason for the change and the potential for averting its ill effects.

Table 9-7 Obesity Standards for Caucasian Americans*

| Age (years) | Skinfold Measurements (minimum triceps skinfold thickness in millimeters indicating obesity)** | |
	Male	Female
5	12	14
6	12	15
7	13	16
8	14	17
9	15	18
10	16	20
11	17	21
12	18	22
13	18	23
14	17	23
15	16	24
16	15	25
17	14	26
18	15	27
19	15	27
20	16	28
21	17	28
22	18	28
23	18	28
24	19	28
25	20	29
26	20	29
27	21	29
28	22	29
29	23	29
30–50	23	30

Source: Christakis G. Nutritional assessment in health programs, Table 6. *American Journal of Public Health* November 1983; 63(2):23.
* Adapted from Seltzer CC, Mayer J. A simple criterion of obesity. Postgrad Med 1965; 38:A101–107.
** Figures represent the logarithmic means of the frequency distributions plus one standard deviation.

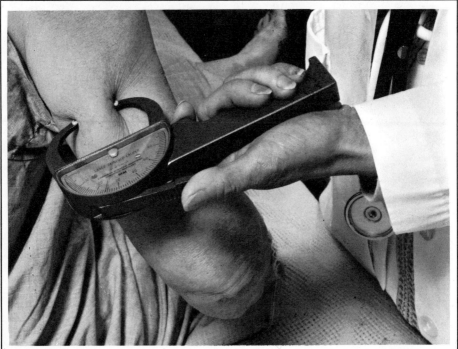

Figure 9-1
Proper measurement of triceps skinfold thickness using calipers is a reliable way to assess obesity.

Nutritional Anemia

The most common nutritional anemia in older adults is iron deficiency anemia. Transferrin saturation below 15%, hemoglobin below 12 mg/100 mL (10 mg/100 mL for women), and hematocrit below 37 vol% (31 vol% for women) are indicative of iron deficiency anemia.

Inadequate protein intake may influence anemia, even without iron deficiency, since protein forms the *globin* part of hemoglobin. Dietary evaluation will usually show marginal protein intakes. Serum albumin levels reflect protein nutriture, but it takes a long period of deprivation before these levels drop significantly (below 3.5 g/100 mL) (Beattie and Louie 1983).

The occurrence of macrocytic anemia, due to folate deficiency, is a possibility in the older adult, especially in alcoholics. Serum and red cell folate levels are necessary to determine whether a macrocytic anemia is due to folate deficiency. Folic acid is present in many foods, but deficiencies may develop after periods of food deprivation such as following surgery or during a period of depression. Estrogen medications have been reported to lower blood folate levels.

Constipation

Bowel habits are related to diet because fluids and fiber promote proper elimination. Unfortunately, many older adults have come to rely on laxatives for "regularity." Nutritional assessment includes questions about the use of self-prescribed medications that interfere with nutrient absorption, and analysis of dietary intake for fiber content. Using bran as a fiber supplement may interfere with mineral absorption.

Poor Appetite and Weight Loss

In many patient care situations, the only attempt at nutritional assessment is a vague statement regarding poor appetite in the client's record. Use weight change or skinfold thickness as significant indicators of weight loss. Skinfold thickness is a measure of loss of body fat as well as a measure of excess fat. Table 9-8 gives skinfold thickness measures indicative of weight loss.

Gradual weight loss without any demonstrable physical reason is indicative of impending death for some older persons (Margie 1977).

Osteoporosis and Osteomalacia

Osteoporosis is thought to be related to calcium deficiency, although it is probably a disease of multiple etiology. (See Chapter 14 for a discussion of osteoporosis.) Assessment of dietary intake, use of mineral supplements, and clinical evaluation of possible malabsorption are useful steps.

Osteomalacia may be caused by insufficient dietary vitamin D intake, inadequate endogenous production of vitamin D, or malabsorption. Assessing dietary intake of vitamin D (primarily from fortified milk), exposure to

Table 9-8 Triceps Skinfold (Adults, Sexes Separate)

Sex	Triceps Skinfold (mm)				
	Standard	90% standard	80% standard	70% standard	60% standard
Male	12.5	11.3	10.0	8.8	7.5
Female	16.5	14.9	13.2	11.6	9.9

Source: Reproduced with permission of Nutrition Today magazine, PO Box 1829, Annapolis, Maryland 21404, (c) March/April, 1975.

sunlight (which allows endogenous production), use of supplements (cod liver oil), and reviewing history of small bowel disease will help in evaluating the risk of developing osteomalacia.

Drug-induced Nutritional Deficiencies

Alcohol is probably the major drug affecting nutritional status. Alcoholics are at risk of protein, vitamin, mineral, and trace element deficiencies, particularly thiamin, riboflavin, niacin, folic acid, zinc, and magnesium. Evidence of chronic heavy alcohol intake should trigger close dietary evaluation as well as clinical and laboratory investigation of body levels of these nutrients. Questions about alcohol use should be part of any dietary assessment.

Self-prescribed or over-the-counter drugs affect absorption and use of nutrients. Mineral oil, a commonly used laxative, interferes with fat-soluble vitamin absorption. Aspirin use may lead to vitamin C deficiency.

Anti-convulsants (like phenobarbital) and methotrexate (used to treat psoriasis) can precipitate folate deficiency. The drug used to treat tuberculosis, INH (isoniazid), can cause vitamin B_6 deficiency (Roe 1985).

There are many similar drug/diet interactions of which you should become aware. Chronic drug use should signal a close look at clinical, laboratory, and other data for evidence of a potential for nutrient deficiencies.

9   Chapter Summary

I. Age-related nutritional requirements
   A. Basically, older adults' nutritional needs are the same as other adults', with decreases in the RDA for calories, thiamin, riboflavin, niacin, iron
   B. Lesser quantity but higher quality of food; fewer "empty calories"

II. Assessment
   A. Clinical assessment
      1. Signs of malnutrition
   B. Anthropometric assessment
      1. Measurement of physical parameters of body

   C. Biochemical assessment
      1. Measurement of various substances in body fluids and tissues
   D. Dietary assessment
      1. Food intake
      2. Eating habits
      3. Socioeconomic influences

III. Pathologies
   A. A variety of factors can increase the older adult's risk of nutritional disorders, including problems involving the following:
      1. Dental and oral status
      2. Bowel function and habits

3. Muscular status
4. Chronic disease
5. Drugs
6. Mood
7. Personal habits
8. Institutionalization
B. Obesity
1. Weight in excess of 20% above desirable range
2. Skinfold measurement above normal
C. Nutritional anemia
1. Below normal transferrin saturation, hemoglobin, hematocrit, and serum albumin
D. Constipation
E. Poor appetite and weight loss
F. Osteoporosis
G. Osteomalacia

IV. Related nursing diagnoses
A. Activity intolerance
B. Constipation
C. Diarrhea
D. Fluid volume deficit
E. Fluid volume excess
F. Altered health maintenance
G. Potential for infection
H. Potential for injury
I. Knowledge deficit
J. Noncompliance
K. Altered nutrition: less than body requirements
L. Altered nutrition: more than body requirements
M. Altered oral mucous membrane
N. Self-care deficit
O. Altered thought processes

READINGS AND REFERENCES

Beattie BL, Louie VY. Nutrition and health in the elderly. In: *Clinical Aspects of Aging*, 2nd ed. Reichel W (editor). Baltimore: Williams and Wilkins, 1983, pp 248–70.

Butterworth CE. The skeleton in the hospital closet. *Nutrition Today* March/April 1974; 9:24.

Exton-Smith AN, Scott DL (editors). *Vitamins for the Elderly: Report of the Proceedings of a Symposium Held at the Royal College of Physicians, London on May 2, 1968*. Bristol, England: John Wright & Sons, 1968.

First Health and Nutrition Examination Survey, United States 1971–1972. Dietary Intake and Biochemical Findings. Pub. No. (HRA) 74–1219–1. Washington, DC: National Center for Health Statistics, 1974.

Food and Nutrition Board: Recommended Dietary Allowances, 9th ed. Washington, DC: National Academy of Sciences, 1980.

Goodhart RS, Shils ME. *Modern Nutrition in Health and Disease*, 5th ed. Philadelphia: Lea & Febiger, 1973.

Harper AE. Recommended dietary allowances for the elderly. *Geriatrics* May 1978; 33(5):73–75, 79–80.

Lappe FM. *Diet for a Small Planet*. New York: Ballantine Books, 1971.

Malasnos L et al. *Health Assessment*, 3rd ed. St. Louis: Mosby, 1986.

Margie JD (editor). *Nutritional Problems of the Elderly. Dialogues in Nutrition*. Bloomfield, NJ: Health Learning Systems, 1977.

Posner BM. *Nutrition and the Elderly*. Lexington, MA: Lexington Books, 1979.

Robinson NB. Dietary needs in later life. In: *Nursing Care of the Older Adult*. Hogstel MO (editor). New York: Wiley, 1981.

Roe DA. Therapeutic effects of drug-nutrient interactions in the elderly. *Journal of American Dietetic Association* 1985; 85:174–181.

Rossman I. Anatomy of aging. In: *Clinical Geriatrics*, 3rd ed. Rossman I (editor). Philadelphia: Lippincott, 1986, p 11.

Watt BK, Merrill AL. *Composition of Foods: Raw, Processed and Prepared*. USDA Handbook No. 8. US Government Printing Office, December 1963.

Yen PK. What is an adequate diet for the older adult? *Geriatric Nursing* May/June 1980; 1:64.

10 Assessment of the Nervous System

Constance Joan Meyd, RN, MS

The nervous system is responsible for our communication with the environment and its many components—both in the way we perceive the world around us and in the appropriateness with which we respond to those perceptions. Acts ranging from retreating from painful stimuli to thinking through elaborate mathematical equations depend on this system. The status of the nervous system influences the degree to which we are able to enjoy the pleasures of our environment, protect ourselves from harm, maintain intellectual stimulation, accurately perceive reality, and behave and speak in a normal manner. Thus, when age-related changes affect the nervous system, the impact can be profound for the many activities of daily life. To understand fully the older adult's complete function and interaction with the world, a keen assessment of the nervous system is essential.

REVIEW OF THE NERVOUS SYSTEM

The purpose of the nervous system is to receive, process, and respond to information. Cells in the nervous system are specialized for this task.

Neurons

There are estimated to be billions of neurons that are specialized for efficient, swift conduction of impulses. Neurons have numerous processes whose function is to convey information in one direction only. Processes conveying information toward the cell body are termed *afferent*—usually these are dendrites. Dendrites are numerous and can branch profusely. Processes conveying information away from the cell body are termed *efferent*—these are always axons. Each neuron has a single axon. An axon usually has an insulating substance, myelin, wrapped around it. The myelin is interrupted at regular intervals by nodes of Ranvier. During impulse conduction, the impulse "jumps" from node to node. The speed of conduction is much more rapid than if the impulse were to travel along the entire axon surface.

Neurons transfer their information to other neurons, glands, smooth muscles, or skeletal muscles by way of a chemical synapse. Each axon ends in an enlarged area (bouton) that contains the chemical neurotransmitter

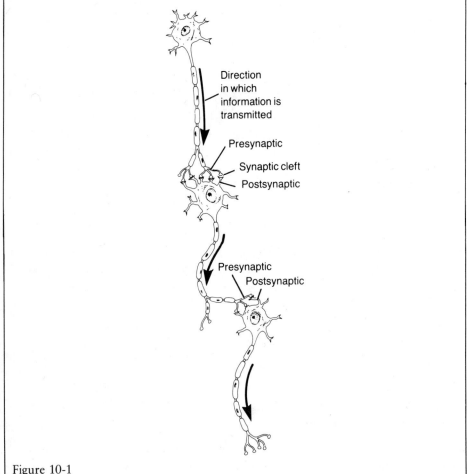

Figure 10-1

Typical neuron and synaptic ending. Source: Spence AP, Mason EB. *Human Anatomy and Physiology*, 2nd ed. Redwood City, CA: Benjamin/Cummings, 1983.

substance. Examples of neurotransmitters are catecholamines (dopamine and norepinephrine), serotonin, and acetylcholine. When an electrical impulse reaches the bouton, the transmitter is released into the synaptic cleft (Figure 10-1). The transmitter diffuses across the cleft and causes excitation or inhibition of the postsynaptic membrane. To get an idea of the potential for communication among neurons via synapses, consider the fact that a single neuron can receive up to 100,000 synapses!

Neurons that serve a single function are grouped together. Groups of neurons in the brain and spinal cord appear gray and are termed gray matter. Fibers (axons) running together are called tracts or white matter. The white appearance is due to the myelin sheath. The brain and spinal cord are collectively referred to as the central nervous system (CNS). Groups of neurons outside of the CNS are termed *ganglia*, and the bundles of axons are termed *nerves*. The peripheral nervous system (PNS) includes the cranial nerves, the spinal nerves, and their respective ganglia.

Brain

The brain is composed of the *cerebral hemispheres, brain stem*, and *cerebellum*. The organization of the hemispheres can be seen in the motor-sensory division. The lateral hemisphere has two obvious surface markings: the central sulcus or fissure and the lateral fissure (Figure 10-2). Although not absolute, the area in front of the central sulcus is primarily motor; the area behind and inferior is primarily sensory. The grooves on the surface are sulci and the area of brain between two sulci is a *gyrus*. Flattening of the gyri can occur with aging.

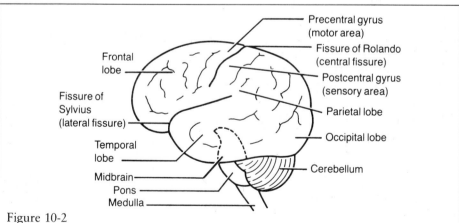

Figure 10-2

Lateral view of the brain. Source: Holloway NM. *Nursing the Critically Ill Adult*. Menlo Park, CA: Addison-Wesley, 1984.

Table 10-1 Divisions of the Brain

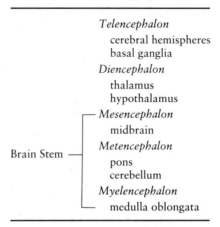

The overall schema of the divisions of the brain is given in Table 10-1. The lobes of the brain are as follows:

- *Frontal lobe*: concerned with voluntary motor function and higher intellectual functions; contains the *motor strip* (precentral gyrus)
- *Parietal lobe*: perception and integration of touch, pain, temperature, proprioception; contains the *sensory strip* (postcentral gyrus)
- *Temporal lobe*: special senses of taste, smell, hearing, speech integration
- *Occipital lobe*: vision only

The *basal ganglia* are groups of neurons deep in the hemispheres that are concerned with the smoothing out of movements begun by the motor strip. These ganglia are the master control for an "automatic pilot" for the maintenance of posture, and for the initiation and termination of movement. An important pathway from the brain stem (midbrain red nucleus) projects to the basal ganglia striatum. This rubrostriatal pathway uses dopamine as the neurotransmitter. Loss of dopamine neurons results in Parkinson's disease, a fairly common disease of the older adult. Deep to the cerebral cortex and to the basal ganglia is the *diencephalon*, which contains:

- *Thalamus*: relay station for all sensory input to the cortex (except for olfaction)
- *Hypothalamus*: center for autonomic nervous system control and for pituitary gland control

Brain Stem

The brain stem is divided into three portions: *midbrain, pons,* and *medulla.* Through this compact area pass all fibers to and from the spinal cord. In the brain stem are the nuclei for cranial nerves (CN) III through XII (see Table 10-2), the centers for cardiorespiratory function, and the important but diffuse reticular activating system (RAS). The RAS filters information from the periphery and decides what information will be allowed to pass to the hemispheres. In this manner the RAS controls states of consciousness, including drowsiness and sleep.

Closely related anatomically and functionally to the brain stem is the cerebellum, which has the function of coordinating information concerning balance and movement.

Meninges, Ventricles, and Cerebrospinal Fluid

The brain has a jellylike consistency. If it sat inside the skull without cushioning, it would not be able to withstand day-to-day movement. The meninges and the cerebrospinal fluid provide this support for the brain.

The brain and spinal cord are covered by three membranes. The outermost membrane is the tough *dura mater*. It folds back on itself in two areas: the falx cerebri at the midline between the two hemispheres, and the tentorium cerebelli, the shelf-like area between the occipital lobes and the cerebellum. The tentorium cerebelli divides the anterior from the posterior fossa. Brain above this tentorial shelf is termed *supratentorial*; brain below is termed *infratentorial*. Infratentorial and posterior fossa are used frequently to refer to pathology in the cerebellum and/or brain stem. The dura mater has a nerve supply from the trigeminal nerve (CN V) and to the draining veins that traverse it. Stretching of these veins or of the dura may result in headache.

The *arachnoid* is a thin sheet of delicate collagenous tissue. This membrane is the most probable source of meningiomas, a common type of benign brain tumor. The *pia mater* is a delicate membrane that clings to the surface of the brain and spinal cord, following all the contours. Between the arachnoid and pia is the *subarachnoid space* within which cerebrospinal fluid (CSF) circulates. Arachnoid granulations (villi) jut into the dural venous sinuses, and from these CSF is reabsorbed. The *subdural space* is a potential space. Normally there is no substance between dura and arachnoid.

The meninges extend along the olfactory nerve (CN I) as it lies on the cribriform plate. Skull fractures in this area can result in the drainage of cerebrospinal fluid through the nose. The meninges also extend along the optic nerve (CN II). Increased pressure within the skull results in decreased venous drainage of the retina, the choked disc, or papilledema.

The cerebrospinal fluid is a clear fluid produced by the choroid plexus within the ventricles. The ventricular system (Figure 10-3) is composed of the two lateral ventricles, one in each hemisphere: a midline third ventricle and the fourth ventricle. CSF is produced in all four ventricles and circulates from the ventricles over the hemispheres to be absorbed in the arachnoid villi. The lateral ventricles open into the third ventricle via the interventricular foramen.

Table 10-2 Cranial Nerves

Number	Nerve	Function	Testing
I	Olfactory	Sense of smell	Smell tobacco, coffee (don't use pungent substance)
II	Optic	Vision	Visual acuity—Snellen's chart Visual fields—confrontation Funduscopic—ophthalmoscope
III	Oculomotor	Pupillary constriction	Pupil size, shape, reaction to light, and accommodation
		Elevation of upper lid	Relationship of lid to pupil
		Most of extraocular muscles (EOMs)	Pursuit movements
IV	Trochlear	Downward, inward movement of eye	Pursuit
V	Trigeminal	Motor—temporal and masseter muscles (chewing)	Attempt to open closed jaw
		Lateral movement of jaw	
		Sensory—facial (includes corneal)	Light touch with pin Corneal reflex
VI	Abducens	Lateral movement of eye	Pursuit

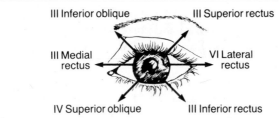

III Inferior oblique   III Superior rectus

III Medial rectus   VI Lateral rectus

IV Superior oblique   III Inferior rectus

The numbers correspond to the cranial nerve number. The names are the muscles resulting in the shown deviation.

Number	Nerve	Function	Testing
VII	Facial	Motor—muscles of facial expression	Keep eyes closed Show teeth
		Sensory—taste on anterior $\frac{2}{3}$ of tongue	Test different flavors
VIII	Acoustic	Hearing (cochlear division) Balance (vestibular division)	Listen to watch tick
IX	Glossopharyngeal	Sensory—pharynx and posterior tongue motor—pharynx	Touch gag, uvula swallowing
X	Vagus	Sensory—pharynx and larynx	Touch gag, uvula
XI	Spinal accessory	Motor—sternocleidomastoid and upper portion of trapezius	Shoulder shrug
XII	Hypoglossal	Motor—tongue	Protrude tongue and move it side to side

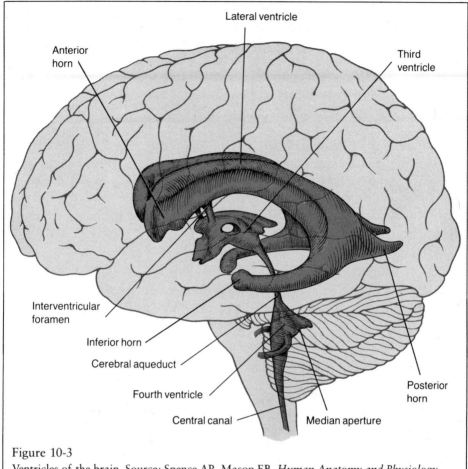

Figure 10-3
Ventricles of the brain. Source: Spence AP, Mason EB. *Human Anatomy and Physiology*, 2nd ed. Redwood City, CA: Benjamin/Cummings, 1983.

The third ventricle is at the diencephalic midline area, and it opens via the aqueduct of Sylvius into the fourth ventricle. The fourth ventricle is at the pons–medulla level. Three openings, one midline and two lateral, allow CSF to circulate out of the ventricular system and into the subarachnoid space from which it is reabsorbed. CSF flows down to surround the spinal cord as well as circulating up around the brain. There is about 150 mL of CSF present. The pressure is up to 180 to 200 cm of water pressure. CSF pressure will vary with intracranial pressure.

Blood Supply to the Brain

Four major arteries supply blood to the brain: the *common carotid arteries* anteriorly and the *vertebral arteries* posteriorly.

Anterior Circulation: The common carotid artery bifurcates at the angle of each side of the jaw to form the internal and external carotid arteries, which supply each hemisphere. The internal carotid artery enters the skull and gives off its first important branch, the ophthalmic artery, which supplies the eye. It then branches to form the middle cerebral artery and the anterior cerebral artery. These latter two arteries supply the major portion of the hemisphere on that side.

Posterior Circulation: The vertebral arteries travel through the foramen transverserium in the upper six cervical vertebrae. They enter the skull through the foramen magnum and join together at the level of the pons to form the basilar artery. There are main branches to supply the upper cervical spinal cord, brain stem, and cerebellum. The posterior cerebral artery is the bilateral terminal branch, which supplies the occipital lobes and inferior temporal lobes.

Circle of Willis

The union of the anterior and posterior cerebral arteries forms an anastomosis at the base of the brain, known as the circle of Willis (Figure 10-4).

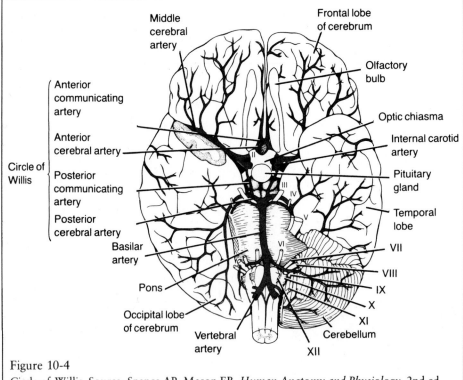

Figure 10-4

Circle of Willis. Source: Spence AP, Mason EB. *Human Anatomy and Physiology*, 2nd ed. Redwood City, CA: Benjamin/Cummings, 1983.

Between the anterior and posterior circulation and the two anterior cerebral arteries, there may be three communicating arteries: the anterior communicating artery and the two posterior communicating arteries. These arteries are not present and/or patent in all individuals. Normally blood does not flow through the circle from left to right or right to left. However, if blood flow is gradually decreased in a proximal portion, blood can shunt from one side to the other. An example would be an atherosclerotic plaque in the internal carotid artery resulting in decreased blood flow to its hemisphere. The communicating arteries will provide blood supply through the opposite internal carotid artery or from the posterior circulation.

Spinal Cord

The spinal cord is primarily a complex pathway for conveying information to the brain and sending information to the periphery. The spinal cord segments also maintain reflex control (Figure 10-5). These reflexes are important because they allow us to go about our intellectual business without worrying about what our arms and legs are doing. We can walk and talk at the same time. We can do this because the "automatic pilot" of the basal ganglia, cerebellum, and the brain stem act on the spinal cord segments.

There are 32 spinal cord segments: 8 cervical, 12 thoracic, 5 lumbar, 5 sacral, and 2 coccygeal. In the adult, differential growth of the bony vertebrae results in the spinal cord ending at lumbar vertebrae two. Below this level is the *cauda equina*, which is the nerve roots of the lower segments.

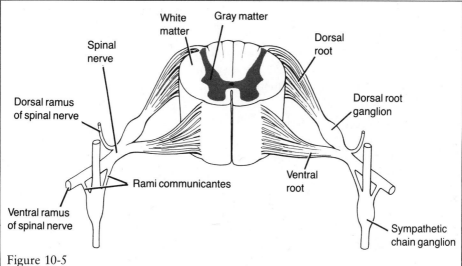

Figure 10-5

The spinal cord. Source: Spence AP, Mason EB. *Human Anatomy and Physiology*, 2nd ed. Redwood City, CA: Benjamin/Cummings, 1983.

The cervical cord controls the neck and arms; the thoracic cord controls the trunk; and the lumbar-sacral cord controls the legs. Each segment gives rise to a mixed spinal nerve that innervates a specific area of the body. Major portions of the autonomic nervous system are present in the spinal cord. The sympathetic nervous system has its outflow from the thoracic cord. The parasympathetic system is craniosacral. In the head, cranial nerves III, VII, IX, and X contain parasympathetic fibers; in the body, the parasympathetic outflow is in the sacral nerves. The most important parasympathetic portion is in the pelvic nerves to the bowel and bladder.

AGE-RELATED CHANGES IN THE NERVOUS SYSTEM

Despite numerous descriptive data on the nervous system in old age, *no* evidence exists to show that structural abnormalities correlate with behavioral changes in the older adult. Atrophy of gyri with widening of the sulci and dilation of the ventricles are commonly seen with aging, although these findings do not occur consistently. Grossly normal brains are seen in demented persons as well as atrophied brains in persons who were neurologically intact when they died.

It is clear that neuronal loss is a natural consequence of aging. Neurons do not divide, so that cell loss is permanent and inevitable. An overall decrease in brain weight occurs by 5% to 17%. Areas most affected by cell loss include the frontal and temporal lobes of the cerebral cortex. These areas are determinants of personality, motor activity, and speech—all play a key role in determining who we are and how we express ourselves. Simple reaction time (psychomotor speed) is decreased with age, resulting from several changes including (a) vision impairment due to a decrease in the transparency of the lens, decrease in the pupil size, and changes in the vitreous humor and retina, which decrease the input to the brain; (b) a decrease in the number of axons in the nerves, particularly the fast-conducting axons; and (c) changes at the synapses that slow conduction. All of these changes combine to result in delayed reaction time.

Learning ability is not lost with age although factors such as slower response and reaction time, poor vision, reduced hearing, and lack of motivation can interfere with the learning process.

Histologic changes include an increase in intracellular pigments and a decrease in protein synthesis. The so called "senile plaque" occurs in both normal and senile individuals, thus its significance is unclear. A decrease in deep tendon reflexes occurs as well as a decrease in the rate of conduction velocities in peripheral nerves.

ASSESSMENT OF THE NERVOUS SYSTEM

A nurse's time is not without limits. A thorough assessment of every portion of the nervous system would limit appropriate assessment of other body systems due to the amount of time required. With practice and judgment, you can make decisions about which areas to assess in each client. The assessment presented here is complete. Emphasis is on those areas of the nervous system most often disturbed in the older adult. All evaluations should be done under optimal conditions. Eyeglasses, hearing aids, and other prostheses should be in place. The room should be well lighted and the client should be in a comfortable position.

Speech and Language

Communication involves two different processes: the use of symbols (language) and articulation by the motor apparatus (speech). It is important to distinguish the two processes. The causes and necessary interventions for speech and language problems are different as well.

Dysarthria is a problem with articulation. The problem may be with motor control of the tongue, pharynx, lips, or a combination of these controls. The speech may be slurred, mumbled, distorted, but all the words used are correct. Subtle dysarthria can be elicited by having the client repeat syllables: la, la, la (tongue); ga, ga, ga (pharynx); me, me, me (lips). Phrases can also be used: "Methodist Episcopal," "Fifth artillery brigade."

Dysphasia (aphasia) is an impairment of the integrative use of symbols. The mildest form is paraphasia, the substitution of one word for another. You may notice that the client uses a similar yet not quite correct word. Ask the client to name objects: point to your watch or shoe and ask the client to name parts. An example of paraphasia is calling the watch hand a pendulum, or the watch band a bracelet.

Most dysphasias involve both a receptive and expressive component. In asking the client to name objects, you have judged the client's understanding of what you want. If you judge there is a receptive component, ask the client to follow some commands such as point to your left arm and point to the key (see commands in level of consciousness section). Receptive problems are associated with posterior brain lesions: the more posterior the lesion, the greater the receptive problem. If the dysphasia is predominantly expressive, the lesion is more anteriorly placed. In general, lesions are mixed.

Assess the client's ability to read and write. Have him or her read a newspaper or magazine passage. Ask the client to write his or her name, a short passage, or a sentence such as "This is a lovely day in May." Of course, some knowledge of the client's literacy and educational level is crucial in interpreting the response to these tasks.

Olfactory Nerve

Cranial nerve I is the olfactory nerve. To assess olfaction, the sense of smell, test each nostril separately by occluding the other. Use a substance that is strong but not pungent, such as coffee or tobacco. Oil of wintergreen or peppermint are not good choices as they are irritative, and the client may respond to the irritation, not the smell. Keep in mind that many local processes in the nose can result in loss of the sense of smell. If the sense of smell is absent in both nostrils, the cause is not likely in the nervous system. A normal response is that an odor is detected. Identification of the odor is not necessary.

Optic Nerve

Cranial nerve II is the optic nerve. The majority of the causes of decreased vision in older adults are due to local disease of the eye rather than optic nerve or nervous system disease.

Visual acuity can be tested by several different ways. The most objective is the Snellen chart. For most purposes, determining if the client can read printed matter is sufficient. Make sure the client's eyeglasses are on for testing, and test one eye at a time. Have the client count fingers held before him or her if unable to read, and if unable to count fingers, ask him or her to describe perceived objects and light. The most common cause of decreased visual acuity is presbyopia, a refractive error secondary to age-related changes in the lens. Presbyopia can be corrected with eyeglasses.

Visual fields are tested by determining if the client can perceive objects held at different positions before him or her. Although the most accurate determinations are obtained by an ophthalmologist with the use of a target screen, you can derive gross determinations of visual field in the following manner. Seat the client comfortably in a chair or on the edge of the examining table and position yourself opposite him or her, approximately 3 feet away, with your eyes level with the client's. Stretch your arm midway between you and the client and point a finger toward the sky. Laterally extend your arm until your finger leaves your field of vision. As the client and you stare directly into each other's eyes, gradually bring your finger into the peripheral field. Using your index finger as the test object and yourself as a control, ask the client to indicate when he or she sees your finger. Systematically repeat the test for all points along a 360° area in the visual field. Older adults often display a reduction in their peripheral vision.

Particular attention should be paid to two types of lesions that may be present in the older adults: scotoma and homonymous hemianopsia. *Scotoma* is a blind area in the visual field and often accompanies glaucoma. *Homonymous hemianopsia* is bilateral blindness in one-half of the visual field; for example, the right half of each eye. The client who has had a cerebrovascular accident may experience homonymous hemianopsia. Clients affected by these conditions may be unaware of their presence.

Funduscopic examination is beyond the scope and skills of most nurses performing basic assessment. For information in this area, refer to a physical diagnosis text.

Extraocular Movements

Cranial nerves III, IV, and VI are the oculomotor, trochlear, and abducens nerves. They are usually grouped together because, acting in concert, they control the extraocular movements (EOMs) of the eyes. Have the client look straight ahead; observe whether there is any deviation of the eyes. Using your finger as a target, ask the client to follow it as you move to the extremes of horizontal and vertical movement (Figure 10-6). The eyes should move together (conjugate) and no jerking movement should occur. There may be some restriction of upward gaze (Carter 1986). Ask the client to inform you of double vision in any field of gaze. Table 10-2, in its section on Cranial Nerve VI, includes an illustration of the specific nerves involved for each position of gaze.

The oculomotor nerve (III) has several other important functions, including the light reflex and control of the relationship of the lid to the pupil. Both of these functions must be examined. To check pupillary response to

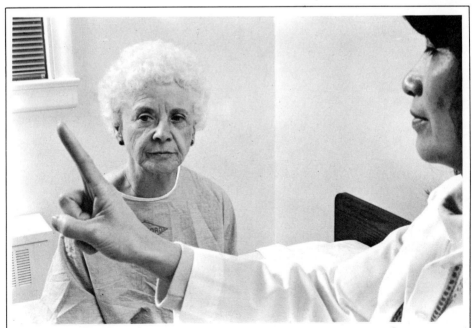

Figure 10-6
As they follow a moving object, the eyes should move together without any jerking movements.

light, begin by looking at both pupils. Normally, both will be the same size. Small pupils are common in older adults. Be sure to ask the client if he or she uses any eyedrops to avoid misinterpreting deviations as pathologic. Unequal pupils (anisocoria) may be normal, particularly if the difference is less than 1 millimeter. Check the direct light reflex by shining a light into the eye, bringing the flashlight from the side of the patient rather than the front. Recall that the light reflex is dependent on an intact optic nerve, thus a blind eye will not react directly to light. Constriction of the pupil is the normal response to light; it also will occur as the near, or accommodation, reflex. There may be some sluggishness of the light reflex.

In order to check for *ptosis* (drooping) of the eyelid, ask the client to stare straight ahead. Look at the relationship of the upper lid to the pupil. In general, the lid should not cover the pupil at all.

Trigeminal Nerve

The cranial nerve V, or the trigeminal nerve, is the sensory nerve of the face and also the motor nerve to the muscles of mastication. Using a wisp of cotton and a pin, gently touch the face to determine if the client, with his or her eyes closed, can differentiate between the two (Figure 10-7). Test the face at three

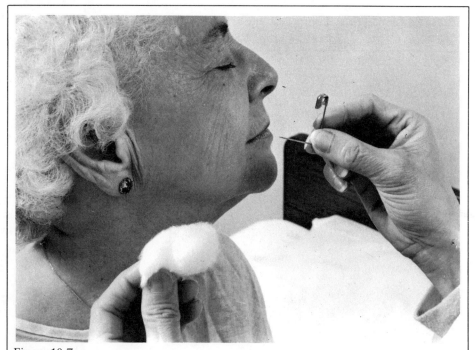

Figure 10-7
If the trigeminal nerve is intact, the client should be able to differentiate between the touch of a cotton wisp and a pin on various areas of the face.

levels: the forehead, the cheek, and the chin. Ask the client to compare the right side with the left. Testing the muscles of mastication can be done by asking the client to open his or her mouth slightly and to resist your efforts to close it.

Facial Nerve

The facial nerve, cranial nerve VII, is the nerve that controls the muscles of facial expression. Examine the client's face for symmetry. Observe if one side of the mouth droops or appears flattened, and if both sides of the face move when the client talks. Ask the client to smile or show the teeth by raising the lips. Instruct the client to close both eyes tightly and to keep them closed while you attempt to open them.

There are two important types of *facial nerve lesions*. Peripheral nerve lesions occur commonly as a Bell's palsy and present as paralysis of the upper and lower face on the same side. On the affected side, the client will be unable to close the eye and the mouth will droop. The second type of facial paralysis is more common in older adults. It is the upper motor neuron lesion of stroke in which asymmetry and paralysis occur about the mouth. The upper portion of the face remains unaffected, however, and the client can close both eyes normally.

Hearing

The vestibulocochlear nerve, cranial nerve VIII, is concerned with hearing and balance. In general, problems with hearing can be divided into two types: conductive hearing loss and sensorineural hearing loss. With *conductive hearing loss*, the problem lies in the passage of sound through the canal, ossicles of the middle ear, or the tympanic membrane. With *sensorineural hearing loss*, the problem is associated with the inner ear receptors or the nerve itself.

Evaluation of hearing competency is a process conducted throughout the entire examination. It may be detected through interview that the client has trouble hearing normal speech, compensates by reading lips, or loses the conversation when the nurse's voice drops to a soft whisper. To obtain a gross determination of auditory acuity, the nurse can occlude one of the client's ears, and at a distance of 1 to 2 feet away, begin to speak with a whisper. The client should not be able to see the nurse's mouth. If necessary, the nurse should gradually increase the volume of his or her voice until the client is able to hear. High-frequency losses can be tested with the use of a ticking wrist watch. The nurse should gradually move the watch away from the ear and ask the client to indicate when it can no longer be heard.

Using a tuning fork to test air conduction and bone conduction can also be helpful. Air conduction refers to the transmission of sound through the ear canal, tympanic membrane, and ossicular chain to the cochlea and finally to the auditory nerve. Bone conduction refers to the auditory nerve receiving sound after it has traveled through the bones of the skull to the cochlea. The *Weber test* uses bone conduction to determine hearing deficits. In this test, a vibrating tuning fork is placed on the vertex of the skull or on the forehead. In conduction deafness, the sound is referred to the deafer ear whereas in perceptive deafness the sound is referred to the more functional ear. The *Rinne test* uses both air and bone conduction. In this test, the vibrating tuning fork is brought close to the auditory meatus, until the sound is no longer heard, and then it is applied to the mastoid bone. Normally, the client will not be able to hear the sound when the fork is placed on mastoid bone; if the client does hear the sound better by bone than air, the Rinne test is negative and a conductive loss may be present. Professional audiometric examination is advisable when loss is suspected.

Gag Reflex

The glossopharyngeal and vagus nerves are cranial nerves IX and X. These two nerves are the sensory and motor innervation to the pharynx and palate. Observe the pharynx as the client opens his or her mouth. Ask the client to say "ah." The uvula should rise and both sides of the palatine arches should rise symmetrically. The gag reflex is normally symmetrical.

Spinal Accessory Nerve

The spinal accessory nerve, cranial nerve XI, supplies the sternomastoids and the trapezius. To test the function of this nerve, ask the client to shrug his or her shoulders. Observe for symmetry. Lag of one side is abnormal.

Hypoglossal Nerve

The hypoglossal nerve, cranial nerve XII, controls the movement of the tongue. Ask the client to stick out his or her tongue and to move it from right to left several times. Observe for deviation.

Coordination and Cerebellar Testing

Test the client's coordination by using point-to-point tests. For the arms, have the client touch your finger and then his or her nose and then your finger again. Move your finger to several different positions. Test in both arms. Observe for smoothness of movement to and from the target. Does tremor appear near the target? Does the client point past the target? For the legs, have the client lie down and run his or her heel up and down the shin. Repeat with the opposite extremity. Observe for uneven, jerky movements.

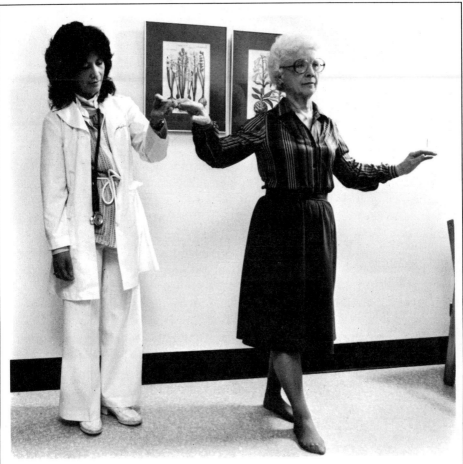

Figure 10-8
The client may need to hold your hand for assistance when you test coordination of tandem walking.

Test the client's ability to make *rapid alternating movements*. Have the client rapidly tap his index finger on his thigh and/or on the first proximal interphalangeal joint. Observe for a smooth regular tapping.

Test the client's performance of *tandem walking*. Have the client walk heel to toe. Some older adults may require the examiner's assistance to perform this test. Have the client hold your hand for assistance (Figure 10-8).

Sensation

Sensation is the most difficult area of the nervous system to test. The client's subjective responses must be carefully evaluated. Explain in detail to the client what you will be doing and in what order. For each modality tested, apply stimuli in a random, unpredictable fashion and ask the client to keep both eyes closed.

Determine if the *primary sensations* are present. The primary modalities are touch, pain, temperature, vibration, and joint position sense. All clients should be screened for touch sensation. Use a cotton wisp or the light touch of your index finger. Touch at least two distant areas on each extremity. Ask the client to report absence of sensation and to compare analogous areas on both right and left extremities. Also compare proximal with distal areas on each extremity. Peripheral neuropathy is common in older adults and tends to have a distal, symmetrical distribution. If an area of loss or change is reported, map out the area of loss. Drawings are useful for recording.

If the primary sensations are intact, determine if the client can distinguish two *simultaneous stimuli*. Touch the client lightly on two places, one on the right, the other on the left. For example, touch the right forearm and the left hand. The client should be able to report accurately the two areas touched. Try several different combinations.

Test the client's *stereognosis* (cortical sensation). Ask the client to identify objects in his or her hand. Test one hand at a time—do not allow the client to pass the object from hand to hand. Coins, keys, and paper clips are suitable objects. Normally one can distinguish the types of coins from each other. Inability to distinguish objects by touch is called astereognosis. Testing of cortical sensation is only valid if touch is intact.

Reflexes

Although they are not difficult to elicit, deep tendon reflexes are not tested routinely by nonphysician examiners. With practice, you can learn to use the reflex hammer. Reflexes are involuntary motor responses to stretching the muscle. The absolute magnitude of the response is not as significant as symmetry and correlation with other observations. In order to elicit reflexes, the client must be relaxed. The optimal amount of tension must be produced in the muscle by proper positioning. In general, the muscle should be struck about midway between its maximal and shortest length. An adequate stretch stimulus must be applied. Reflexes are graded as follows:

0 absent
1 decreased
2 normal
3 increased
4 spasticity

Grade four reflexes are often associated with clonus, which is a sustained contraction and relaxation of the ankle. Clonus often is observed after a stroke: the client may find that his or her foot involuntarily taps on the floor when weight is put on the affected leg.

Superficial reflexes are easier to assess. The sensory input for the corneal reflex occurs through the previously discussed trigeminal nerve. The corneal reflex is elicited by lightly touching the cornea of the eye with a wisp of clean cotton. Gauze should not be used because it can cause abrasions of the cornea. The normal response is a brisk eye blink.

The most common pathologic reflex is the *plantar response* or Babinski's reflex. Stroke the plantar (sole) surface of the client's foot. The normal response is flexion of the toes. The abnormal response is extension and fanning of the toes.

DISORDERS OF THE NERVOUS SYSTEM

The most common nervous system problems of the older adult are:

- Mental status change
- Loss of acuity of the special senses (related to primary changes in the receptors rather than to changes in the nervous system itself)
- Loss of sensation in the extremities
- Weakness or paralyses in the extremities

Changes must be evaluated within the context of the life situation. Losses in physical ability and changes in mental status may be a direct outgrowth of economic and social losses, and therefore require astute evaluation.

Mental Status

Most older adults normally maintain intellectual function sufficiently to continue to manage their own affairs and function in society. There does appear to be an increasing dependency on the environment for maintaining reality contact. Knowing that the sun shines through the bedroom window at ten o'clock each morning, that the rustling of the leaves is only the mailman making his delivery, and the banging from the other room is the old radiator helps older adults maintain a sense of security and orientation to their surroundings. Knowing that a half-turn of the knob sets the oven on 350° and knowing the layout of the home that has been lived in for forty years enables an individual to function without sharp vision. It is the known that maximizes the older adult's ability to function despite sensory deficits. At the other extreme, it is the new or unknown that causes sensory deficits to be pronounced and more incapacitating. Relocation to a new apartment or admission to a hospital presents the older adult with an unfamiliar environment that is devoid of the sights and sounds that have served as security and have been adapted to. The reaction to this unknown may be confusion. As with all the changes with aging, there is a wide variation in response and adaptation. The extremes of complete loss of contact with reality and complete orientation regardless of the environment are easily recognized. Most of the population fits somewhere in between these extremes. Confusion or dementia is an abnormal state characterized by loss in memory, judgment, intellectual functions, and by lability and changes in affect. (Chapter 11 provides a broader review of problems with mental function.)

Meningitis

Meningitis is said to be "one of the most silent neurologic abnormalities of old age" (Carter 1986). Due to the difficulty in identifying this disorder, there is a 50% mortality rate from meningitis in the elderly population.

Older persons with meningitis may not complain of the classic stiff neck usually associated with this problem. However, when evaluating range of motion, you will note that rigidity affecting flexion of the head is present; rotation is not affected. The client may complain of a slight headache and be lethargic, drowsy, and disoriented to place and time. Temperature may be only slightly elevated and vomiting may not occur until later, as the infection progresses. A lumbar puncture is warranted whenever meningitis is suspected.

Transient Ischemic Attacks

Occlusive cerebrovascular disease causes a sudden disruption to neurologic functioning known as transient ischemic attack (TIA). Factors such as hypertension, hypotension (often secondary to drug therapy), anemia, cigarette smoking, inactivity, and diabetes contribute to TIA.

A variety of signs and symptoms accompany TIA, including: dizziness, aphasia, personality changes, falling, diplopia, hemiparesis, unilateral loss of vision, motor weakness, and amnesia. The TIA can last from minutes to hours, with recovery of function usually occurring within twenty-four-hours. Since TIAs are often warnings of a major stroke, a full diagnostic evaluation (including scans, skull x-rays, and echoencephalography) is planned when a TIA has occurred, and aggressive treatment to prevent future attacks is instituted.

Parkinson's Disease

Parkinsonism is the second most common neurologic disease of the elderly, affecting 1 in 100 individuals over age 55. This slowly progressing degenerative disease causes muscle rigidity, tremors, slow muscle movements, lethargy, and depression. Postural and gait disturbances and autonomic nervous system disorders, such as sweating, oily skin, and drooling, follow later. In addition to clinical signs, a positive Myerson's sign is present in which tapping on the client's forehead or glabella causes repetitive and synchronous blinking (whereas the eyes of the person without Parkinson's disease stop blinking after the first several taps). Levodopa often is effective in the management of symptoms for nondrug-induced Parkinsonism.

Vision

Loss of acuity of the special senses is a concomitant of the aging process. Presbyopia begins to occur around age forty and is inescapable. This farsightedness in a previously nearsighted person may be interpreted as "second sight." More bothersome to the older adult is glare. Vision in dimly lighted areas and at night is worse. Peripheral vision decreases, narrowing the range of the visual field. Depth perception is altered, responsible for many of the falls experienced by older adults as they encounter changes in surface level. Yellowing of the lens alters perception of the low-tone colors: blues, greens, and violets. Thorough examination by an ophthalmologist is an important component of the older adult's total assessment.

Visual acuity also may be altered by cataracts. A *cataract* is opacification of the lens of the eye, which causes blurred vision and decreased light perception. A cataract may be seen as an opacity or whiteness of the pupil. Smaller or less dense cataracts require inspection with an ophthalmoscope. It is sometimes said that a cataract must be "ripe" to be removed, but this is not the case. Cataracts that interfere with vision should be considered for removal.

Glaucoma is increased pressure within the eye and may also alter visual acuity. Most cases in the elderly are chronic open-angle (simple). The intraocular pressure is measured with a tonometer, an instrument requiring special training in its use. Glaucoma is typically asymptomatic until it is detected with tonometry measurement or when significant loss of vision has occurred. Blurred vision, halos around lights, pain in the eye, and conjunctivitis are symptoms of glaucoma. Enlargement of the normal blind spot, or scotoma, occurs if untreated. If glaucoma is suspected, tonometry must be performed.

Hearing Disorders

A common *hearing deficit* with age is presbycusis, the loss of ability to hear high frequency sounds: the f, s, sh, and ph family of sounds. Conversation can be distorted to the affected person and result in what may appear to be inappropriate or confused behaviors. This sensorineural type of hearing loss does not respond to the use of a hearing aid, as does a conductive loss. A complete audiometric evaluation is essential to differentiate the type of hearing loss present, and to guide realistic care planning.

Other Sensory Losses

Although visual and hearing losses are the most common and obvious sensory problems experienced by the older adult, problems can exist with the other special senses. Taste buds are lost, primarily affecting the sweet and salt flavors, and this may result in poor nutrition by the ingestion of excess salt, sugar, and carbohydrates to compensate for this loss. Tactile sensations of pain, pressure, and temperature are altered. The combined effects of the losses of the various special senses can result in profound misperceptions of the environment and significant threats to the older adult's safety and well-being.

Mild loss of sensation in the extremities to touch, pain, pressure, and temperature is common in older adults and relates to the loss of axons in their peripheral nerves. Careful consideration must be given, however, to other causes of sensory loss such as diabetic neuropathy.

Mild, generalized reduction in muscle power can occur in the older adult for a variety of reasons, such as loss of muscle mass, arthritic processes, and nutritional deficiencies. Focal changes are weaknesses in one body part, for example, hemiparesis, monoplegia, and facial weakness. Focal changes are not normal and should alert you to search further or to refer the client for neurologic evaluation.

10 Chapter Summary

I. Age-related changes
   A. No proven correlation between structural changes and behavior; changes are inconsistent
   B. Atrophy of gyri with widening of sulci
   C. Dilation of ventricles
   D. Loss of neurons
   E. Brain weight decreases 5% to 7%
   F. Simple reaction time decreases
   G. Impaired vision
      1. Less transparent lens
      2. Decreased pupil size
      3. Changes in vitreous humor
   H. Impaired hearing
      1. Decreased ability to hear high-frequency sounds

   I. Reduced olfaction
   J. Decreased tactile sensation
   K. Slower conduction of impulses; delayed reaction time
   L. Development of "senile plaque"
   M. Deep tendon reflexes decreased
   N. Slowed conduction velocities in peripheral nerves

II. Assessment
   A. Speech and language
   B. Cranial nerves
      1. Cranial nerve I: olfactory
         a) Test olfaction in each nostril
         b) Note if problems are unilateral or bilateral: if unilateral, the cause is

most likely not in
nervous system
2. Cranial nerve II: optic nerve
   a) Visual acuity: Snellen
      chart objective test
   b) Visual field
   c) Funduscopic examination
3. Cranial nerves III, IV, and
   VI: extraocular movements
   of the eyes
   a) Coordinated movement
      of eyes
   b) Pupillary response to
      light
   c) Relationship of lid to
      pupil
4. Cranial nerve V: trigeminal
   a) Sensory nerve of face and
      motor nerve to muscles
      of mastication
5. Cranial nerve VII: facial
   nerve
   a) Symmetry of face
6. Cranial nerve VIII: hearing
   and balance
   a) Gross screening done by
      testing ability to hear
      wristwatch ticking
   b) Audiometric testing
      performed for the most
      precise determination
7. Cranial nerves IX and X:
   sensorimotor innervation to
   pharynx and palate
   a) When client says "ah,"
      uvula should rise and
      both sides of palatine
      arches rise symmetrically
   b) Symmetrical gag reflex
8. Cranial nerve XI: spinal
   accessory nerve to
   sternomastoids and trapezius
   a) Symmetry when
      shrugging shoulders
9. Cranial nerve XII:
   hypoglossal nerve
   a) Normal, controlled
      tongue movements
C. Coordination—cerebellar
  testing

1. Point-to-point tests
2. Rapid alternating
   movements
3. Tandem walking
D. Sensory system
1. Primary sensations
2. Ability to distinguish two
   simultaneous stimuli
E. Reflexes
1. Symmetrical motor response
   to stretch of muscle
2. Grades of reflexes:
   0 absent
   1 decreased
   2 normal
   3 increased
   4 spasticity
3. Corneal reflex
4. Plantar reflex (Babinski)

III. Disorders
  A. Speech and language
    1. Dysarthria
      a) Problem with articulation
      b) Altered motor control
         of organs of speech:
         no problem with
         selection and use of
         words
    2. Dysphagia (aphasia)
      a) Problems with integrated
         use of symbols
      b) Can be receptive,
         expressive, or both
  B. Cranial nerve
    1. Cranial nerve I
      a) Bilateral loss of sense of
         smell can indicate
         impairment of nerve
    2. Cranial nerve II
      a) Presbyopia: decreased
         visual acuity secondary
         to age-related changes
      b) Decreased visual field
    3. Cranial nerves III, IV,
      and VI
      a) Jerking or inability of
         eyes to follow moving
         object
      b) Ptosis

4. Cranial nerve V
   a) Inability to detect facial sensations; problems with mastication
5. Cranial nerve VII
   a) Bell's Palsy: paralysis of upper and lower face on same side
   b) Upper motor neuron lesion of stroke: asymmetry and paralysis near mouth while upper portion of face is normal
6. Cranial nerve VIII
   a) Conductive hearing loss: problem with canal, ossicles, or tympanic membrane
   b) Sensorineural loss: problem with inner ear receptors or nerve
7. Cranial nerves IX and X
   a) Problem with gag reflex
8. Cranial nerve XI
   a) Unilaterally when shrugging shoulders
9. Cranial nerve XII
   a) Problems with tongue movements

C. Sensory System
   1. Peripheral neuropathy common in older adult, tends to have distal, symmetrical distribution
   2. Astereognosia: inability to distinguish objects by touch alone

D. Reflexes
   1. Clonus: sustained contraction and relaxation
   2. Absence of corneal reflex: eyes fail to blink quickly when touched
   3. Abnormal plantar response: extension and fanning of toes when sole of foot is stroked

E. Loss of acuity of special senses
   1. Age-related visual changes
      a) Presbyopia
      b) Glare more bothersome
      c) Poor vision in dim areas and at night
      d) Decreased peripheral vision
      e) Yellowing of lens
   2. Age-related hearing loss
      a) Decreased ability to hear high-frequency sounds
   3. Other age-related sensory loss
      a) Mild loss of sensation to touch, pain, pressure, and temperature

F. Meningitis
   1. Difficult to identify early, high mortality rate as a result
   2. Complaint of stiff neck may not be present
      a) Rigidity of neck on flexion present

G. Transient Ischemic Attack
   1. Disruption to neurologic function lasting from minutes to hours
   2. Recovery usually within one day
   3. Evaluation required to determine cause and prevent future attacks

H. Parkinson's disease
   1. Slowly progressing degenerative disease
   2. Muscle rigidity, slow movements, lethargy, depression, disorders of autonomic nervous system
   3. Positive Myerson's sign

IV. Related nursing diagnoses
   A. Activity intolerance
   B. Anxiety
   C. Pain
   D. Impaired verbal communication
   E. Ineffective individual coping
   F. Diversional activity deficit
   G. Fear
   H. Altered health maintenance

I. Impaired home maintenance
management
J. Potential for infection
K. Potential for injury
L. Knowledge deficit
M. Impaired physical mobility
N. Noncompliance
O. Altered nutrition: less than
body requirements
P. Altered oral mucous membrane
Q. Powerlessness

R. Self-care deficit
S. Personal identity disturbance
T. Sensory/perceptual
alterations
U. Sexual dysfunction
V. Impaired skin integrity
W. Sleep pattern disturbance
X. Impaired social interaction
Y. Social isolation
Z. Altered thought processes

READINGS AND REFERENCES

Angevine JB. *Principles of Neuroanatomy*. New York: Oxford University Press, 1981.

Carter AB. Neurologic aspects of aging. In: *Clinical Geriatrics*, 3rd ed. Rossman I (editor). Philadelphia: Lippincott, 1986, p 327.

Gastone C, Daly RF. Effects of aging on visual evoked responses. *Archives of Neurology* July 1977; 34:403–407.

Kokemen K, Bossemeyer R. Neurological manifestations of aging. *Journal of Gerontology* 1977; 32:411–419.

Locke S, Galaburda AM. Neurological disorders of the elderly. In: *Clinical Aspects of Aging*. Reichel W (editor). Baltimore: Williams & Wilkins, 1978.

Malasanos et al. *Health Assessment*, 3rd ed. St. Louis: Mosby, 1986.

Mayo Clinic. *Clinical Examinations in Neurology*. Philadelphia: Saunders, 1976.

McGreer P et al. Aging and extrapyramidal function. *Archives of Neurology* January 1977; 34:33–35.

Schiebel A. Aging in human motor control system. *Sensory Systems and Communications in the Elderly* 1979; 10:297–304.

Takahashi K. A clinicopathologic study on the peripheral nervous system of the aged. *Geriatrics* March 1976; 31:123–133.

11 Assessment of Mental Status

Mary Jane Lucas, RN

PURPOSE OF THE MENTAL STATUS EXAMINATION

The mental status examination consists of a structured interview to identify abnormal status. Specific areas examined include emotional symptoms and cognitive deficits that may seriously interfere with the older client's ability to cope with life stresses and deal with problems in an appropriate and effective way. The purpose of the examination is to detect evidence of mental disorders and abnormal mental experience to enable the nurse to begin to formulate the care plan for the client.

INTRODUCTION OF THE MENTAL STATUS EXAMINATION

Performing the examination in a quiet and private setting is important and you must be relaxed, unhurried, and comfortable with the material. You and the client should be seated comfortably and you should introduce the examination with no apologies, as a routine part of the comprehensive assessment. Some clients may need reassurance that this aspect of the assessment is done on all examined persons and that it does not necessarily mean that anyone thinks that the client is "crazy." Emphasize that the information you gather will be helpful to the client in planning long-term care.

    Various factors can interfere with an accurate assessment of mental status. The client may view the examination as insulting or embarrassing.

Significant differences such as age and role may exist between you and the client. Additionally, the older adult may be experiencing an acute physical or psychologic disorder that can temporarily alter the true mental status. For example, febrile stress, fluid and electrolyte imbalances, malnutrition, drug reactions, and even the stress of being in an unfamiliar environment or situation can cause acute confusion. The mental status assessment of the older adult obtained during that period may have no resemblance to the mental status apparent after the pathophysiology has been treated or the situation has been adapted to. These are aspects that must be considered when performing the examination.

THE EXAMINATION

The following approach is suggested as a guideline for a full mental status examination. There are other forms that can be used, some of which are shorter instruments that have been developed to test the client's cognitive and emotional states. Examples of these reliable instruments are the Mini Mental Status (Folstein et al 1975), the Symptoms Check List 90 (Derogatis et al 1974), the General Health Questionnaire (Goldberg 1972), and the Raskin (Raskin 1960). These instruments can serve as a means of screening and evaluating the impact of treatment on the individual's intellectual functioning and emotional states. The full mental status examination includes a number of components based on observation and direct formal questioning. Remember that vision, hearing, and other deficits can affect the examination.

General Appearance and Behavior

Note the dress, grooming, posture, mobility, facial expressions, and gestures that the client exhibits. Does the client appear to be his or her stated age? What is the client's state of mental alertness?

Involuntary, rhythmic movements of the tongue, mouth, face, and limbs can be associated with tardive dyskinesia and indicate a history of psychotropic medication use. When this finding is evident, the client should be asked about prior psychiatric treatment or hospitalization. It should be remembered that the client with tardive dyskinesia does not have a decline in intellectual function; therefore, communication should respect the intellectual level of the individual.

Speech

Note the client's tone of voice, and rate and wording of speech. Is the language and content coherent and relevant? Take note of unusual words, jargons, phrases, and the ability to articulate.

Mood and Self-Attitude

Note the client's mood (cheerful, sad, bored, or hostile) and note if there are frequent changes in mood, known as mood lability. Mood lability will be manifested by alternating periods of crying and laughing. Ask the client directly if he thinks he has been a good person, and ask how the client feels about himself. These questions will elicit a sense of self-attitude, particularly if there has been a recent significant change.

Delusions and Hallucinations

Ask directly about delusions and hallucinations of all types, including auditory, visual, tactile, and olfactory. Note the presence of misinterpretations of statements, disorders of perception, and somatic preoccupations. Does the client claim to hear voices? Does the client believe anyone is trying to harm him or her? Is the client frightened? Is the client compelled to heed the voices? Does the client feel comfortable and at home with these thoughts and feelings? Explore the quality, quantity, and content of these thoughts and how the client perceives them.

Depression and Mania

Ask directly about feelings of hopelessness, extreme sadness, and the presence of suicidal thoughts and ideas. If such ideas are present, ask about plans and the availability of the means with which to commit suicide. Ask specifically about sleep disturbances, particularly early morning awakening, appetite, weight loss, and constipation. Also ask the client if he or she feels euphoric, unusually happy, and especially important.

Neurotic Symptoms

Question the client about nervousness, tenseness, palpitation, hyperventilation, swallowing difficulties, excessive worry, and fear of impending disaster, all of which may indicate anxiety. To detect phobias, ask directly about unusual or irrational fears that may prevent the client from doing what he or she wants to do. Determine if there are obsessions or compulsions by inquiring if there are recurring or unwanted thoughts or behaviors that interfere with daily life.

Cognitive Tests

Determine if the client knows the present date, time, and season, and if the client knows where he or she is. Test the client's recent memory by asking him or her to repeat the names of three objects after you and to remember them for a few minutes. Meanwhile, have the client subtract 7 from 100 continuing through five answers (or if arithmetic or educational level is limited, this can be changed to subtracting 3 from 20, continuing through five answers). Then ask the client to repeat the three objects that you asked him or her to remember earlier. Determine if the client can follow a three-stage command such as, "lift your right arm, close your eyes, and stick out your tongue." If the client is literate, have him or her read a sentence and do what it says, and also write a sentence for you.

To demonstrate abstract or concrete thinking, the client can be asked to interpret a simple proverb such as "people in glass houses shouldn't throw stones" or "a bird in the hand is worth two in the bush." Present a situation that would require simple judgment in problem solving. For example, ask the client's opinion of this statement, "John's pants were too small for him, so he took them off over his head."

A person with cognitive deficits may react to intellectual testing with tears, frustration, irritations, or anger. This reaction is known as a "catastrophic reaction." If such catastrophic reactions occur, give the client reassurance; the examination may need to be interrupted temporarily to make the client more comfortable.

The examination should take 30 to 40 minutes. Encourage the client when he or she does well and correct the client when he or she makes mistakes in cognitive tasks, such as stating the date or time. After completing the examination, ask the client for any particular questions or comments. Remember that the mental status examination must be supplemented by the rest of the physical assessments and the psychosocial history. The mental status examination is only meaningful within this context.

Periodic reassessment is beneficial not only because the older adult's mental status can alter rapidly, but also because mental status can be an indicator of the effectiveness of treatment and the general health status. It must be remembered that the stress associated with admission to a hospital or nursing home, or adjustment to a new setting can cause the client to perform poorly during the mental status evaluation. This could indicate a reaction to the situation and not the typical cognitive function of the client. If dysfunction is apparent during the initial assessment it may be wise to repeat the evaluation after the client has had a chance to adjust. At no time should the client be labelled dysfunctional based on a single mental status examination.

PSYCHIATRIC DISORDERS

Psychiatric clinical syndromes fall into four categories:

1. Syndromes of confusion (dementia and delirium)
2. Affective disorders and schizophrenia
3. Anxiety and personality disorders

4. Syndromes of reactive and transient situational disorders, and a variety of abnormal behaviors such as drug abuse and medical complaining

These psychiatric disorders need to be recognized so that appropriate treatment can be applied and strategies can be planned for the amelioration of symptoms.

Dementia

Dementia, formerly referred to as organic or chronic brain syndrome, is a progressive decline in cognitive function as a result of primary degenerative diseases of the brain or cerebrovascular disturbances to the brain. The prevalence of dementia increases with each decade in late life.

Alzheimer's disease is believed to be responsible for a majority of dementias. In this disease, the brain atrophies with a widening of sulci, narrow convolutions, lateral ventricular enlargement, reduction in white matter, cortical neuronal loss, senile plaque, and neurofibrillary tangles in the cortex. Because these findings can only be confirmed on autopsy, the diagnosis of Alzheimer's disease is a diagnosis of exclusion, meaning that only after scans and other diagnostic measures have ruled out other causes can the dementia be attributed to Alzheimer's disease. Before the Alzheimer's disease label is placed on a client it is important that diagnostic tests be performed to eliminate other potential causes.

The next most significant cause of dementia is ischemic cerebral lesions, known as multi-infarct dementia. A small percentage of dementias are caused by less common disorders such as:

- Wernicke's encephalopathy, secondary to alcoholism
- Pick's disease, characterized by the presence of the Pick cell, in which cerebral atrophy is confined to the frontal temporal regions of the cerebral cortex and senile plaque and neurofibrillary tangles are present
- Creutzfeldt-Jakob disease, a rapidly progressing neurologic disorder in which there is destruction of neurons in the cerebral cortex, overgrowth of ganglia, abnormal cellular structure of the cortex, hypertrophy and proliferation of astrocytes, and a spongelike appearance of the cerebral cortex
- Sjögren's syndrome, an autoimmune disease associated with extreme dryness of glands, vasculitis, and, in some victims, declines in cognitive function that mimic Alzheimer's disease.

Trauma, Parkinson's disease, brain tumors, and drug intoxication are among the other less common causes of dementia.

The onset of symptoms of dementia tends to be gradual, sometimes taking years before being noticed by others in contact with the affected individual. Typically there is a disturbance in memory, impaired abstract thinking, decreased conceptual thought, disorientation, decreased coping ability, changes in affect, decreased attention span, impaired judgment, and catastrophic reactions. Social functioning tends to decline, and as the condition progresses basic self-care measures become increasingly difficult. In the early stage, persons with dementia may be aware of their cognitive decline and suffer depression; in turn, depressed persons who are not eating or sleeping well and who have a disinterest in life may mimic demented individuals. Astute differential diagnosis is crucial: neurologic dysfunction and impairments in intellectual function are typically not present in the depressed person. Also, the demented individual usually will attempt to answer questions or complete tasks during the examination and can be influenced by suggestions, whereas the depressed person's affect is not influenced by suggestion and he or she may not even attempt to answer questions or complete tasks presented by the examiner.

An important aspect of evaluating the individual with dementia is to determine how the family is coping with the disease. Coping with and caring for a person with dementia can be a tremendous task. Families may need assistance in locating resources to assist them and in identifying when the client's care demands exceed the family's capacity to fulfill them.

Delirium

Delirium is an acute confusional state in which there is a disturbance in cerebral circulation. Anything that disrupts homeostasis can be responsible for delirium; potential causes include dehydration, malnutrition, congestive heart failure, hyper- or hypoglycemia, hyper- or hypothermia, hyper- or hypocalcemia, anemia, infection, medications, hypoxia, and emotional stress. The confusion will mimic that seen in demented persons, with the major exceptions being a rapid onset and an altered level of consciousness (ranging from mild drowsiness to hypervigilance).

A thorough physical evaluation is essential when delirium is present to detect the underlying cause. Prompt treatment of the underlying cause usually reverses the problem and spares the client permanent dysfunction.

Depression and Mania

Depression, a common disorder in older adults, is characterized by a mood disturbance with the vegetative signs of anorexia, constipation, weight loss, and disturbed sleep, especially early morning awakening. Mental confusion may be present as a result of malnutrition. The client will describe feelings of guilt, self-blame, sadness, hopelessness, and helplessness. Somatic delusions and paranoid ideas may be present. Suicide is a frequent and serious risk in older adults with depression. In fact, it has been reported that older adults account for approximately 25% of all reported suicides in the United States. Some suicidal impulses may be subtle; direct questions regarding suicidal intent are an essential component of the mental status examination, including an assessment of the lethality of impulses or plans and the availability of means.

Manic states are characterized by hyperactivity, euphoria, extreme loquaciousness, hostility, feelings of grandiosity, and paranoia. While the etiology of these disorders is yet unknown, the effects of unrecognized and prolonged periods of depression and/or mania can be life threatening for the older adult.

Anxiety

Neurosis is considered a functional illness, the etiology of which lies in the interaction of an individual's personal predisposition, life experiences, and stress. Anxiety can be manifested by tenseness, nervousness, palpitations, and hyperventilation, or by phobias, obsessions, compulsions, and hypochondriasis. Excessive nervousness and feelings of sadness and demoralization are common symptoms. The older adult is particularly vulnerable to anxiety states. Hypochondriasis may accompany these disorders and is very common in the older adult.

Personality Disorders

Those who suffer from personality disorders have neither structural nor functional changes in any organ system resulting from this problem. These disorders are characterized by long-term, habitual, maladaptive styles and patterns of behavior, particularly in relation to others. These behaviors primarily cause distress in other people while creating little anxiety in the affected person. Examples of these traits may include inadaptability, self-centeredness, self-dramatization, overdependence on others, intentional stubbornness and overefficiency, social instability, and avoidance of close relationships. It is important to recognize that personality disorders are generally life-long and, in older adults, can compound any other mental illness and physical illness. This fact produces considerable difficulty in the medical and nursing management of such individuals.

Transient and Situational Disorders

Transient and situational disorders are characterized by a disruption in an individual's life that causes suffering and distress in reaction to real and external stressful life situations. These reactions may be characterized by sadness, tearfulness, anxiety, minor sleep disturbances, and minor somatic symptoms, such as heavy breathing or sighing. They are transient in nature and the symptoms do not become protracted or prolonged. One's usual coping mechanisms are adequate for dealing with these real life problems.

11 Chapter Summary

I. Age-related changes
   A. Personality consistent throughout life span
   B. Intelligence unaltered
   C. Short-term memory poorer; long-term memory relatively unchanged
   D. Learning ability unaltered although other factors may interfere with learning
   E. Decline in mental status not a normal consequence of aging process

II. Assessment
   A. Introduction of examination
      1. Introduce mental status examination as routine part of total assessment
      2. Provide comfort, quiet, and privacy
      3. Be aware of client's reactions, attitudes, and impressions of examination
   B. Areas of examination
      1. General appearance and behavior
         a) Note dress, grooming, posture, mobility, facial expressions, gestures, mental alertness, and overall impression made
      2. Speech
         a) Note tone of voice, rate of speech, use of language, ability to articulate
      3. Mood and self-attitude
         a) Note mood

         b) Mood lability may be manifested by alternating periods of crying and laughter
         c) Explore client's self-perception
      4. Delusions and hallucinations
         a) Specifically ask about auditory, visual, tactile, and olfactory types
         b) Note quality, quantity, and content of thoughts
      5. Depression and mania
         a) Ask about sleep disturbances, appetite, weight loss, constipation, feelings of euphoria or hopelessness, and helplessness
         b) Directly question as to presence of suicidal thoughts and plans
      6. Neurotic symptoms
         a) Anxiety may be manifested through feelings of nervousness, hyperventilation, difficulty swallowing, excessive worry, and fear of impending disaster
         b) Phobias are unusual or irrational fears that interfere with life
         c) Obsessions and compulsions are indicated by recurring or unwanted thoughts or behaviors that interfere with life

7. Cognitive tests
   a) Orientation
   b) Memory
   c) Counting backwards
   d) Retention
   e) Three-stage command
   f) Judgment

III. Disorders
   A. Dementia
      1. Alteration in cognitive functioning in presence of normal state of consciousness
      2. Potential causes: Alzheimer's disease, arteriosclerosis, Creutzfeldt-Jakob disease, and Parkinson's disease
      3. Symptoms include alterations in intellect, judgment, memory, orientation, comprehension, and emotional stability
   B. Delirium
      1. Alteration in cognitive functioning and other psychiatric symptomatology in presence of altered state of consciousness
      2. Causes: disruption of physiologic homeostasis
   C. Affective disorders
      1. Depression: mood disturbances with vegetative signs of loss of appetite and weight, and disturbed sleep
      2. Mania: state of hyperactivity, euphoria, extreme loquaciousness, hostility, paranoia, feelings of grandiosity
      3. Causes unknown
      4. Affective disorders can be life-threatening to the older adult: 25% of all suicides involve older adults
   D. Anxiety
      1. Functional illness
      2. Demonstrated through tenseness, nervousness, palpitations, hyperventilation, phobias, obsession
      3. Hypochondriasis may accompany anxiety
   E. Personality disorders
      1. Functional illness
      2. Characterized by long-term habitual, maladaptive styles and patterns of behavior: inadaptability, self-centeredness, self-dramatization, overdependence on others, intentional stubbornness, social instability, avoidance of close relationships
      3. Generally a life-long problem
   F. Transient and situational disorders
      1. Reaction to real and external stressful life situations
      2. Characterized by sadness, tearfulness, feelings of loss, minor somatic symptoms
      3. Symptoms are temporary

IV. Related nursing diagnoses
   A. Activity intolerance
   B. Anxiety
   C. Constipation
   D. Pain
   E. Impaired verbal communication
   F. Ineffective individual coping
   G. Ineffective family coping
   H. Diversional activity deficit
   I. Altered family processes
   J. Fear
   K. Grieving
   L. Altered health maintenance
   M. Impaired home maintenance management
   N. Potential for injury
   O. Knowledge deficit
   P. Noncompliance

Q. Altered nutrition: less than
    body requirements
R. Altered nutrition: more than
    body requirements
S. Powerlessness
T. Self-care deficit
U. Personal identity disturbance
V. Sensory-perceptual alterations

W. Sexual dysfunction
X. Sleep pattern disturbance
Y. Impaired social interactions
Z. Social isolation
AA. Spiritual distress
BB. Altered thought processes
CC. Altered tissue perfusion
DD. Potential for violence

READINGS AND REFERENCES

Blazer DG. *Depression in Late Life*. St. Louis: Mosby, 1982.

Brody E. *Mental and Physical Health Practices of Older People*. New York: Springer-Verlag, 1982.

Butler RN, Lewis MI. *Aging and Mental Health: Positive Psychosocial and Biomedical Approaches*, 3rd ed. St. Louis: Mosby, 1982.

Care of the Mentally Ill in Nursing Homes. Addendum to national plan for the chronically mentally ill. Rockville, MD: Department of Health and Human Services. National Institute of Mental Health, September 1980.

Charles R, Truesdale M, Wood EL. Alzheimer's disease: Pathology, progression, and nursing process. *Journal of Gerontological Nursing* February 1982; 8(2):69–73.

Derogatis RS et al. The Hopkins Symptom Checklist: A measure of primary symptom dimensions. *Pharmacopsychiatry* July 1974; 7:79–110.

Eisdorfer C, Fann WT. *Treatment of Psychopathology in the Aging*. New York: Springer, 1982.

Finkel SI. Psychiatric consultation in a community serving the elderly. *Hospital and Community Psychiatry* August 1980; 31:551–554.

Folstein MF, Folstein SE, McHugh PR. Mini-mental state. A practical method for grading the cognitive state of patients for the clinician. *Journal of Psychiatric Research* 1975; 12:189–198.

Gaitz CM. Identifying and treating depression in an older patient. *Geriatrics* 1983; 38(2):42–46.

Goldberg D. *The Detection of Psychiatric Illness by Questionnaire*. London: Oxford University Press, 1972.

Goodstein RK. The diagnosis and treatment of elderly patients: Some practical guidelines. *Hospital and Community Psychiatry* January 1980; 31:19–24.

Henig RM. *The Myth of Senility: Misconceptions About the Brain and Aging*. New York: Anchor Press, 1981.

Issacs AD, Post F. *Studies in Geriatric Psychiatry*. New York: Wiley, 1978.

Kennedy CC. Use of health assessments for placing patients for geropsychiatry. *Journal of Gerontological Nursing* May 1981; 7(5):273–279.

LaPorte HJ. Reversible causes of dementia: A nursing challenge. *Journal of Gerontological Nursing* February 1982; 8(2):74–80.

Lucas MJ, Steele C, Bognanni A. Recognition of psychiatric symptoms in dementia. *Journal of Gerontological Nursing* 1986; 12(1):11–15.

Ludwick R. Assessing confusion: A tool to improve nursing care. *Journal of Gerontological Nursing* August 1981; 7(8):474–477.

Maloney JP, Bartz C. Aging and memory loss. *Journal of Gerontological Nursing* July 1982; 8(7):402–404.

McNab A. Screening an elderly population for psychological well-being. *Health Bulletin* July 1980; 38(4):160–162.

Miller P. Interrupting the depression cycle . . . so prevalent among the elderly. *Geriatric Nursing* July/August 1980; 1:133–135.

Pavkor GR, Walsh J. For nursing homes: A mental health charting instrument. *Journal of Gerontological Nursing* January 1981; 7(1):13–20.

Pierce PM. Intelligence and learning in the aged. *Journal of Gerontological Nursing* May 1980; 6:267–270.

Rabins PV, Folstein MF. The demented patient: Evaluation and care. *Geriatrics* 1983; 38(8):99–106.

Raskin AJ (editor). Replication of factors of psychopathology of hospitalized depressives. *Journal of Nervous and Mental Disease* 1960; 148:87–88.

Richardson K. Hope and flexibility—your keys to helping O.B.S. patients. *Nursing 82* June 1982; 12(6):65–69.

Shaw J. A literature review of treatment options for mentally disabled old people. *Journal of Gerontological Nursing* September/October 1979; 5:36–42.

Wilkinson IM, Groham-White J. Dependency rating scales for use in psychogeriatric nursing. *Health Bulletin* January 1980; 38:36–41.

Wolanin MO, Phillips LF. *Confusion: Prevention and Care.* St. Louis: Mosby, 1981.

Wolanin MO, Phillip LR. Who's confused here? *Geriatric Nursing* July/August 1980; 1:122–126.

12 Assessment of the Urinary System

Charlotte Eliopoulos, RNC, MPH

Alterations in the function of the urinary system are a noticeable part of the aging process for most adults. Renal changes can threaten the maintenance of homeostasis and the proper excretion of drugs and other substances, resulting in serious consequences to total body health. The dependence of every body system on adequate urinary system function demands that a careful evaluation of this system be an essential component of every older adult's assessment.

Not only are urinary problems threatening to physical health, they also can profoundly affect the older adult's psychosocial well-being. Persons voiding throughout the night may not have the energy or interest to participate in activities of daily living to the fullest extent. Incontinence can seriously threaten self-esteem, socialization, and participation in routine family and community events. To many persons, urinary problems have sexual connotations, creating guilt and embarrassment in the affected individual. People with urinary disorders may feel self-conscious of the odors, appliances, and inconveniences associated with their problem. The full impact of urinary problems on social function and psychologic well-being should be explored during the assessment of this system.

REVIEW OF THE URINARY SYSTEM

The profound work of the urinary system is conducted by two kidneys, two ureters, the bladder, and the urethra (Figure 12-1).

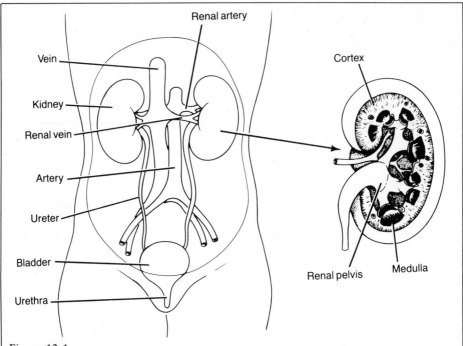

Figure 12-1
The urinary system. Source: Matta MS, Wilbraham AC. *Atoms, Molecules, and Life: An Introduction to General, Organic, and Biological Chemistry.* Redwood City, CA: Benjamin/Cummings, 1981.

Kidneys

The *kidneys* are bean-shaped organs located on either side of the vertebral column in the posterior portion of the abdominal cavity behind the peritoneum. Most of the kidney lies in the upper quadrant with a portion of the lower segment extending to the lower quadrant. The kidneys are surrounded by adipose tissue, which allows movement of the kidneys with diaphragmatic movement. The ribs and back muscles offer good protection to the kidneys.

The kidneys function as a filter for the 500 to 1000 mL of blood that passes through these structures every minute. The kidneys' complex tubular function regulates the body's acid–base balance; removes excess glucose, sodium, and other essential elements from the blood to maintain a health level; and eliminates drugs and other foreign substances from circulation. From each kidney extends a ureter, a tube approximately 10 to 12 inches in length. Ureters transport urine from the kidneys to the bladder.

Bladder

The *bladder* is a reservoir for urine, lying in the lower midline of the abdomen behind the pubis. Distention of the bladder muscles causes nerve receptor stimulation and arouses the urge to void; this normally occurs when approximately 300 mL have accumulated in the bladder. Urgency and discomfort are experienced when levels of about 700 mL of urine are present in the bladder. Urine passes from the bladder through a single tube, the *urethra*, and then exits out to the exterior of the body. The female's urethra is 1 to $1\frac{1}{2}$ inches long and the male's is 6 to 7 inches long.

Urine

Urine is the watery nitrogenous waste excreted from the urinary system. Approximately 95% of urine is water; the remainder is various inorganic and organic substances. Urine is usually acidic but may be alkaline if a vegetarian diet is ingested. The normal range of specific gravity of urine is from 1.002 to 1.040. Glucose normally is not found in urine, although a high carbohydrate intake or stress can cause glycosuria (presence of glucose in the urine) without indicating pathology. Likewise, acetone (ketone) bodies are not a normal constituent of urine but can result from a low carbohydrate diet or from increased activity in a healthy person. Pus, blood, albumin, and casts are abnormal components of urine.

AGE-RELATED CHANGES IN THE URINARY SYSTEM

The renal system experiences a variety of degenerative changes with age. Not only are nephron units lost, but renal tissue growth declines as we grow older, resulting in a reduction in kidney size. Atherosclerosis and other disease processes that more frequently occur in the geriatric population compound these degenerative changes. Among the effects of these renal changes is the slowing of filtration functions. The glomerular filtration rate begins to decline in the second decade of life and continues, so that by age 90 it is half of what it was at age 20 (Feinstein 1986). Renal plasma flow also decreases. Blood urea nitrogen (BUN) levels increase to 21 mg% at age 70. The kidneys' ability to concentrate urine is decreased by changes in tubular function.

Perhaps the most noticeable effects of the system's aging are changes that are experienced by the bladder. Bladder capacity decreases, causing frequency and nocturia to be common experiences for the elderly. Emptying of the bladder is more difficult due to a weakening of bladder muscles. This can result in the retention of large volumes of urine: some older bladders can retain 100 mL of urine after voiding.

ASSESSMENT OF THE URINARY SYSTEM

Although the most specific determination of the urinary system's status is achieved through laboratory and radiology studies, you can learn much about the system by obtaining a good history. However, you might not obtain this history easily from the older adult. Frequently, the client is embarrassed when discussing urinary problems, especially if such problems include dribbling of urine or incontinence. The client may also have misconceptions concerning the relationship of the urinary system to sexual function, thus creating anxiety, guilt, and reluctance in discussing urinary system disorders. There also are those who have become so accustomed to frequency, nocturia, and other urinary disorders that they identify them as normal and fail to inform the interviewer of their existence. Thus, you are challenged to structure an interview so that the older adult will feel at ease in discussing urinary system function in order to provide complete, accurate data.

Signs and Symptoms

Specific questions pertaining to the pattern of voiding should be asked, including the frequency of voiding during daytime and night hours, and the amount voided at each time. It is not unusual for older adults to void every two hours during daytime hours and once during the night due to decreased bladder capacity. More frequent voiding or sudden increases in frequency of voiding can be associated with infection, lesions, drugs, an unusual increase in fluid consumption, diabetes mellitus, hypocalcemia, and anxiety; a referral for more discrete diagnostic work is appropriate under these circumstances.

Older individuals may complain of needing to void approximately one-half hour after going to bed even when they have voided just prior to lying down. This is an actual phenomenon with many older adults due to improvement in renal circulation when changing from an upright to a recumbent position.

Some urinary retention is an outgrowth of the aging process. This problem can be intensified by certain medications, prostatic enlargement, and, in females, fecal impaction. A neurogenic bladder can be responsible for urinary retention also. Some older adults can give clues to retention problems through comments such as "I feel as though I still have to void right after I go to the bathroom" and "It seems as though I'm always holding back some urine when I void." A distended bladder is a good indicator of urinary retention. This problem should be detected and corrected early to minimize the risk of infection.

Stress incontinence and dribbling of urine after voiding are other possible results of weaker bladder muscles. Multiparous women frequently experience these disorders. Data pertaining to these problems can be elicited through questions such as "Do you leak urine when you cough or sneeze?" "How long do you wait on the toilet for your urine to stop dripping after you void?" and "Do you lose control of your bladder if you wait too long to go to the bathroom?"

Urinary incontinence is not a normal consequence of the aging process but rather a sign of some disorder. A neurogenic bladder associated with diabetic neuropathy, cerebral cortex lesions, and myasthenia gravis can cause incontinence. Prostatic enlargement, calculi, and tumors can be responsible for mechanical problems that cause incontinence. Urinary incontinence can result from temporary situations such as urinary tract infections and drug therapy. Obviously, potential interventions are directly related to the root of the problem. For example, if an infection is causing the incontinence, efforts would focus on treating the infection rather than just initiating a bladder training program. Therefore, a medical evaluation is warranted when urinary incontinence exists.

Urine Sample

The urine sample usually provides a good insight into the urinary system's function and general health status. However, interpretation of the urine sample in older adults must include consideration of age-related factors that influence the urine's characteristics.

Specific gravity of urine, which indicates the kidney's ability to concentrate urine, ranges from 1.005 to 1.025 in the general adult population. Decreased tubular function causes lower specific gravity values to be common among many older adults. It should be remembered that urine is most concentrated in the early morning.

Changes in tubular function also alter the manner in which elements, such as proteins, are reabsorbed from the filtrate. Although protein is considered an unusual finding among younger adults, a 1+ proteinuria with the absence of sediment is of no diagnostic significance among older adults. When problems are suspected, a 24-hour urine collection for total protein is recommended. Casts, crystals, and red and white blood cells are abnormal elements in urine; these are identified by microscopic examination of the urine.

Many healthy older adults have a lower renal threshold for glucose. Thus, glucosuria is not necessarily indicative of pathology in older adults and as a sole finding does not warrant extensive diagnostic evaluation. If diabetes mellitus is suspected as being responsible for glucosuria, a glucose tolerance test that uses age-related gradients is recommended (Table 12-1).

Altered renal function not only causes glucosuria to be present without hyperglycemia but can cause individuals to be hyperglycemic without any evidence of glucose in the urine. Blood values are the best indicator of altered glucose levels.

The acidity or alkalinity of urine is assessed through the pH reaction. A freshly voided specimen is normally acidic in young age groups, but can range

Table 12-1 Glucose Tolerance with Aging

	PLASMA GLUCOSE (mg/dL)				
	Normal			Probable Diabetes	Diabetes
Age	Fasting	1 Hour	2 Hours	2 Hours	2 Hours
0–30	110	185	165	166–185	>185
30–40	112	191	175	176–195	>195
40–50	114	197	185	186–205	>205
50–60	116	203	195	196–215	>215
60–70	118	209	205	200–235	>235
70–80	120	215	215	216–245	>245

Source: Krupp MA, Chatton MJ. Current Medical Diagnosis and Treatment. Table 19-4, p 753. Copyright 1980 by Lange Medical Publications, Los Altos, CA. As adapted from Prout TE. *Diabetes Mellitus*, 4th ed. American Diabetes Association, 1975.

between a 4.6 to 8 pH in older adults. The urine will be alkaline and appear cloudy if a proteus infection is present or if the specimen is more than several hours old.

The concentration of urine determines its color. The color will be light if the urine is dilute; dark if it is concentrated. Discolored urine indicates a deviation from normal. Yellow-brown or green-brown urine can result from an obstructive bile duct system or jaundice; red or rust-colored urine usually indicates the presence of blood; orange-colored urine may be due to the presence of bile or the ingestion of Pyridium; smokey-colored urine can indicate hematuria or the presence of sperm or droplets of prostatic fluid; and dark-brown or black urine can be associated with hematuria or carcinoma.

Urine normally has a faint aromatic odor. The ingestion of certain foods, such as asparagus, can give a different odor to urine; thus when odorous urine is present, it is advisable to explore what foods and medications have been ingested that day. Infections may cause the urine to smell foul or ammonialike.

DISORDERS OF THE URINARY SYSTEM

Urinary Tract Infections

Urinary tract infections are common among older adults, especially those who have indwelling catheters, fluid imbalances, diabetes, neurogenic bladders, urethral strictures, or limited mobility. Often, the classic signs of a urinary tract infection are missed in the older adult. For example, frequency may be viewed as a normal feature for older persons and an elevated temperature may not be recognized if the nurse is unaware that fever levels can be different for older adults. (Remember, normal body temperatures for older adults can be 95°F or 96°F, which means that a temperature of 99°F indicates a significant elevation.) Extremely odorous urine can be associated with a urinary tract infection also. Urinary retention, incontinence, and hematuria can result from an advanced urinary tract infection.

Incontinence

Although the prevalence of urinary incontinence increases with age, it is not a normal outcome of aging. Its presence should always warrant a thorough evaluation.

Stress incontinence tends to occur more frequently among women who have had multiple pregnancies and results from a weakness of the supporting pelvic muscles. The client will report a loss of urine when she coughs, sneezes, laughs, or exercises. If good sensation and voluntary control over urine flow exist, the client can be taught pelvic muscle exercises that can aid in controlling stress incontinence.

Urge incontinence is the sudden need to void due to spasm or irritation of the bladder wall. Urinary tract infection, bladder tumor, prostatic hypertrophy, vaginitis, and diverticulitis are among the causes of this type of incontinence.

Overflow incontinence results from the retention of urine, associated with drug therapy or obstruction of the bladder neck.

Neurogenic incontinence occurs when there is a loss of sensation to void or lack of bladder control due to a neurologic condition. Causes of this type of incontinence include tabes dorsalis, diabetic neuropathy, cerebral cortex lesion, and multiple sclerosis.

Often, older adults do not report their incontinence because they erroneously believe this to be a normal condition in advanced age, or they fear institutionalization or other negative consequences. This problem should be explored during every assessment and referred for evaluation if it exists. Urinalysis, cystoscopy, cystometry, and intravenous pyelogram are among the diagnostic measures that may be utilized.

Renal Calculi

Calcium and other elements that form calculi are usually present in urine. Maintenance of normal urine concentration and pH helps to prevent these elements from clustering into stones. Unfortunately, some of the common conditions among frail older adults—namely, immobility, dehydration and infection—promote calculi formation. Symptoms of this problem often mimic those of a urinary tract infection and also include pain and hematuria. Obstruction caused by a stone is a significant risk. Any obstruction should be corrected early to avoid infection and potential renal damage.

Acute Glomerulonephritis

Older adults who have a history of chronic glomerulonephritis are at high risk of developing episodes of acute glomerulonephritis. Early signs of this disorder may be vague and misleading. For example, fever, nausea, vomiting, fatigue, anorexia, abdominal pain, and anemia may be among the initial clinical manifestations. As the disease continues, oliguria, hypertension, headaches, generalized edema, and signs associated with cerebral edema will develop. The urine sample of the client with glomerulonephritis may reveal an elevated sedimentation rate, proteinuria, and hematuria.

Pyelonephritis

The most commonly prevalent renal disorder of older women is pyelone-phritis. Urinary obstruction is considered responsible for most cases of pyelonephritis. Early signs of the acute stage of this problem include dull back pain, gastrointestinal upset, frequency of urination, dysuria, bacteriuria, and pyuria. Fever may or may not be present in older adults with this disease. Chronic pyelonephritis causes anorexia, weight loss, fatigue, polyuria, and the signs of uremia. Individuals with both glomerulonephritis and pyelonephritis should be encouraged to be periodically evaluated for the recurrence of infection.

Carcinoma of the Bladder

Bladder cancer has a high incidence among older adults, especially those with a history of chronic urinary tract infection and cigarette smoking. Symptoms of this problem resemble those of a urinary tract infection. In addition, painless hematuria is the classic sign associated with bladder cancer.

Although alterations in urinary system function commonly give rise to complaints of frequency, retention, dribbling, and other uncomfortable and embarrassing signs, these complaints should not be ignored or under-estimated. Astute investigation of complaints, a complete review of the function of the urinary system, and regular urinalysis can be most valuable in detecting serious problems early and preserving this extremely important system's function. Reversible urinary tract disorders left untreated may result in discomfort, social isolation, depression, and ostracism of the older adult. Optimal function of the urinary system is crucial to good physical and social health.

12 Chapter Summary

I. Age-related changes
  A. Decreased bladder capacity
    1. Frequency of urination
    2. Nocturia
  B. Weakened bladder muscles
    1. Retention of urine
    2. Stress incontinence
    3. Dribbling
  C. Decreased tubular function
    1. Lower specific gravity
    2. Proteinuria of 1+ may be normal
    3. Lower renal threshold for glucose
      a) May be little correlation between blood glucose level and level spilled in urine

II. Assessment
  A. Voiding pattern
    1. Frequency
    2. Amount
  B. Retention of urine
    1. Feeling of fullness
    2. Distended bladder
  C. Continence of urine
    1. Stress incontinence
    2. Postvoiding dribbling
  D. Urine sample
    1. Specific gravity
    2. Protein
    3. Glucose
    4. pH reaction
    5. Color
      a) Yellow-brown or green-brown: obstructive bile duct or jaundice
      b) Red or rust-colored: presence of blood
      c) Orange colored: presence of bile or ingestion of pyridium
      d) Smokey colored: hematuria or presence of sperm or prostatic fluid
      e) Dark brown or black: hematuria or carcinoma
    6. Odor
    7. Microscopic evaluation

III. Disorders
  A. Urinary tract infection
    1. Common among older adults with indwelling catheters, fluid imbalances, diabetes, neurogenic bladder, urethral stricture, immobility
    2. Signs: alkaline, odors, and cloudy urine
      a) Fever may be missed due to presence of lower body temperature in older adults
    3. Advanced infection can cause urinary retention, incontinence, and hematuria
  B. Incontinence
    1. Stress: weakness of pelvic muscles
    2. Urge: sudden need to void due to bladder wall irritation or spasm
    3. Overflow: obstruction of bladder neck or drug-related retention
    4. Neurogenic: lack of sensation to void or inability to control bladder elimination
  C. Renal calculi
    1. Associated with immobility, dehydration, infection
    2. Signs resemble urinary tract infection and include pain and hematuria
  D. Acute glomerulonephritis
    1. Primarily occurs among older adults with chronic glomerulonephritis
    2. Early signs can be missed
    3. Advanced signs: oliguria, hypertension, headaches,

generalized edema, cerebral edema
4. Urine sample: elevated sedimentation rate, proteinuria, hematuria

E. Pyelonephritis
1. Most frequent cause: urinary obstruction
2. Early signs: dull back pain, gastrointestinal upset, frequency, dysuria, fever
3. Chronic pyelonephritis causes anorexia, weight loss, fatigue, polyuria, signs of uremia
4. Urine sample: bacteriuria, pyuria

F. Carcinoma of the bladder
1. Associated with history of chronic urinary tract infection and cigarette smoking
2. Signs can resemble urinary tract infection and include painless hematuria

IV. Related nursing diagnoses
A. Anxiety
B. Pain
C. Potential for infection
D. Knowledge deficit
E. Noncompliance
F. Self-care deficit
G. Personal identity disturbance
H. Sexual dysfunction
I. Impaired skin integrity
J. Sleep pattern disturbance
K. Impaired social interaction
L. Social isolation
M. Altered patterns of urinary elimination

READINGS AND REFERENCES

Bates B. *A Guide to Physical Examination*, 4th ed. Philadelphia: Lippincott, 1987.

Breschi L. Common lower urinary tract problems in the elderly. In: *Clinical Aspects of Aging*, 2nd ed. Reichel W (editor). Baltimore: Williams and Wilkins, 1983, pp 302–318.

Brink C. Assessing the problem. *Geriatric Nursing* November/December 1980; 1(4):241–250.

Feinstein EI. Renal disease in the elderly. In: *Clinical Geriatrics*, 3rd ed. Rossman I (editor). Philadelphia: Lippincott, 1986, p 217.

Freed SZ. Genitourinary disease in the elderly. In: *Clinical Geriatrics*, 3rd ed. Rossman I (editor). Philadelphia: Lippincott, 1986, pp 352–362.

Frentz GD, Bell DP. Managing urinary tract infections in the geriatric population. *Geriatrics* 1983; 38(11):42–50.

Jaffe JW. Common lower urinary tract problems in older people. In: *Clinical Aspects of Aging*, 2nd ed. Reichel W (editor). Baltimore: Williams and Wilkins, 1983.

Kendall AR, Stein BS. Stress urinary incontinence. *Geriatrics* 1983; 38(5):69–79.

Segura JW. Guidelines for diagnosing and treating urinary tract infections. *Geriatrics* September 1978; 33(9):87–88.

Shapiro WB, Porush JG, Kahn AI. Medical renal disease in the aged. In: *Clinical Aspects of Aging*. Reichel W (editor). Baltimore: Williams and Wilkins, 1978.

Whitman S. Curbing incontinence. *Journal of Gerontological Nursing* April 1987; 13(4):35–40.

Willington FL (editor). *Incontinence in the Elderly*. New York: Academic Press, 1976.

Willington FL. Urinary incontinence: A practical approach. *Geriatrics* June 1980; 35:41–48.

13 Assessment of Sexual Function

Charlotte Eliopoulos, RNC, MPH

Perhaps the most neglected area of any assessment involves sexual function. Embarrassment, ignorance, and anxiety often interfere with the client's open discussion of sexual matters, thus leaving a gap in the nurse's understanding of the total person. Frequently, nurses lack the knowledge and skills necessary to assess sexual function adequately; they may believe that sexual matters are personal and have no place in the health assessment. Not to be overlooked is the reality that nurses are human beings with their own attitudes and values that influence their comfort, ability, and willingness to discuss sex with their clients.

The situation becomes more complicated when the assessment of sexual function involves an older adult. Many nurses have difficulty discussing sex with persons who are their senior or who remind them of their parents or grandparents. They may find humor in the fact that the older adult is concerned about sexual function and may play down the significance of the concern. They may be repulsed by the image of sexual intimacy between older adults and label them as "dirty," "perverse," or "lecherous." Their own misunderstandings may lead them to counsel clients incorrectly, informing them that sex is not possible, normal, or necessary in old age. Too often, nurses, who otherwise conscientiously explore every detail of the client's health status, do not consider the older adult's sexual function and interest at all.

Introspection of feelings and attitudes about sex is essential for nurses who are engaged in assessing older adults. Talking with colleagues, sexual counselors, and older friends can assist in identifying and clarifying misconceptions. Realistic insight can be gained by exploring the growing pool of literature pertaining to sexual function in old age. The interrelationship between sexual function and health status in general demands that assessment of sexual function be an integral and essential part of every individual's health evaluation.

SEXUAL HISTORY

Eliciting sexual histories from older adults is not always a smooth process. Today's older adults are of a generation socialized to view sex as a private, almost secretive matter. They did not have, unlike today's younger generation, the advantages of sex education classes, the candid exposure of sex through the media, and the general openness about sex. Instead, they often were taught that discussing (and even thinking about) sex was immoral and improper. It stands to reason, therefore, that older adults may be reluctant to discuss openly their sexual functions with anyone—much less the nurse!

Some older adults feel embarrassed and guilty about their sexual interests. An older widow, for instance, may believe she is "bad" for being sexually active with someone who is not her husband. A male older adult may shudder to think of what his children and grandchildren would think about him if they knew that he masturbated while fantasizing about his young neighbor. An older couple may think they are selfish and abnormal because they prefer their intimacy to an opportunity to have their grandchildren visit for summer vacation. Older adults often suffer from the conflict between the sexual interest they normally feel and societal expectations for them to behave as "sexless, sedate, and safe."

Special skill and sensitivity are obviously required for the nurse interested in collecting a sexual history. You should portray an open, nonjudgmental attitude. The manner in which you phrase questions will communicate a great deal to the client—for example, "Do you experience any difficulties with intercourse?" versus "I guess sex isn't a concern of yours anymore, is it?" Also, the amount of information the client shares will be greatly determined by whether the information is managed with respect, dignity, and confidentiality, or with ridicule, indiscretion, and condemnation.

The client deserves an explanation of why you are asking for a sexual history and how you will use it. Comments such as "I want to be sure that your new medication hasn't altered your sexual function" and "Some changes do occur with age, but they can be managed to help you continue your sexual activity" can open the door to a discussion of sexual function. The client should understand that problems in sexual function can give you clues to major health problems, such as diabetes, depression, alcoholism, drug reactions, and gynecologic disorders.

Incorporating the sexual history in the assessment of the urinary system may be useful. Most persons closely associate these systems together, making them a logical combination during the health assessment. Of course, as problems related to other systems are discussed, the opportunity may arise to investigate the sexual history; for example, if a client states that her husband has lost interest in sex since he has retired, or that she experiences discomfort from her hiatus hernia at bedtime.

An important part of collecting the sexual history is identifying and correcting misconceptions regarding sexual function. Older clients may demonstrate the need for tactful education through comments such as "Naturally I stopped being interested in sex after menopause," "I can't have an erection because I have prostate trouble," "My hysterectomy caused me to stop having intercourse," "I can't have sex with a heart condition," and "Older people aren't supposed to be interested in sex."

THE OLDER FEMALE

Several standard items are included in the sexual history of the female:

- *Pregnancy history*: Attempt to outline the dates and outcomes of each pregnancy, for example, "1935: aborted pregnancy at three months due to accident; 1937: gave birth to healthy son, uneventful pregnancy."
- *Menstrual history*: Determine the onset and cessation of the menstrual period with a brief description of the pattern of menstrual periods. A general description of menopause may provide useful data, for example, "Client claims to have experienced a severe menopause 1946–1955, forcing her to quit her job and cease sexual intercourse."
- *Gynecologic examination history*: Review the frequency of gynecologic examination and record the date of the last exam recorded. Explore significant events, such as surgery or treatment of prolapsed uterus.

Age has a profound effect on the female's genitalia. The vulva gains an atrophic appearance due to a reduction in vascularity, elasticity, and subcutaneous fat. A loss of pubic hair and a flattening of the labia occur. Vaginal epithelium is thinner and less vascular. The vaginal environment is more alkaline, drier, and altered in the type of flora present. Upon inspection, the vagina appears pink, dry, and smooth with fewer rugae. The cervix and uterus become smaller in size—sometimes the uterus shrinks to the extent that it cannot be palpated during the gynecologic examination. The fallopian tubes and ovaries atrophy, and ovulation and estrogen production cease in old age. Breasts atrophy and sag.

Since the vulva is more fragile it is more easily irritated. Question the client for the presence of vulvar soreness and pruritis. This irritation may be revealed through the presence of rawness, redness, and scratch marks on examination. Vulvar lesions should be identified: half the cases of cancer of the vulva occur in older women.

Alterations in the vaginal canal predispose the older woman to *vaginitis*. Many older females believe vaginitis to be a problem of younger, more sexually active females and often don't consider their symptoms to be associated with this infection. Assess for the presence of vaginal discharge, odor, irritation, and itching.

The older woman may be asked if she experiences *dyspareunia*. The drier, more delicate vaginal walls can make intercourse very uncomfortable and unpleasurable for many older women. When this problem is noted, the client may be counseled in the use of lubricating jellies and creams. If the client indicates that such a lubricating agent is used, ensure that it is water soluble, rather than petroleum jelly, which risks blocking the entrance of the urethra and causing urinary tract problems.

Vaginal bleeding is an abnormal experience for older women, indicative of carcinoma and other disorders. When establishing the date for the last menstrual period, ask the client if she has experienced any episodes of bleeding or even slight spotting since her last period. Investigate the amount and duration of the bleeding, as well as its relationship to other factors, such as intercourse. Older women receiving estrogen therapy may experience vaginal bleeding due to the endometrium continuing to be responsive to hormonal stimulation in old age.

Prolapsed uterus is a frequent disorder detected among older females, especially those who have had multiple pregnancies. Urinary system symptoms may indicate a prolapsed uterus; such symptoms may include urinary frequency, retention, and recurrent urinary tract infections. Back pain and constipation can be associated with this problem. Symptoms directly related to the reproductive system include a sense of pelvic pressure or "heaviness," and a protrusion of the anterior wall outside the vulva.

Although *cervical cancer* reaches its peak during the middle years and declines in incidence in old age, it can be a problem affecting the older woman. Leukorrhea and vaginal bleeding are early manifestations of carcinoma of the cervix. Ensure that the client receives a pap smear at least annually, and incorporate the results of this test in the total health assessment.

Ovarian cancer peaks in the late seventh decade of life, reinforcing the importance of regular gynecologic examination.

Breast cancer increases in incidence with age and is the major cause of cancer death among older women. Regular breast examination is crucial, and the most effective technique is self-examination of the breast (Figure 13-1). Assess the client's knowledge of this procedure and plan to instruct her if she is unfamiliar with breast examination. The client is more apt than you to detect

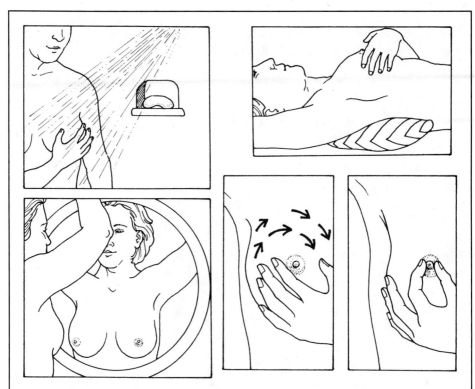

Figure 13-1

Breast self-examination. Examine breasts while bathing or showering; hands glide easily over wet skin. Fingers flat, move them gently over every part of each breast. Use right hand to examine left breast, left hand for right breast. Check for lumps, hard knots, or thickening. Before a mirror, inspect breasts with arms at sides and raised over head. Observe for changes in contour of each breast, swelling, dimpling of skin, or changes in nipple. To examine right breast while lying down, place a pillow under right shoulder. Place right hand behind head. With left hand, fingers flat, palpate at the top outermost portion of the breast in a clockwise direction. At the completion of a circle, move in an inch and repeat and keep repeating until reaching the nipple. Slowly repeat procedure on left breast. Gently squeeze the nipple and observe for any discharge.

early changes in her breasts. In fact, most cases of breast cancer are detected by clients themselves. In addition, older women should have annual mammograms. Signs of breast cancer include a nontender breast mass, asymmetry of the breasts, dimpling of the skin, nodular axillary masses, and nipple retraction and bleeding. Normal age-related shrinkage and fibrotic changes to the breast can cause nipple retraction that mimics cancer.

THE OLDER MALE

The male's reproductive system suffers less pronounced changes with age than does the female's. The size and firmness of the testes decrease with age.

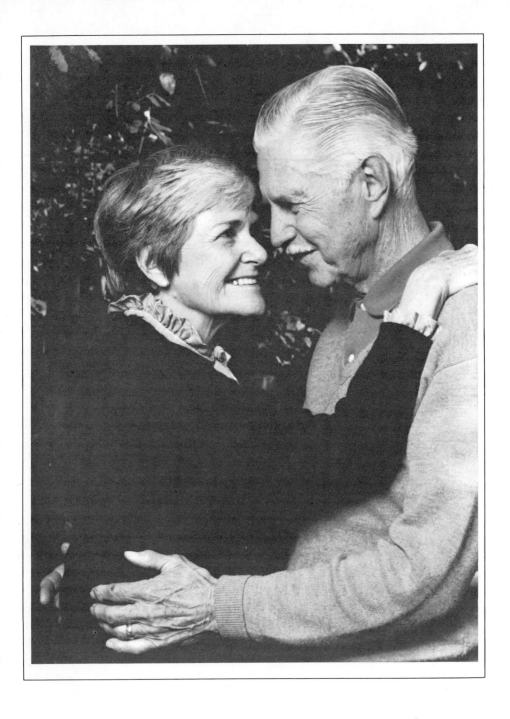

Testosterone continues to be produced in old age although in lesser amounts. The penis maintains its ability to become erect. More direct physical stimulation and time are required for the older man to achieve an erection, but he can maintain his erection for a longer period of time before ejaculation than the younger man. Ejaculations are slower and less forceful in older men, and ejaculation will not necessarily occur during each intercourse, especially if intercourse occurs frequently.

The male's genitalia has the advantage of being easily examined. Inspect the *penis* for ulcers, chancres, nodules, and other abnormalities. If the client is uncircumcised, retract the foreskin and note any lesions and discharge that are present. Urethral discharge can be caused by urethritis, prostatitis, or gonorrhea.

Look for irritation, nodules, ulcers, and inflammation of the *scrotum*. Pressure on the testes produces pain; however, gentle palpation should not be uncomfortable unless inflammation, infection, or bleeding is present. Enlargement of the scrotum or testes indicates a problem, such as epididymitis, orchitis, and carcinoma.

Most older men have some degree of *prostatic enlargement*. In fact, in older men the prostate is the most frequently diseased organ and the most common site of malignancy (Freid 1986a). This condition causes a gradual narrowing of the prostatic urethra, manifested through symptoms such as urinary frequency, hesitancy, retention, nocturia, dysuria, dribbling, decreased force of urinary stream, and less forceful ejaculations. The size of the enlargement does not necessarily correlate with the degree of urinary dysfunction. Clients with prostatic enlargement require biannual examination and close follow-up not only to detect and manage the recurrent urinary tract infections they frequently experience, but also to ensure that carcinoma does not exist.

Although it can be a potential outcome, impotency is not guaranteed by prostatic disorders or surgery. Medical consultation concerning the individual client's problem is advisable to ensure that realistic, accurate counselling can be conducted.

PROBLEMS IN SEXUAL FUNCTION

The age-related physical changes experienced by both sexes do not prevent sexual function nor alter the libido and pleasure derived from sexual activity. More time may be required for the male to become fully erect and greater attention to the female's more fragile vaginal canal may be necessary, but these can be incorporated into sensitive foreplay activities rather than be viewed as obstacles to a full sexual experience. Touching, caressing, hugging, and sharing intimacy with another human being remains important in the later years of life.

Occasions may occur, however, when circumstances and health problems do interfere with sexual function. Thus, when sexual dysfunction is identified, it is necessary to explore possible causes. Specifically appraise the nature and prognosis of the problem, and realistically advise the client.

Sexual dysfunction can result from *disease processes*. Diabetes, for instance, can reduce vaginal lubrication in females, and cause premature ejaculation and impotency in males. Arthritic problems can limit positions and mobility during intercourse. Shortness of breath and reduced energy levels during intercourse can result from cardiovascular and respiratory illnesses. These disease processes do not necessitate the cessation of sexual function. Often, counselling as to alternative positions and technique, and the real impact of sex on the illness (and vice versa) can prove highly beneficial.

Erectile dysfunction can be the first sign of intermittent claudication in persons with diabetes mellitus or arteriosclerosis. Often, this can be manifested by the "steal syndrome," in which the erection disappears after coital movements due to blood flow being sufficient to achieve erection but insufficient to sustain it during coital activity (Freid 1986b).

Drugs can alter sexual function in varying degrees among individuals. Drugs known to reduce libido and potency include diuretics, tranquilizers, sedatives, alcohol, tricyclic antidepressants, and some of the antihypertensives. The older client has a right to be informed of the sexual consequences of specific drugs and to decide if he or she desires to risk alterations in sexual function for the benefit of drug therapy.

Long periods of *abstinence* can create sexual function problems. The vaginal canal may become tighter and less flexible, resulting in dyspareunia; local estrogen creams can be prescribed to treat this problem. Males may experience impotency in attempting to reinitiate intercourse. Encourage patience and perseverance. Initial problems in reestablishing sexual relationships do not mean that continued attempts should be discouraged.

Other factors also affect satisfying sexual relationships in old age. *Overeating* and *fatigue* can reduce sexual interest and activity. *Depression* and other *mental health problems* can result in sexual dysfunction. Psychologic factors, such as the *preoccupation with health, work, or money, insecurity over the lack of privacy*, and *concern about what others may think* also can limit sexual activity. The absence of a partner and the limited opportunities to meet a new partner also produce considerable obstacles.

It must be recognized that sexuality encompasses more than a physical sex act. The way older persons feel about their own identity and how they perceive others to feel about them are important to their sexual health. During the assessment, you should search for clues regarding your clients' sexual self-concepts. Do they believe they are worthy of others' affections or that no one could possibly find them attractive and desirable? Are they able to give and receive affection openly or are they inhibited? Is maintaining practices that reinforce a feminine or masculine image important to them? Each person's sexual interest, attitudes, practices, and satisfactions will be different; your task is not to judge but to understand these factors to gain insight into the whole individual.

The touching, sharing, compassion, and warmth provided by an intimate relationship can be significant to older persons in providing essential security and support to face the multiple losses commonly experienced with aging. Sexual function, sexual identity, and expressions of intimacy should be encouraged and maintained among older adults. When problems in sexual function are noted among older adults, exert every effort to diagnose and treat these problems accurately. Sex counselors, social activities, penile prostheses, cosmetics, plastic surgery, and other interventions to promote sexuality should be options available for older clients.

13 Chapter Summary

I. Age-related changes
  A. Female
    1. Vulva has atrophic appearance due to reduction in vascularity, elasticity, and subcutaneous fat
    2. Loss of pubic hair
    3. Flattening of labia
    4. Thinner, less vascular vaginal epithelium
    5. Vaginal environment more alkaline, drier, altered in type of flora
    6. Cervix and uterus shrink
    7. Atrophy of fallopian tubes and ovaries
    8. Cessation of ovulation and estrogen production
    9. Dyspareunia
    10. Sagging breasts
  B. Male
    1. Decreased size and firmness of testes
      a) No cessation in testosterone production
    2. More time needed to obtain erection
    3. Slower, less forceful ejaculations
    4. Some degree of prostatic enlargement

II. Assessment
  A. Female
    1. Pregnancy history
    2. Menstrual history
    3. History of gynecologic care
    4. Inspection of vulva and vaginal canal
      a) Lesions
      b) Discharge
      c) Irritation
      d) Vaginal odor
      e) Itching
    5. Sexual activity
      a) Availability of partner
      b) Interest, preference
      c) Ease of intercourse
  B. Male
    1. Inspection of genitalia
      a) Ulcers, chancre, nodules, irrigation, urethral discharge, swelling
      b) Circumcision
    2. Prostate examination

3. Sexual activity
   a) Availability of partner
   b) Interest, preference
   c) Potency

III. Disorders
   A. Female
      1. Vulvar lesions
      2. Vaginitis
      3. Vaginal bleeding
      4. Prolapsed uterus
         a) Signs include: urinary frequency, retention, recurrent urinary tract infection, back pain, constipation, pelvic pressure, protrusion of anterior wall outside vulva
      5. Cervical cancer
         a) Signs: leukorrhea, vaginal bleeding
      6. Breast cancer
         a) Signs: nontender breast mass, asymmetry of breasts, dimpling, nodular axillary masses, nipple retraction, and bleeding
   B. Male
      1. Urethral discharge
         a) Associated with urethritis, prostatitis, gonorrhea
      2. Ulcers, chancres, nodules on penis
      3. Scrotal swelling or pain
         a) Associated with epididymitis, orchitis, carcinoma
      4. Prostatic masses
      5. Impotency
         a) Causes can include: disease, drugs, alcohol, long periods of abstinence, overeating, fatigue, psychologic factors

IV. Related nursing diagnoses
   A. Activity intolerance
   B. Anxiety
   C. Decreased cardiac output
   D. Pain
   E. Altered family processes
   F. Fear
   G. Grieving
   H. Potential for infection
   I. Knowledge deficit
   J. Impaired physical mobility
   K. Impaired gas exchange
   L. Personal identity disturbance
   M. Sensory/perceptual alterations
   N. Sexual dysfunction
   O. Altered thought processes

READINGS AND REFERENCES

Bates B. *A Guide to Physical Examination*, 4th ed. Philadelphia: Lippincott, 1987.

Burnside I. *Sexuality and Aging*. Los Angeles: University of Southern California Press, 1975.

Butler R, Lewis M. *Sex after Sixty*. New York: Harper and Row, 1976.

Comfort A. Sexuality in old age. *Journal of the American Geriatrics Society* October 1974; 22(10):440–442.

Falk G, Falk UA. Sexuality and the aged. *Nursing Outlook* January 1980; 28:51–55.

Freid SZ. Genitourinary disease in the elderly. In: *Clinical Geriatrics*, 3rd ed. Rossman I (editor). Philadelphia: Lippincott, 1986, a) p 352, b) p 359.

Glowacki G. Geriatric gynecology. In: *Clinical Aspects of Aging*, 2nd ed. Reichel W (editor). Baltimore: Williams and Wilkins, 1983.

Hafez ES. *Aging and Reproductive Physiology*. Ann Arbor: Ann Arbor Science Publishers, 1976.

Malasanos L et al. *Health Assessment*, 3rd ed. St. Louis: Mosby, 1986.

Masters WH, Johnson VE. *Human Sexual Inadequacy*. Boston: Little, Brown, 1970.

Masters WH, Johnson VE. *Human Sexual Response*. Boston: Little, Brown, 1966.

Moran J. Sexuality: An ageless quality, a basic need. *Journal of Gerontological Nursing* September/October 1979; 5:13–16.

Woods NF. *Human Sexuality in Health and Illness*, 2nd ed. St. Louis: Mosby, 1979.

Wright VC. Carcinoma of the vulva. *Journal of the American Geriatrics Society* May 1976; 14(5):232–235.

14 Assessment of the Musculoskeletal System

Erick Larson, PT

The musculoskeletal system is an amazingly complex system, which millions of dollars have not helped us to duplicate. This system gives us shape and form while allowing an infinite variety of strength, speed, and coordination in our body movement. Imagine the jellylike masses we would all be without our musculoskeletal system! Although frequently misused, this system continues to function throughout a lifetime, without the need for extended rest or replacement.

To appreciate the musculoskeletal system fully, a brief review of its anatomy and physiology will be given. Specific anatomy and physiology textbooks are recommended in the bibliography for more detailed information.

REVIEW OF THE MUSCULOSKELETAL SYSTEM

The Skeletal Structure

Approximately 206 different bones provide levers for the muscles to move, support surrounding tissue, protect various organs, and enclose the blood-forming marrow within certain cavities.

The bones are not dry and rigid as seen in the typical laboratory skeleton. They are enclosed in a vascular membrane (periosteum) and have numerous blood vessels at each end. The bones are also resilient and capable of bending within certain limitations. They are structured for maximum strength and efficiency by having dense compact bone at mid-shaft where the bending stresses occur, and thinner layers of bone at the ends where lighter "spongy" bone exists. This spongy bone is actually a carefully arranged system of trabeculae that supports the compressing weight of the body. The best example of trabeculae occurs in the head of the femur where the trabeculae are similar to the struts and ties of a crane or modern suspension bridge. Bone, however, is more effective than most metals in its ability to resist crushing and tearing.

Bone is constantly changing with the continued deposit of new bone over the whole area (osteoblasts) and the reciprocal process of taking and shaping the bone (osteoclasts). Thus, bone is capable of healing a break and maintaining a smooth functional support system. Bones, however, also will atrophy or cease to grow when the stresses of weight bearing and muscular forces are decreased or eliminated. This atrophy often is evidenced in the bones of limbs that are paralyzed, casted, or rested for prolonged periods. Decalcification and osteoporosis (increased porousness of the bone) are not uncommon in the inactive older adult.

The Muscular System

Approximately 434 muscles in the body cause various parts of the body to move. They range in size from the small orbicularis oris muscle of the eye to the large gluteus maximus of the hip. They all have the common action of contraction. Muscles can only pull; they cannot push.

The muscles that will be discussed are those concerned with posture and movement. These muscles consist of approximately 75 pairs of muscles that must work together in order to accomplish any task. When one muscle contracts, its paired muscle, or antagonist, must relax. If cocontraction occurs, there is no motion.

The large fleshy part of the muscle that can be seen and felt is actually made up of many muscle units. These units consist of bundles of contractile muscle cells or fibers that are bound together to work in a smoothly coordinated fashion. Toward the end of the muscle belly, the contractile cells decrease, but the connective tissue that covers the fibers and bundles continues and becomes muscle tendon. The tendon attaches the muscle to the bone.

A muscle fiber is not simply a mechanism like a rubber band or a spring. The individual fibers must be able to function with the other fibers in the muscle body in order to maintain tone, to contract by gradually increasing tension, and to relax or lengthen. Muscle fibers form a highly complicated system consisting of many checks and balances that are dependent on many factors.

The Nervous System

In order to move, each muscle must receive a signal from the nervous system. This begins (except for reflex arc actions) within the brain and travels through the peripheral nerve to the muscle. Again, it is not as simple as, for instance, an electric impulse to which it is similar. One or more nerves enter the muscle. (Only one will be used in this example.) Each nerve has both a sensory and motor component and each contains a large number of motor axons that serve the bundles of muscle fibers (fasciculus) (Figure 14-1).

As these branches enter the fasciculus, the branch again divides into each muscle fiber. The groups of muscle fibers that are innervated by a motor nerve work as a single motor unit, although they may consist of as few as three in the eye muscles to as many as 400 in the large antigravity muscles. The work of the muscle is astonishing when one considers that there can be over 1,000,000 muscle fibers in one muscle receiving over 1000 nerve fibers.

The muscle fibers contract when a stimulus is received from the nerve fiber. The entire fiber will react to the stimulus; however, the number of muscle fibers and bundles of fibers that react is dependent on the strength of the stimulus. Each branch of the nerve works in a fine, integrated manner, bringing together only the necessary fibers required to perform the task. Thus, one is able to raise a feather or a 50-pound weight with a smooth, coordinated movement. Without this integration, spastic, uncoordinated movements would occur. Remember, the muscles can only respond to the strength and frequency of the stimulus received.

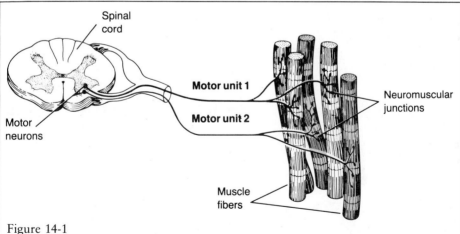

Figure 14-1

Two motor units of a muscle. The groups of muscle fibers that are innervated by a motor nerve work as a single motor unit. Source: Spence AP, Mason EB. *Human Anatomy and Physiology*, 2nd ed. Redwood City, CA: Benjamin/Cummings, 1983.

The muscle fiber is stimulated by a chemical (acetylcholine) that causes the contraction. The muscle would remain in a contracted state if another chemical (cholinesterase) did not mediate the effect of the stimulator. Thus, in order to have movement, there must be conduction by the nerve to the motor endplate, stimulation and mediation of the fibers, and a healthy muscle fiber.

Movement

The nervous system is complicated further by the mechanism of moving. The skeleton is basically a support structure with no movement. The neuro-muscular system provides movement once it is attached to the skeletal system. Thus, a series of levers consisting of links and hinges is produced, appropriately classified as first, second, and third class levers.

A first class lever has a fulcrum between the force (F) and the resistance (R). Figure 14-2 illustrates the use of a first class lever involved in raising the face. For movement to occur, there must be a difference in (a) the resistance times the length of distance between the fulcrum and the resistance (resistance

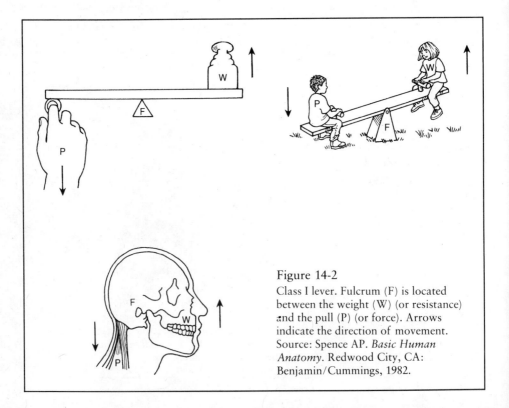

Figure 14-2

Class I lever. Fulcrum (F) is located between the weight (W) (or resistance) and the pull (P) (or force). Arrows indicate the direction of movement. Source: Spence AP. *Basic Human Anatomy*. Redwood City, CA: Benjamin/Cummings, 1982.

arm or RA), and (b) the force times the force arm (FA), which is the distance between the fulcrum and the force. For stability, this is commonly referred to as

$$R \times RA = F \times FA$$

The tricep is a first class lever. However, the FA is very short. Thus, the force has to be greater than the resistance to counteract the length of the resistance arm. The following equation illustrates this concept.

$$R \ (1 \ lb) \times RA \ (10'') = FA \ (1'') \times F \ (10 \ lb)$$

A second class lever has the fulcrum at the end of the force and resistance arm. The resistance is between the fulcrum and the force. The gastrocnemius and soleus are examples of a second class lever, with the body weight acting as the resistance (Figure 14-3). Using approximate figures, imagine the effort

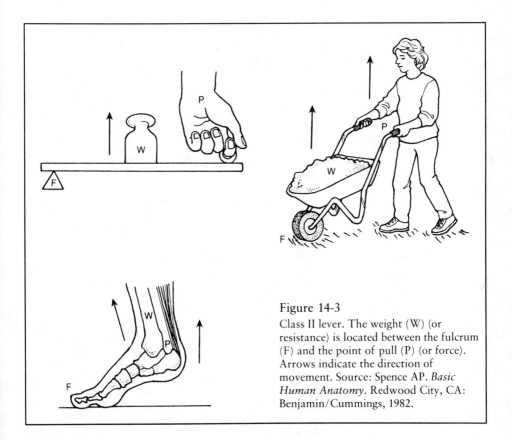

Figure 14-3

Class II lever. The weight (W) (or resistance) is located between the fulcrum (F) and the point of pull (P) (or force). Arrows indicate the direction of movement. Source: Spence AP. *Basic Human Anatomy*. Redwood City, CA: Benjamin/Cummings, 1982.

needed for a 100 lb person to stand on his or her toes:

$$\text{RA } (5'') \times \text{R } (100 \text{ lb}) = \text{FA } (1'') \times \text{F } (500 \text{ lb})$$

A third class lever also has the fulcrum at the end, with the force applied between the fulcrum and the resistance (Figure 14-4). This lever is the most inefficient for lifting but the most efficient for speed. It is also the most common lever in the body. The biceps is a good example of a third class lever.

Thus, if a person's arm weighed 3 lb and was lifting a 5-lb weight, the total resistance would be 8 lb (actually slightly less because the weight distribution

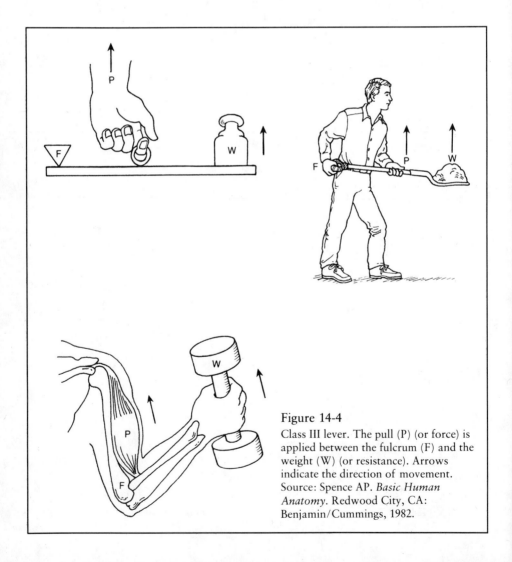

Figure 14-4

Class III lever. The pull (P) (or force) is applied between the fulcrum (F) and the weight (W) (or resistance). Arrows indicate the direction of movement. Source: Spence AP. *Basic Human Anatomy*. Redwood City, CA: Benjamin/Cummings, 1982.

of the arm is not in one place). Assuming the biceps attached 1″ from the fulcrum and the weight was 10″ from the fulcrum, the amount of force necessary to hold the weight would be:

$$F \times FA = R \times RA$$
$$F \times 1'' = 8 \times 10''$$
$$F = 80 \text{ lb}$$

This basic review points out the forces that are acting against the older adult during a physical assessment. In the example given, it should be noted that the fulcrum must receive all of the force; thus, the elbow joint would also be receiving 80 lb of pressure. The example only included one motion, assuming the fulcrum was stable. However, the human body is a series of levers and fulcrums, one acting on and depending on another. It was also assumed that the movement was smooth without any resistance at the fulcrum and, of course, without pain. In reality, the joint may have some degree of degeneration that causes resistance and pain when stressed.

AGE-RELATED CHANGES IN THE MUSCULOSKELETAL SYSTEM

Skeletal Changes

Not too long ago the common thinking was that if proper nutrition and exercise were maintained no consistent bone loss would occur in individuals, with the possible exception of postmenopausal women who were inactive and did not consume dairy products. However, this thinking has changed. We now know through research that adult bone loss takes place in both sexes, and it is not a sudden phenomenon brought about by hormonal changes but starts earlier in life around the age of 40 (Goldman and Rockstein 1975).

The causes of bone loss are not specifically known but are thought to include diet, hormonal changes, physical activity, and possibly RNA activity that is thought to be part of a great age control mechanism that affects bone, muscle, nerve, and other body functions.

The effect of this bone loss is simple: the bones become weaker. A loss of bone mass occurs; therefore, the vertebrae are not as firm and may become compressed. The long shaft bones, such as the femur, lose the cancellous structure, thus becoming less resistant to bending and more susceptible to breakage. Although neither of these conditions is life threatening, they can become debilitating and painful.

Due to a reduction in cartilage along the spinal column there is a 1.2 cm reduction in height every 20 years through adulthood (Jacobs 1981). Cartilage loss and fibrillar degeneration begin to appear in the knee joint in the second decade of life. There is a backward tilting of the head, reducing the occiput to shoulder distance.

Neuromuscular Changes

The impairment of motor capacity starts in one's thirties and declines rapidly with old age (Buerger and Tobis 1976). Again, a wide variability among different individuals exists and nothing is absolute. The heart's decreased efficiency in providing oxygen to the muscle has a direct effect on the muscle's ability to maintain a sustained work load. In addition, be aware that both diet and environmental factors are conditions that affect muscle function.

In the older adult, an approximate 15% slowing of nerve conduction time exists, which, although not overly significant in everyday activity, when combined with other changes will affect overall reaction. Additional factors involving strength play an important part in everyday activity. Buerger and Tobis identify four areas that contribute to the generalized weakening that occurs with age (Buerger and Tobis 1976):

1. A slowing of the impulse conduction along the motor units, especially at the distal regions of the axon, causing prolongation of the contraction time.

2. A decrease in the synthesis and release of the mediator, which will directly affect the contraction time and contribute to the interference with the smooth flow of continuous motor performance, that is, coordination. The decrease in the transmitter synthesis at the very latest stages of the aging process leads to a slowing of neuromuscular contact and random fallout of muscle fibers. Interestingly, this process is done randomly so that there are always some fibers to be activated, and although the transmitter release is decreased markedly in the senile motor units, it is not lost completely as in denervation. Also, there are no signs of terminal axon degeneration.

3. The motor unit size decreases, leading to a decrease in the amount of tetanic tension in the muscle fibers. This decrease in the tone of the muscle fibers leads to a decrease in the diameter of the fibers, which results in a decrease in the muscle strength.

4. A decrease in the glycolytic enzymes occurs, leading to a decrease in the oxidate activity. This results in increased fatigability and a greater need for rest.

Thus, the older client fatigues easily, has a slower reaction time due to a decrease in the nerve conduction and muscle tone, and may not display smooth, coordinated movement. You must be aware of these effects so you do not fatigue your client. For example, activities should be designed to allow for short periods of exercise, rather than one long session, followed by an adequate time for rest.

The aging process cannot be stopped, but it can be slowed. As noted, there often are several cumulative problems occurring with age that in themselves create a handicapping inefficiency. A decrease in speed, strength, reaction time, resistance to fatigue, and coordination are typical. What is not known or addressed in aging studies, for indeed it would be difficult and require a longitudinal study, is the effect of motivation and life-style on these aging processes.

ASSESSMENT OF THE MUSCULOSKELETAL SYSTEM

In assessing a "normal" 20- to 30-year-old individual, one could expect that there would be, for the most part, one specific diagnosis or complaint of the musculoskeletal system that could be easily identified. Through a series of objective tests, the strength, range of motion, sensation, and function could be evaluated and an accepted plan of action developed for that individual. The older individual is much more challenging due to the multiple social, medical, and environmental factors that complicate the assessment process. Although the same basic procedures are followed, your skill and knowledge as a nurse determines the assessment's effectiveness and completeness.

Whenever possible, do the musculoskeletal assessment in the client's home to enable the client to be rested and relaxed so you can make a more normal determination of strength and ability. If this is not possible, be sure that the client is not stressed or rushed from one place to another without any chance to rest during the examination. The entire process of preparing for an examination, leaving a familiar surrounding, and being transported or walking to an examining area are very fatiguing exercises. If a secondary complication involving the cardiovascular system exists, these efforts become more taxing. A musculoskeletal assessment is a tiring exercise. Allow time during and after the assessment for rest.

Obtain a history from both the medical record and the client. Be aware that various aches and pains may be exaggerated or ignored and attributed to "getting old." An awareness of other complicating chronic conditions is helpful also.

First, observe the client (Figure 14-5). Watch the client walk in the house or to the examining room. Walk with him or her to where the assessment is to take place. Watch how the client moves, sits, and talks. Is there a deviation from the midline while sitting, weight bearing, or during the swing phase of walking? Accompanying the client while he or she walks should put the person at ease, help to correlate the history with actual findings, and assist in narrowing the area to assess initially. The key to intervention is *function*.

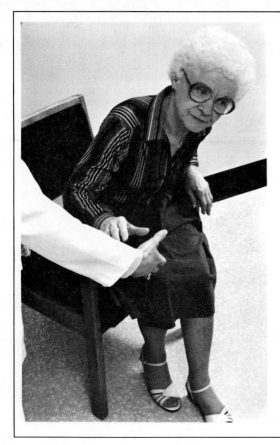

Figure 14-5
Observing the client's mobility can give valuable insight into the status of the musculoskeletal system.

Second, review the area of complaint. This may be a slow, tedious process, but it is vitally important. Skill and diligence are necessary in order to separate the various complaints. The time you take to do this also allows the client to rest.

Third, proceed with the physical assessment. This includes range of motion and muscle evaluation.

Range of Motion (ROM)

Evaluation of range of motion is relatively simple and usually painless. Both active (how far the person can independently move the extremities) and passive (how far the nurse can move the extremities) movements are included. Is there a difference? It is not critical that the ROM is 100% in all motions, but it is important that the client is able to move sufficiently to carry out normal living activities. For example, a 20-year-old would be expected to have 180° range of motion in shoulder flexion. An 80-year-old may be expected to have that motion also if he or she routinely must reach into a cupboard above his or her head. However, 90° may be sufficient in order to dress and cook if necessary materials are on the lower shelves.

Range of motion should include all motions of the joints. Frequently, rotation of the hip and shoulder are forgotten or overlooked. A client may have full flexion, but the inability to rotate externally may cause an increase in pain or an inability to get dressed independently. In assessing passive ROM, be sure to give support above and below the joint so that as much pressure as possible is taken away from all the interconnecting joints (Figure 14-6).

Muscle Evaluation

Kendall has best described how a normal test can and should be done (Kendall and Kendall 1971). With slight modifications, the technique is correct for older adults.

Because of the physiologic changes previously mentioned, you should expect some weakness. There are no specific guidelines as to an acceptable degree of weakness, but the amount of weakness should partially relate to functional ability. Also, there may be some difference in the upper extremities, with the dominant hand and arm slightly stronger. However, the lower extremities should have equal strength. If a consistent weakness on the nondominant side occurs, you should not assume normalcy, for this could indicate some neurologic involvement. There should be some correlation between any identified weakness and either an existing diagnosis or complaint.

Arthritic persons frequently demonstrate weakness for at least two reasons. The first reason relates to pain. If pain is present in the joint, then the person is not going to exercise the muscle and increase the pain. Secondly, the bony changes associated with arthritis will cause a change in the direction of the pull and/or a stretching of the tendon, making the force even more inefficient.

The muscle evaluation should consist of two parts, the first being an isometric contraction with the muscle contracted to its shortest position. In this position, apply resistance to cause the muscle to "give a little." A 100% or normal grade muscle will hold its position. This procedure tests the muscle's total strength in holding its shortest position. Secondly, with the muscle relaxed, apply maximum resistance throughout the active range. The muscle contraction should be smooth and steady and actually increase in strength near the end of the range. This procedure tests the person's ability to maintain a continuous strong contraction throughout the range and is a practical assessment in determining functional ability.

Manual muscle testing will identify specific problem areas that relate directly to and affect function. A weakness of one muscle will directly affect the neighboring muscle's ability to function effectively. However, you should not rely entirely on individual muscle testing for the total evaluation. A muscle

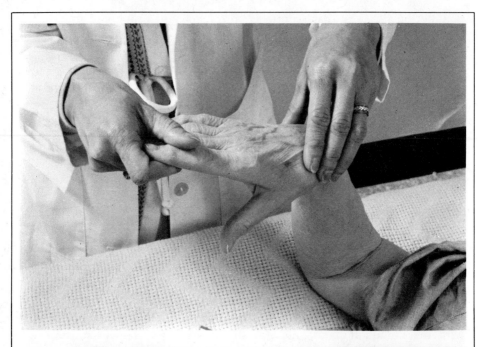

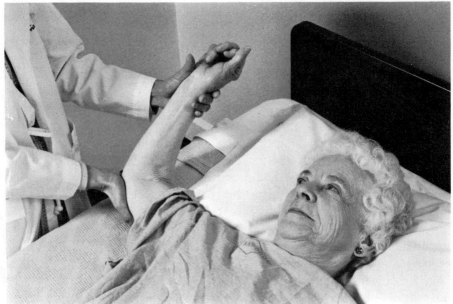

Figure 14-6

Provide support above and below the joint when performing passive range of motion. See also photograph at top of next page.

Figure 14-6—(*Continued*)

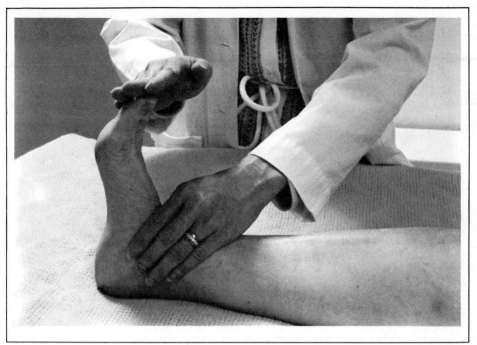

test on the lower extremities of an older person may indicate that the muscles are too weak to attempt stairs, but the person actually may climb two flights of steps daily. This is due to the interrelationships of the muscles and joints as well as the adaptations made by the individual which, when working together, are greater than the sum of the individual parts. A muscle evaluation can test one muscle at a time or a group of muscles. Although the tests may indicate weaknesses, you must determine if the adaptation made by the individual is stable or whether the weakness will lead to progressive functional disability.

Standing tests include walking up and down stairs, preferably home steps; walking forward, backward, and sideways; crossing one leg in front of the other while moving sideways, tested in both directions; standing on one foot; walking on toes; and walking on heels. These activities help you to obtain a more accurate picture of the functional muscle strength of the lower extremities.

You cannot disassociate the musculoskeletal system from the nervous system. Sensation, balance, vision, and other neurologic functions all have a direct effect on musculoskeletal assessment.

In assessing the musculoskeletal system, you must use not only your hands, but also your eyes. Watch the person's face for grimaces of pain or anticipated pain. You must be gentle but firm, and most of all you must have patience.

To assess the head and neck, observe active motion in flexion, extension, rotation, and lateral flexion to both sides. Rarely will there be a need for testing strength or testing passive motion beyond the active range.

In assessing the shoulder and arms, observe the scapula by standing behind the person as he or she leans and pushes against a wall or your hand. The scapula should not bulge back. This is important because if the scapula cannot stabilize, the humerus will not be able to go through the full motion even if strength is normal.

The extensor muscles of the shoulder and elbow are most important, for they assist in standing and give support when using a cane, crutches, or walker. Be sure to check shoulder depression (latissimus dorsi) by pushing the shoulders down against resistance at the elbow.

Check internal and external rotation, actively and passively. There should be only a minimal (5° to 10°) increase passively.

To assess hands, check for equal strength in both flexion and extension, combined with coordination and fine pinch. Also, observe the interosseous for atrophy or wasting.

To assess the trunk, observe for proper postural alignment and movement. Again, it is rarely necessary to do any resistance; the weight of the body is sufficient in determining adequate strength.

Whenever doing a leg assessment, observe for pain signals. Pain may be due to muscle spasms of the low back muscles, arthritis of the hip or vertebrae, bony deformity of the vertebrae, or tight hip or back muscles. Depending on the cause, hip movement can facilitate pain in the back, the hip, and the leg. The hip muscles directly affect trunk positioning during ambulation. Observe them before the evaluation.

Active hip flexion through the normal range is sufficient. There is no need to give resistance to hip flexion due to the increased pressure this places on the lumbar vertebrae for stabilization. Straight leg raising is done to observe for muscle tightness and/or low back pain. This movement should always be done passively.

Closely observe hip extension. Is there complete extension or is there a hip flexion contracture? Is the trunk steady and upright during ambulation? Can the person walk up and down stairs easily? Many older persons will not be able to tolerate the prone position used to test the hip extensors; therefore, it is important to identify any problems before doing specific tests. The same is true for the hip abductors; however, they are easier to isolate while standing than the hip extensors. Simply have the person stand upright on one foot. If the trunk remains steady and straight, the hip abductors are stabilizing. If the trunk shifts in either direction, the abductor is not stabilizing, thus resulting in an unsteady gait pattern.

When assessing the knee, assure that it has complete extension. This evaluation should be done passively and, more important, actively with resistance. Can the knee be held straight? Can the person extend the knee smoothly against an equal amount of pressure? Does the muscle strength decrease during the last 5° of extension? The last 5° are critical in walking and climbing stairs, and in stabilizing the knee and preventing the legs from "buckling."

When evaluating the ankle, determine strength and steadiness. Observe the kind of shoes that the client is wearing. High heels or ill-fitting shoes may be the only cause for an unsteady gait.

Manual resistance will indicate inequality, but body weight is the true test. Have the client walk on his or her toes or rise up on toes ten times (plantar flexors testing); walk on heels holding toes up (dorsi flexors testing); and walk sideways (ankle evertors testing). If weakness or uncoordination is suspected, be sure to be close to the client to prevent a fall. The ankle is supporting the entire body weight each time a step is taken, and if the ankle cannot stabilize, the client will fall.

Gait

Ask the client to walk down a corridor so that you can fully evaluate gait. Observe arm swinging: Is it present and symmetrical? Are the arms postured in flexion? Observe leg follow-through: Is the gait free and easy? Are the steps too small? Is the base widened? Does the client weave or appear unsteady (ataxic)? Is footdrop present? Does circumduction occur at the hip? Does the client have difficulty getting started, as though stuck to the floor? Can the client turn and stop with ease? Some of the common abnormalities of gait are described in Table 14-1.

DISORDERS OF THE MUSCULOSKELETAL SYSTEM

Muscle Cramps

Muscle cramps are a common occurrence in older adults. Although unusual muscle use frequently causes these painful, involuntary muscle contractions, muscle cramps also occur during resting states among older adults. This problem also can result from poor peripheral circulation, peripheral nerve disease, hypoglycemia, uremia, and deficiencies of calcium and sodium. Muscle cramps can also occur among healthy older adults who have no unusual clinical findings.

Tremors

Observation should be made for abnormal movements. *Tremor* is rhythmic, alternating movement of a body part. Jerking movements of an extremity are not tremor. To evaluate tremor, observe the client sitting or lying quietly and with the arms extended in front of him or her. Is tremor present? Does it go away with movement?

Table 14-1 Abnormalities of Gait

Gait	Characteristics	Potential Disorder
Ataxic	Weaving, uncoordinated, uneven steps; foot may be raised high and then fall, with entire sole striking against floor	Cerebellum disease; severe alcohol or barbiturate intoxication
Equine	Slow, cumbersome steps; foot raised high with thigh against abdomen	Peroneal paralysis
Festinating	Body rigid and bent forward; arms lean forward and do not swing with steps; steps are short, shuffling and often on tiptoes; gait starts slowly and continues to increase; gait may be difficult to stop without client confronting an obstruction	Parkinsonism
Flat-footed	Sole and arches depressed and touch floor surface; toes everted; legs may be bowed	Acute or chronic flat-footedness
Footslapping	Broad base gait; foot raised abnormally high; foot dropped with sole slapping against floor; client may carefully watch where foot will be placed	Peripheral nerve disease; paralysis of pretibial and peroneal muscles
Hemiplegic	On affected side, arm flexed and held close to body; leg swings out laterally and is brought forward; footdrop may be noted, recognized by foot being dragged or knee lifted abnormally high	Hemiplegia
Scissors	Legs held close together and crossing during steps	Spastic paraplegia; paresis associated with organic brain disease; cerebral palsy
Spastic	Stiff, jerking, uncoordinated gait; legs held together stiffly; hips and knees slightly flexed; toes drag	Spastic paraplegia; multiple sclerosis; spinal cord tumor
Waddling	"Duck-like" gait; feet wide apart; exaggerated lateral leaning with steps because one hip is excessively elevated and the other depressed; lumbar lordosis may be present	Muscular dystrophy; double congenital hip displacement; weakness of gluteus medius muscle

Common types of tremor include the following:

- *Physiologic*: This is the normal tremulousness associated with being nervous. It can be accentuated with alcohol or drug withdrawal, and in hyperthyroidism.
- *Parkinsonian tremor*: This is a resting tremor occurring in the fingers, hands, feet, lips, or head. It is absent or greatly diminished with activity and is accompanied by muscular rigidity and difficulty in initiating movement.
- *Benign, familial, or postural tremor*: This tremor is absent or minimal at rest and is increased by motion. It is often prominent in the head and asymmetrical in the arms. It is strongly familial. No other neurologic signs are present. The so-called "senile" tremor is often of this type.
- *Cerebellar or intention tremor*: This is absent at rest and becomes apparent with motion. It is usually associated with other cerebellar signs, such as ataxia.

Osteoporosis

Osteoporosis is a metabolic disorder that reduces bone density through the loss of mineral and protein in the bone matrix. Most of the recent public attention to this problem has revolved around the role of calcium deficiency in causing this problem; however, inactivity, estrogen or androgen deficiency, and hyperthyroidism are also potential causes. Approximately 25% of women and 20% of men over age 70 are believed to be affected with osteoporosis.

More often than not osteoporosis is asymptomatic until it has significantly progressed. Bone pain or a fracture may be the first indication of the disease. The lumbar and thoracic vertebrae tend to be involved more than the long bones or skull. As the disease progresses, kyphosis, spinal deformities, limitations of spinal movement, and a reduction of height are present. At least 25% of the calcium content of the bone has to be lost before demineralization of the bone is shown on x-ray (Spencer, Sontag, and Kramer 1986).

Photon absorptiometry is a diagnostic technique used to measure the mineral content of the long bones (usually the radius is used), although sometimes the measurement of the bone used does not always reflect the condition of the overall skeletal mass. Calcium tolerance testing may be performed, whereby the ability of the skeleton to retain intravenously infused calcium is measured. Urinary calcium excretion may be evaluated also. Confirmation of the diagnosis is done by bone biopsy.

With all the media attention to osteoporosis and the recommendations for calcium supplements, it could be useful to question clients about their use of calcium supplements. Once osteoporosis is present, calcium supplements will not be useful in restoring lost bone. Also, excessive calcium ingestion can cause health problems, such as confusion. Clients' misperceptions of calcium supplements should be clarified.

Osteoarthritis

Years of wear and tear on the joints lead to the deterioration and abrasion of joint cartilage, known as osteoarthritis (Figure 14-7). Chronic joint trauma, obesity, and excessive joint use predispose individuals to this form of arthritis. This condition increases in incidence with age and is a fairly common problem in the older population.

Osteoarthritis primarily affects the weight-bearing joints with stiffening and a gradual development of aching pain. Bony nodules may develop on the affected joint and crepitus may be present on joint motion. Symptoms are associated with the affected joint and are not systemic.

The client's history of symptoms and x-ray findings confirm the diagnosis of osteoarthritis. Blood abnormality is not associated with this type of arthritis.

Rheumatoid Arthritis

Although it does not affect as many older adults as osteoarthritis, rheumatoid arthritis is a serious problem because of its deforming and debilitating effects. Older persons may develop this condition as a new problem in old age. However, it is more likely that they developed it in earlier years, especially during their third and fourth decades when the incidence of rheumatoid arthritis peaks. This disorder affects more women than men, and persons with a positive family history are also more susceptible.

The small joints of the hands and feet are the joints most often affected, although virtually any joint may be involved. The affected joint is red, warm, stiff, and painful. It typically shows subcutaneous nodules over bony prominences and atrophy of the surrounding muscles (Figure 14-7). In time, flexion contractures develop, adding further to the client's disability. Systemic symptoms also are present, including low-grade fever, fatigue, malaise, weakness, weight loss, anemia, and tachycardia.

Examination of synovial fluid and x-rays help in the diagnosis of rheumatoid arthritis. Also useful is laboratory evaluation of the blood for anemia, increased globulins, decreased albumin, elevated erythrocyte sedimentation rate, and positive C-reactive protein, all associated with this disorder.

Whenever musculoskeletal problems exist, you should assess the client's ability to manage the pain that accompanies these disorders. A full exploration of medication use, heat application methods, activity restrictions, and other measures related to these disorders is essential to determine the treatment

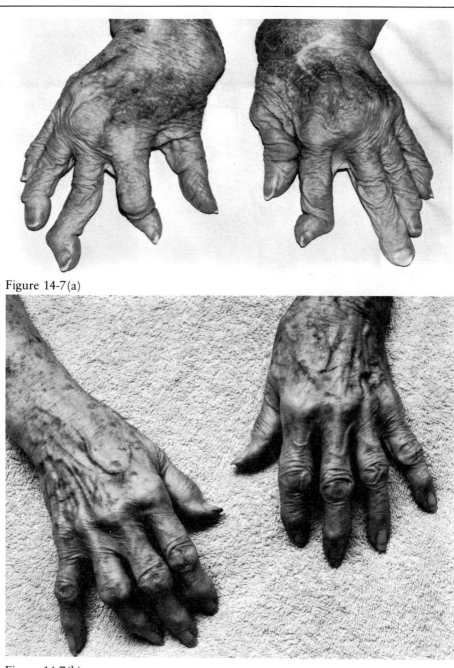

Figure 14-7(a)

Figure 14-7(b)

Rheumatoid arthritis (a) is much more deforming and debilitating than osteoarthritis (b).
Source for photograph b: Bluestone R. *Practical Rheumatology: Diagnosis and Management.* Menlo Park, CA: Addison-Wesley, 1980.

regimen's appropriateness. The client may be creating problems secondary to the management of pain, such as aspirin abuse, skin injury from heat application, and contractures from restricted mobility.

Clients with musculoskeletal deformities, tremors, gait disturbances, and limited function may reduce their interaction with society due to fear of being ridiculed, rejected, or even victimized. Musculoskeletal problems can significantly impact the older adult's ability to engage in normal daily activities. You should explore the clients' ability to climb stairs, get in and out of chairs, prepare meals, dress, and be mobile. The difficulty in completing tasks that persons with normal functions take for granted (such as crossing a street when the light changes, boarding a bus quickly, or negotiating several packages when in a crowded store) may lead older persons to withdraw from activity and become socially isolated. Additionally, older adults may become depressed and frustrated if unable to participate in normal activities within one's home or community due to the disability, deformity, and discomfort associated with musculoskeletal disorders. During the assessment, you must consider the impact of these problems on the total well-being of the older individual.

14 Chapter Summary

I. Age-related changes
   A. Loss of bone, starting at fourth decade of life
   B. Weakening bone
   C. Impairment of motor capacity, starting in third decade of life
   D. Generalized muscle weakness
   E. Decreased muscle strength
   F. Slower reaction time
   G. Poorer coordination
   H. Increased muscle fatigability

II. Assessment
   A. History from medical record and client
   B. General evaluation of function
   C. Review complaints
   D. Physical assessment
      1. Range of motion
         a) Active and passive movements for all joints
         b) 100% range of motion not as critical as ability to perform normal living activities
      2. Muscle evaluation
         a) Isometric contraction with muscle contracted to its shortest position. Apply resistance to determine if muscle will hold its position. Normal grade muscle will hold its position.
         b) Range of motion: Apply resistance throughout active range of motion to determine ability to maintain continuous strong contraction throughout range
      3. Primary areas of assessment
         a) Head and neck: flexion,

extension, rotation, and lateral flexion to both sides

b) Shoulder: rotation and strength of scapula and extensor muscles

c) Hands: equality of strength in flexion and extension; coordination of fine pinch

d) Trunk: postural alignment and movement

e) Hip: flexion, rotation, and stabilizing of abductors

f) Knee: extension

g) Ankle: strength and steadiness

h) Gait: ease, steps, coordination

III. Disorders

A. Muscle cramps
1. Involuntary muscle contractions
2. Causes: unusual muscle use, poor peripheral circulation, peripheral nerve disease, hypoglycemia, uremia, deficiencies of calcium and sodium.

B. Tremors
1. Physiologic tremor: due to nervousness, hyperthyroidism, alcohol or drug withdrawal
2. Parkinsonian tremor: resting tremor, diminished with activity
3. Benign, familial, or postural tremor (senile tremor): minimal at rest, increased with activity
4. Cerebellar or intention tremor: absent at rest, apparent with motion; usually accompanies other cerebellar signs

C. Osteoporosis
1. Reduction in bone density due to loss of mineral and protein in bone matrix
   a) Contributing factors: calcium deficiency, reduction in estrogen or androgen, inactivity, hyperthyroidism
2. May be asymptomatic until bone pain or fracture occur
   a) 25% calcium content of bone must be lost before loss is apparent on x-ray

D. Osteoarthritis
1. Deterioration and abrasion of joint cartilage
2. Predisposing factors: senescence, chronic joint trauma, obesity, excessive joint use
3. Primarily affects joints bearing weight
4. Signs: joint pain and stiffness, bony nodules (Heberden's nodes), crepitus
5. No systemic effects

E. Rheumatoid arthritis
1. Deforming, debilitating disease
2. Higher incidence in women and those with family history of disease
3. Primarily affects small joints of hands and feet
4. Local signs: joint is red, warm, stiff, painful; subcutaneous nodules over bony prominences; atrophy of surrounding muscle; flexion contractures
5. Systemic symptoms: low-grade fever, fatigue, malaise, weakness, weight loss, anemia, tachycardia

IV. Related nursing diagnoses
A. Activity intolerance
B. Pain
C. Impaired home maintenance management

D. Potential for injury
E. Knowledge deficit
F. Impaired physical mobility
G. Self-care deficit
H. Personal identity disturbance

I. Sexual dysfunction
J. Impaired skin integrity
K. Sleep pattern disturbance
L. Impaired social interaction

READINGS AND REFERENCES

Buerger AA, Tobis JS (editors). *Neurophysiologic Aspects of Rehabilitation Medicine.* Springfield, IL: Charles C. Thomas, 1976.

Chusid J, McDonald J. *Correlative Neuroanatomy and Functional Neurology.* Los Altos, CA: Lange, 1980.

Devas M. *Geriatric Orthopedics.* New York: Academic Press, 1977.

Finch CE. *Handbook of the Biology of Aging.* New York: Van Nostrand Reinhold, 1977.

Fries JF. *Arthritis.* Reading, MA: Addison-Wesley, 1979.

Goldman R, Rockstein M. *The Physiology and Pathology of Human Aging.* New York: Academic Press, 1975.

Guyton RN. *Textbook of Medical Physiology,* 6th ed. Philadelphia: Saunders, 1981.

Imms FJ, Edholm OG. Studies of gait and mobility in the elderly. *Aged Aging* August 1980; 10(3):147–156.

Jacobs R. Physical changes in the aged. In: *Elder Care: A Guide to Clinical Geriatrics.* Devereaux MO et al (editors). New York: Grune and Stratton, 1981.

Kendall HO, Kendall FP. *Muscle Testing and Function.* Baltimore: Williams and Wilkins, 1971.

Mayne I. Examination of the back in the geriatric patient. *Journal of the American Geriatric Society* 1977; 25:559–563.

Paterson CR, MacLennon WJ. *Bone Disease in the Elderly.* New York: Wiley, 1984.

Rasch B. *Kinesiology and Applied Anatomy,* 6th ed. Philadelphia: Lea and Febiger, 1978.

Reichel W (editor). *Clinical Aspects of Aging.* Baltimore: Williams and Wilkins, 1978.

Richards M. Osteoporosis. *Geriatric Nursing* March/April 1982; 3(2):98–102.

Spencer H, Sontag SJ, Kramer L. Disorders of the skeletal system. In: *Clinical Geriatrics,* 3rd ed. Rossman I (editor). Philadelphia: Lippincott, 1986, p 527.

15 Assessment of the Feet

Charlotte Eliopoulos, RNC, MPH

In comparison to listening to breath sounds, palpating for masses, and percussing organ size, examining older adults' feet seems unexciting. However, the condition of the feet is an important part of the total health status and demands adequate attention during the assessment process. Not only can poor foot health be a reflection of general health problems present in older adults, but it can clue you to other potential problems that may be secondary to foot disorders. For instance, poor foot health can cause pain, activity limitation, dependency, altered self-concept, and embarrassing and disabling deformities. Thus, the condition of the feet can significantly affect the older adult's physical, emotional, and social well-being.

THE HEALTHY FOOT

The healthy foot is free from breaks, fissures, calluses, rashes and growths. Flexion, extension, inversion, eversion, and lateral movement, all with ease, are possible. Although the movement will be limited when compared with the fingers, the toes can flex, extend, abduct, and adduct. Toenails are firmly attached and straight in growth; some thickening of the nail may be present. A longitudinal arch, extending from the heel to the toe, and a transverse or metatarsal arch, extending across the foot, exist (Figure 15-1). Pulses may be palpated on the foot's dorsum (dorsalis pedis pulse) and below the ankle's medial maleolus (posterior tibial pulse); both are equal (Figure 15-2). Temperatures of both feet also are equal and consistent with the general body temperature. Some mild pallor is not uncommon. Normally, there is no pain, edema, discoloration, or tenderness of the foot.

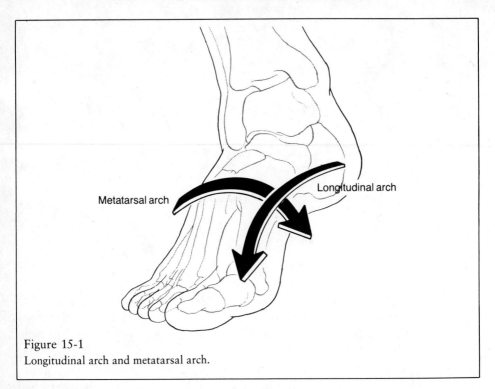

Figure 15-1
Longitudinal arch and metatarsal arch.

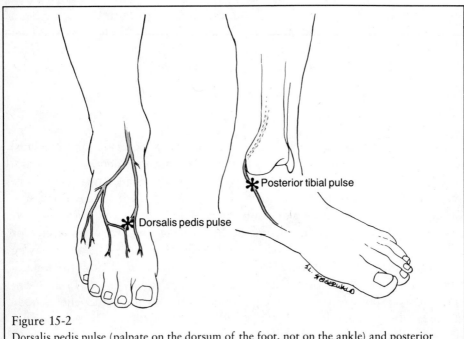

Figure 15-2
Dorsalis pedis pulse (palpate on the dorsum of the foot, not on the ankle) and posterior tibial pulse.

ASSESSMENT OF THE FOOT

Assessment of the foot begins as soon as the client is within your sight by observing gait. Note if the client moves easily or with difficulty. Is there a limp, unsteadiness or evidence of pain? Does the entire foot make contact with the floor? While observing gait (see Chapter 14), observe the fit condition of the shoes. You can learn a great deal about the status of the feet before the client sits down to have the naked foot examined. Are shoes so large that they easily slip off, or are they too tight, thus impairing circulation? Is there evidence of edema where the foot meets the shoe or any pressure areas? Do the shoes reflect wear in specific areas, or have they been cut or altered by the client for better fit? Are the style and heel size safe? Do the shoes offer adequate protection? (Figure 15-3).

As the client removes the shoes for the foot examination, note the stockings. Are they of a constricting nature or are circular garters used? Is there evidence that dye from the stockings has bled onto or irritated the foot? Have the stockings wrinkled within the shoe and left indentations on the foot? At this time, note the general cleanliness and odor of the feet.

Much is gained just through general inspection of the foot. Some of the findings to note are as follows.

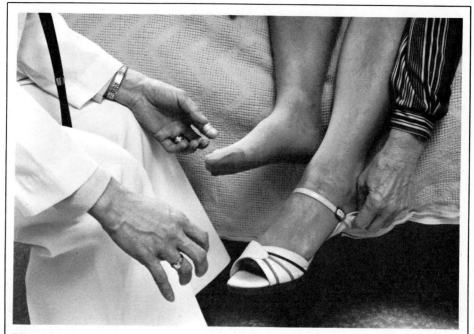

Figure 15-3
While the client takes off his/her shoes in preparation for assessment of the feet, be attentive to the condition and fit of the shoes and stockings.

Discoloration: No redness or cyanosis should be present. Observe the color of the entire foot, including small areas of discoloration on the toes and the undersurface of the foot. Test the blanching in the foot.

Fissures: The heels and the area between the toes are primary locations for fissures. Since dry, cracked, and dead skin areas create excellent sites for bacterial growth, explore evidence of infection if fissures are present.

Corns: A corn is a red, dry, thickened piece of skin usually found over a bony prominence, resulting from chronic pressure on the bony prominence of the toe. The corn is actually cone-shaped with the tip of the cone pointing inward and leading to pain when pressure is placed on it.

Calluses: A callus is a broad-based thickened area of skin that develops from chronic diffuse pressure. It differs from a corn in that it usually forms on an area that normally has thick skin, such as the sole of the foot, and is not painful.

Plantar Wart: A small area on the sole of the foot that looks like a callus but is painful may be a plantar wart. The edges surrounding the thickened skin area will be more defined than a callus, and typically, small dark spots can be seen within the area.

Rash: Rashes can be due to infections or allergic reactions. Note the location and relationship to stockings and shoes. Question the client as to length of time present, itching, and factors associated with its onset.

Structural deformities: Identify displacement and deviations of the toes. Hallux valgus exists when there is medial deviation of the first metatarsal and abduction of the great toe in relation to that metatarsal. A bursa (bunion) may form at the medial side of the metatarsal. A hammertoe (digiti flexus) can occur on any of the lesser toes, although it most commonly involves the second toe. It is identified by hyperextension at the metatarsophalangeal joint with flexion and frequently corn formation at the proximal interphalangeal joint. Another structural problem to note is the presence of overlapping toes. Arthritis-related deformities and contractures should be described.

Toenails: The nail's general thickness, color, care, and pattern of growth are significant. Onychauxis refers to a thickening of the nail, a condition commonly found among older adults. Also common in geriatric populations is fungus toenails, onychomycosis. Onycholysis refers to a loosening of the nail at its distal portion. Ingrown nails, onychocryptosis, exist when the edge of the nail pierces the skin fold; note associated infection. Ask specific questions regarding how the client cuts and cares for the toenails.

Fallen arches: Flat feet can be detected most rapidly when the client is standing. Typically, the longitudinal arch flattens and the medial concave border becomes convex. The entire sole comes in contact with the floor surface. Special shoes with built-up arches can aid in ease of walking and prevention of falls.

Ulcerative lesions: Ulcerations on the foot are usually associated with local pressure. Often, systemic diseases, such as diabetes mellitus and advanced arteriosclerosis, manifest themselves through these lesions. Therefore, diagnostic evaluation for systemic diseases may be warranted if ulcers are present. Conversely, clients with diseases that cause poor peripheral circulation must be observed carefully for ulcer formation.

Palpation of the foot can also give useful insight into foot health. The anterior surface of the ankle joint is palpated for edema and tenderness. Palpate each joint on the foot and the Achilles tendon for nodules and tenderness. Take all joints through a full range of motion.

Palpate the pulses on the foot for rate, strength, and bilateral similarity. To palpate the dorsalis pedis pulse, place several fingers on the dorsum, slightly lateral to the extensor tendon of the great toe. (Be sure not to palpate on the ankle.) The posterior tibial pulse is palpated behind and below the medial malleolus of the ankle. It is not uncommon to experience difficulty in obtaining these pulses. Keeping the fingers in place for a while and varying the pressure used to palpate the pulse may help locate the pulse. During palpation, be aware of the temperature of the feet, comparing one to the other.

THE FEET IN LATER LIFE

Few older adults have healthy feet. Dermatologic problems and structural deformities of the feet are frequent findings and result in significant disability and pain for many older adults. Although not all foot disorders can be eliminated in the older adult, conscientious nursing actions can prevent and improve disorders. Use the assessment as a time to educate the client in healthy foot practices. For instance, if the client uses constricting garters, discuss the impact of this on circulation and advise about alternatives. Similarly, if you detect reddened pressure areas from shoes, give warning to prevent future corns, calluses, and ulcers. Some of the recommendations that you can give to the client include:

- Wear shoes that fit well and offer adequate support and comfort. A wide, low heel offers good support. Avoid wearing for long durations slippers or soft shoes that offer little support.
- Cut toenails straight across, even with the end of the toes.
- Keep feet clean and inspect them daily for breaks, blisters, and discolorations. This is particularly useful for older adults since their decreased sensations may cause them to be unaware of such problems. (A family member or caregiver should inspect the older person's feet if he or she is unable to see or manipulate to do so.)
- Wear clean, well-fitting stockings. Avoid stockings with bleeding dyes.
- Do not walk indoors or outdoors in barefeet.
- Measure water temperature before soaking feet to avoid burns.
- Protect feet from exposure to cold and sun.
- Do not use sharp objects to clean under toenails or to cut off corns and calluses. Avoid commercial preparations to remove corns and calluses.
- Exercise the feet, putting all joints through a full range of motion several times daily.
- See a podiatrist for foot problems and attend to foot problems early.

In an institutional setting, it is wise to include directions for regular foot inspections and arrangements for toenail cutting as routine parts of the older client's care plan. Never forget that good foot health is a significant factor in the older adult's physical, emotional, and social well-being.

15 Chapter Summary

I. Normal findings
 A. No breaks in skin
 B. Foot capable of flexion, extension, inversion, eversion, and lateral movement

C. Toes can flex, extend, abduct, and adduct
D. Arches present
  1. Longitudinal
  2. Transverse or metatarsal

E. Pulses palpable
1. Dorsalis pedis
2. Posterior tibial
F. Temperature consistent with body temperature

II. Assessment
A. Observation
1. Gait
2. Steadiness
3. Evidence of pain
4. Shoes and stockings
5. Edema
6. Discoloration
7. Fissures
8. Dermatologic problems
9. Structural deformities
10. Toenails
11. Arches
B. Palpation
1. Range of motion
2. Pain
3. Tenderness
4. Pulses

III. Foot problems
A. Corns
B. Calluses
C. Plantar warts

D. Rashes
E. Hallux valgus
F. Digiti flexus (hammertoe)
G. Overlapping toes
H. Onychauxis
I. Onychomycosis
J. Onycholysis
K. Onychocryptosis
L. Flat feet
M. Ulcerative lesions
N. Arthritic joints
O. Poor circulation

IV. Related nursing diagnoses
A. Activity intolerance
B. Pain
C. Diversional activity deficit
D. Altered health maintenance
E. Impaired home maintenance management
F. Potential for infection
G. Potential for injury
H. Knowledge deficit
I. Impaired physical mobility
J. Personal identity disturbance
K. Sensory-perceptual alterations
L. Impaired skin integrity
M. Social isolation

READINGS AND REFERENCES

Helfand AF. Foot health for the elderly patient. In: *Clinical Aspects of Aging*, 2nd ed. Reichel W (editor). Baltimore: Waverly Press, 1983.

Helfand AF. Podiatric considerations for the aged patient. *Nursing Homes* 1971; 20:30–31.

Jahss MH. Geriatric aspects of the foot and ankle. In: *Clinical Geriatrics*, 3rd ed. Rossman I (editor). Philadelphia: Lippincott, 1986, pp 567–577.

King PA. Foot assessment of the elderly. In: *Readings in Gerontological Nursing*. Stilwell EM (editor). Thorofare, NJ: Charles B. Slack, 1980.

Schaefer A. Nursing measures to maintain foot health. *Geriatric Nursing* May/June 1982; 3(3):182–183.

Smiler I. Foot problems of elderly diabetics. *Geriatric Nursing* May/June 1982; 3(3):177–181.

16 Integrating Skills: Case Example

Charlotte Eliopoulos, RNC, MPH

The following is a narrative example of an assessment of an older adult. To acquaint you with the client, this example is considerably more extensive than typical written assessments. Many agencies have assessment or history forms that allow nurses to record data more efficiently. You may find it useful to try to develop a problem list and initial plans based on the narrative. Then compare your notes to the nurse's documentation, which follows the case situation. Remember, strive for accuracy, organization, and completeness. Your aim is to determine the best individualized plan of care for the client.

As you have seen, gerontological nursing focuses on the needs of a specific client population, needs embracing a multitude of psychosocial conditions. The older adult frequently comes to you not with just one specific disorder, but with a myriad of health problems such as reduced physical capabilities, depression, poor nutrition, and degenerative diseases. It is hoped that this text has enhanced your understanding of the dynamics and interrelationship of physical, mental, and social function, thus clarifying your role of giving care to the total person. Integrate the skills you've learned. Continue to develop and refine them. Assessment is the initial step in the process of delivering quality nursing care, the key to making a positive difference in the quality of life for the older adult.

CASE EXAMPLE

Marjorie Ellis is a 70-year-old white female. Her address is 632 South Chapel Lane. She has no telephone of her own but is able to use her next door neighbor's telephone whenever necessary. (That number is 728-1901 and belongs to Mrs. Blake.)

Mrs. Ellis came to America from Poland at 8 years of age and retains an accent, although she communicates well in English. Due to family circumstances, she was able to complete only up to the fourth grade of school. She was a domestic worker until marrying her husband in 1928 and has not been employed since then. Mrs. Ellis had a daughter who died in 1948 from peritonitis and has a son, now aged 46, who is unmarried and lives with her. Her husband died from a heart attack ten years ago.

A small pension plan from Mr. Ellis's company and social security benefits give Mrs. Ellis a $320 monthly income. Mrs. Ellis's son is usually unemployed and contributes nothing to the budget. Thus, Mrs. Ellis pays all expenses for herself and her son. Monthly expenses consist of $125 for food, $60 for utilities, and $100 for taxes and maintenance on the house she owns. Occasionally she has a month when utilities and food bills are lower and is able to put some money on the side for medical expenses, gifts, and emergencies. On the other hand, when utility bills are higher, she decreases her food expenditures. She is enrolled in the Medicare program (#000000) and does not receive food stamps or any other form of assistance. In fact, she is adamant about not wanting any "charity."

Although he lives at home, Mrs. Ellis's son offers little assistance to her. Instead, Mrs. Ellis continues to cook, clean, and care for her son, despite her verbalized wish for him to be more responsible. Mrs. Ellis states that her son may work at odd jobs for several months each year, but usually quits or gets fired due to his poor performance, arguments with co-workers, and absenteeism. She claims that he has a drinking problem; in fact, when he needs money for alcohol he argues with Mrs. Ellis until she gives it to him. Her concern over how he would manage independently causes her to continue to allow him to live at home with his current behaviors. This situation causes Mrs. Ellis considerable anxiety and tension.

Mrs. Blake, who is the next door neighbor, provides companionship and emotional support to Mrs. Ellis. Mrs Blake provides transportation and accompanies Mrs. Ellis to shopping centers, church activities, and appointments. Other than a daily visit with her neighbor, Mrs. Ellis has no outside socialization. She refuses to attend the Senior Center and states that most of her friends are deceased or too disabled to visit her. Because she doesn't want to impose on Mrs. Blake, and because her friends are physically limited, Mrs. Ellis seldom socializes with friends.

Mrs. Ellis is an active member of Sacred Heart Catholic Church. She attends church regularly and frequently volunteers to assist in church

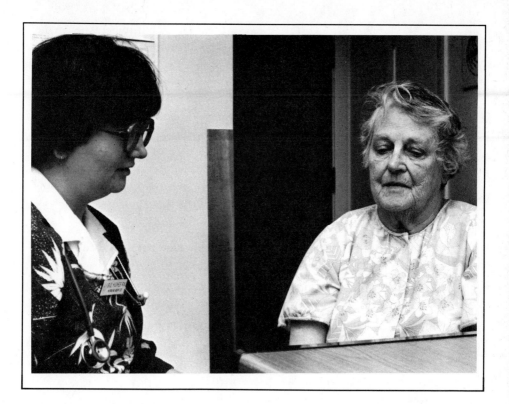

functions. She states that her strong faith helps her deal with the problems she faces, and that she does not fear death but sees it as a time when she can join her husband and daughter in heaven.

To pass her time, Mrs. Ellis reads, knits, and watches television. Her typical day consists of the following schedule:

 7 AM Awakes, watches television

 9 AM Eats breakfast

10 AM Dresses, does housework

12 PM Eats lunch, watches television, naps

 3 PM Visits with neighbor, shops

 6 PM Eats dinner

 7 PM Watches television, naps

 9 PM Bathes

11 PM Falls asleep

Mrs. Ellis claims that this routine has been her pattern for years, although she did awaken earlier when her husband was alive to prepare him for work.

Mrs. Ellis perceives her health as being "good for an old lady." She admits to aches, pains, minor discomforts, and fatigue but believes these are part of growing old. She used to visit Dr. Jones, a local physician, when she needed medical attention or a prescription refilled, but he relocated his practice last year and she has had no health or medical supervision since. She manages colds, falls, indigestion, constipation, and other problems on her own. She has little faith in the medical profession and repeatedly remarks that "people from the old country were able to do as much for the sick as our fancy doctors." Mrs. Ellis has never been hospitalized, nor has she had any type of surgery. She denies any history of fractures; she is unaware of any allergy. Mrs. Ellis is aware that she has some "heart trouble" that her former physician followed. (Medical record shows that an arrhythmia was diagnosed in 1976 for which digoxin and a potassium supplement were prescribed.)

Medications Mrs. Ellis is taking include:

1. Digoxin, one tablet (0.25 mg), taken at 11:00 AM every morning, prescribed by Dr. Jones.
2. Potassium chloride, one tablet two times daily, taken at 8:00 AM and 4:00 PM, prescribed by Dr. Jones.
3. Aspirin, two tablets every two to three hours on days when arthritic discomfort is severe, self-prescribed.
4. Milk of magnesia, one tablespoon every night at bedtime to enable daily bowel movement, self-prescribed.
5. Mylanta, two teaspoons before each meal to manage indigestion, self-prescribed.
6. Tetracycline, one capsule every four hours when fever or cold symptoms are present, self-prescribed, medication was remainder of prescription her son had for an infection.

Adverse reactions to above drugs were reviewed, and Mrs. Ellis denied experiencing any.

Mrs. Ellis's overall appearance showed no gross abnormalities. The skin on Mrs. Ellis's face and extremities was moderately dry; she claims to take a complete bath on a daily basis. Some limited mobility associated with arthritic discomfort was apparent as she transferred to the examining table and as she removed her clothing. Although she can ambulate without difficulty, she has trouble climbing the stairs in her two-story home, which she does several times daily.

Oral temperature was 98°F; apical pulse was 86 beats per minute; and respirations were somewhat shallow, regular, and at the rate of 18 per minute. Blood pressure was 150/86/78 standing, 146/84/76 sitting, and 138/80/72 lying. Height was 5'4", which Mrs. Ellis claims is $1\frac{1}{2}$" shorter than she remembers being.

Mrs. Ellis's current weight of 135 pounds is 25 pounds heavier than the weight she maintained throughout her adult life. She has gained approximately 5 pounds per year in recent years. She admits to a good appetite and a "sweet tooth." Her ability to taste sweet flavors has lessened in recent years. She has no food dislikes or intolerances, other than having trouble digesting highly seasoned foods. Her usual meal pattern is:

7 AM   Coffee (with cream and sugar) and several cookies

9 AM   Soft boiled egg with two pieces of toast or oatmeal with milk, and coffee

11 AM   Coffee

1 PM   Sandwich with two pieces of lunchmeat or leftovers from previous evening's dinner, coffee, several cookies

3 PM   Cookies or one cup of pudding, coffee

6 PM   Small serving of meat (usually fried), potatoes or noodles, applesauce, two slices bread, one slice cake or pie, coffee

9 PM   Large serving of ice cream (two to three scoops) or soda with eight to ten crackers or small bag of potato chips

Sometimes she snacks on cookies, cake, or potato chips when she awakens with nocturia. She denies using alcohol.

Mrs. Ellis averages seven to eight hours of sleep nightly. Occasionally, she may take a $\frac{1}{2}$ hour nap at 4:00 PM (usually on days when she has been shopping or participating in an activity out of the ordinary). She seldom has difficulty falling asleep, although she does state that she is a very light sleeper and awakens several times during the night when she hears her son or noises from the outside. The only time she used sedatives was following her husband's death. Mrs. Ellis remembers uncomfortable side effects from the sedative (sluggishness during the entire day, lack of mental clarity) and discontinued the drug after one month.

Mrs. Ellis has had a complete set of dentures for 25 years. Her last visit to the dentist was ten years ago. The dentures are intact and well cared for; however, they fit loosely and move out of place when she chews and speaks. The friction of the dentures' movement has caused two areas of irritation on her gums: one over the area of the medial incisor and the other over the area of the right first molar. The oral mucosa was otherwise light pink and moist.

Mrs. Ellis's tongue appeared red, smooth, and glossy. There was no deviation, tremor, or limitation of movement, and the ventral surface showed no swelling or varicosities. No tumors were palpated along the tongue, lips, or floor of the mouth. Her uvula and soft palate did rise when she said "ah," and a normal gag reflex was evident. No swelling or exudate was noted from her tonsils. Mrs. Ellis has no problem masticating and swallowing.

No deviation in the shape, size, or color of Mrs. Ellis's nose was noted. Palpation of the soft tissues and nose revealed no tenderness, masses, or displacement of the bone and cartilage. Each naris was patent and capable of identifying odors. The nasal mucosa was red and swollen with a copious, watery discharge present. This acute rhinitis was consistent with Mrs. Ellis's complaints of having a "cold."

Mrs. Ellis's eyelids were able to close completely and no ptosis, lesions, edema, or other abnormalities were present. Several small vessels were noted during inspection of the conjunctiva and a few pigmented deposits were evident on the sclera: both of these findings were within a normal range. Mrs. Ellis was able to read only the top two lines of the Snellen chart with her right eye and the top three lines with her left eye. She was unable to read typewritten letters but was able to see the headlines on the newspaper. She was prescribed eyeglasses 15 years ago and used the same pair until they were lost three years ago. She states that she doesn't feel she needs eyeglasses because television is the only activity she uses her eyes for and she is able to view it quite well. Vision in dim areas is a problem for Mrs. Ellis, and she claims to have trouble judging the depth of stairs and street curbs. She is able to differentiate various colors. Gross evaluation of Mrs. Ellis's visual fields revealed significant impairment on her right side: she denies noticing any change in her visual fields. Extraocular muscle function was normal in all six cardinal positions of gaze. The pupils were equal, round, and responsive to light; the corneal reflex was normal bilaterally.

Throughout the interview, Mrs. Ellis's need to ask the nurse to repeat directions and the cocking of the right side of her head to the nurse indicated

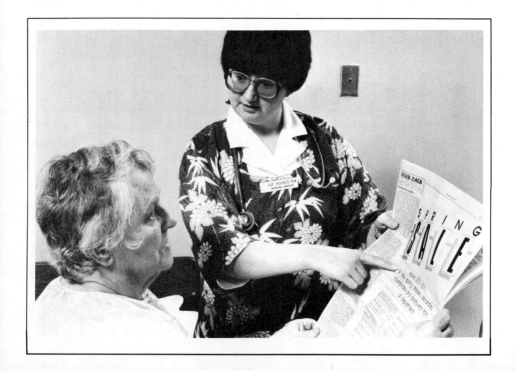

a possible hearing deficit. Mrs. Ellis denied a hearing problem when asked but was unable to hear a wristwatch ticking at her left ear. She admitted to having some discomfort in her left ear and otoscopic examination revealed a significant amount of cerumen present bilaterally. Mrs. Ellis uses cotton-tipped applicators to attempt to remove cerumen. She has never had an audiometric examination. Both auricles were symmetrical, of normal size, and free of swelling, tenderness, or nodules.

Inspection, palpation, and percussion of the chest uncovered no abnormalities. Respirations were shallow, and Mrs. Ellis became dizzy while deep breathing during auscultation of the lungs. She had a mild, nonproductive cough following the deep-breathing activity. Mrs. Ellis gave up smoking ten years ago after a 25-year history of smoking one pack of nonfiltered cigarettes daily. Her one and only chest x-ray was in 1960. She claims that she becomes short of breath when she is faced with unusual activity, such as climbing stairs several times in succession, performing housework, or walking for a long period.

No cardiac abnormalities were detected through inspection and palpation. A soft systolic ejection murmur was heard at the base of the heart and beats were irregular. Arterial and venous pulses and pressures all were within a normal range. The nurse noted some varicosities of the lower extremities, and Mrs. Ellis did admit to experiencing periodic cramps in her legs and feet. Mrs. Ellis's last complete cardiovascular evaluation with electrocardiogram

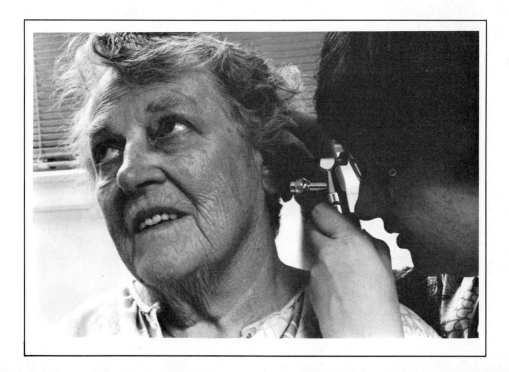

was performed five years ago when her tachycardia was initially diagnosed by Dr. Jones.

Evaluation of the range of joint motion identified several limitations. Mrs. Ellis was unable to lift her right arm above the level of her shoulder, thus interfering with her ability to care for her hair independently and to reach items on high shelves. Limitations in her ability to flex and externally rotate her left hip caused ambulation and transfer problems; bilateral pain

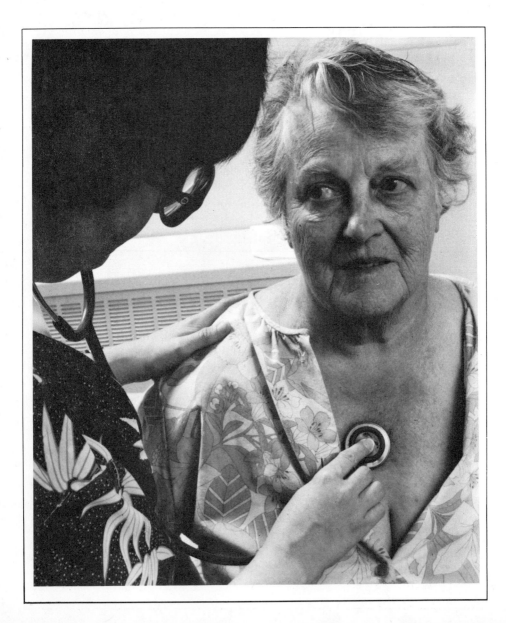

in her knees when they were taken through a full range of motion contributed to this problem also. The digits of both hands possessed bony nodules, and Mrs. Ellis claims that during damp weather they are uncomfortable and limited in movement. On days when her arthritis is bothersome she is unable to button clothing or hold utensils securely. Mrs. Ellis manages her arthritic pain by taking two aspirin every two hours (occasionally two aspirin hourly or three to four aspirin every two hours) and limiting her joint motion. Her muscle contractions were smooth and steady. Some weakness and flabbiness of the muscles were evident in the extremities, but this was not unusual based on the minimal amount of physical activity she experienced. All of her reflexes were normal.

Mrs. Ellis's abdomen was round and flabby with no masses or areas of tenderness. All organs were palpated to be of normal size, and bowel sounds were average. The daily use of milk of magnesia causes Mrs. Ellis to have at least one bowel movement daily; she claims to be unable to have a bowel movement without the use of a laxative. Her bowel movement is of a small amount and soft to watery in consistency. She denies noticing any change in bowel habits. Rectal examination detected severe hemorrhoids that bled during the examination. Mrs. Ellis states that her hemorrhoids bleed several times each week, and that she uses a hemorrhoidal preparation daily.

Typically, Mrs. Ellis voids approximately every three hours, day and night. However, in the past month she has voided smaller volumes of urine every one to two hours, accompanied by urgency and burning. She was most concerned that during the past two weeks she has had several episodes of urinary incontinence and fears that she is experiencing an inevitable consequence of old age. Her urine was odorous, cloudy, and had a 2+ proteinuria.

Both of Mrs. Ellis's children were delivered by a midwife in her home following uncomplicated pregnancies. She suddenly ceased having menstrual periods in 1960 when she was 47 years of age and claims to have experienced some emotional lability and irritability for approximately one year near that time. She has never had a gynecologic examination because she has never had any problems that she felt warranted a gynecologist's attention. She admits to a sense of heaviness and discomfort that started after her second pregnancy. This pelvic pressure caused sufficient discomfort to interfere with satisfying intercourse; she and her husband discontinued sexual activity and assumed separate bedrooms while she was in her 30s. Mrs. Ellis had never found sexual intimacy enjoyable and commented that society has the trouble it does today due to too much concern about sex.

Mrs. Ellis does not know how to examine her breasts. No masses, tenderness, or nipple discharge were present during breast palpation. The sagging, flabby appearance of her breasts was typical for women her age.

Throughout the examination, Mrs. Ellis was alert, responsive, and oriented to person, place, and time. Her speech and language were appropriate.

She perceived herself as being "normal and healthy," and prides herself on having better mental faculties than many other persons her age. She admits to being more forgetful than she was in earlier years (for example, she often forgets if she has taken her digoxin or where she has placed her mail). Her son is her major preoccupation and source of stress. Repeatedly she made comments pertaining to her disappointment in her son, her anger at having to support him, her fear during his drunken outbursts, and the worry he causes her. When confronted with the suggestion that she force her son to be more responsible and accountable for his behaviors (for example, not supplying him with money or requesting that he move from her home), she stated that she couldn't do that because "he'll never be able to make it on his own." Although the source of considerable anger and tension, the behaviors of Mrs. Ellis's son are continually fostered by her. Her interests, activities, and purpose all seem to center on her middle-aged son.

Based on the information obtained during this assessment, the nurse developed the following nursing diagnoses and initial plans.

Nursing Diagnosis	Plan
1. Ineffective family coping related to son's dependency and alleged alcoholism	1a. Attempt to have son attend screening clinic for assessment.
	b. Offer counselling to client and son.
2. Potential altered health maintenance and impaired home maintenance management related to limited finances	2a. Arrange appointment with social worker to review all benefits to which she is entitled.
	b. Encourage the use of all benefits to which she is entitled.
3. Social isolation and diversional activity deficit related to limited social activity and recreation	3a. Identify senior groups in her community, and if acceptable to client, arrange for a member of a local group to visit her.
	b. Arrange appointment with occupational therapist to explore activities appropriate to her capabilities and interests.
4. Activity intolerance related to fatigue; pain related to indigestion	4a. Obtain blood sample for analysis, including complete blood count (CBC),

Nursing Diagnosis	Plan
	digitalis, potassium, and salicylate levels.
	b. Review diet and medications.
5. Knowledge deficit and potential for injury related to excessive administration of aspirin	5a. Discuss pain relief measures for arthritis.
	b. Consult with physician as to alternative analgesics.
6. Knowledge deficit related to laxative dependency	6a. Initiate program to wean client from laxatives.
	b. Educate as to the differences in elimination patterns in advanced age, the hazards associated with laxative use, and natural measures to facilitate bowel elimination.
7. Knowledge deficit and potential for injury related to self-prescription of drugs	7a. Discuss hazards of taking nonprescribed or other persons' drugs.
8. Activity intolerance, impaired physical mobility, potential for injury, and pain related to limited joint mobility	8a. Refer to arthritis clinic for evaluation.
	b. Consult with physical therapist for exercise plan.
	c. Discuss safety measures (eg, proper shoes to prevent falls) and promote safe transfer and stair-climbing methods.
9. Ineffective breathing pattern and altered tissue perfusion (cardiopulmonary) related to poor lung expansion	9a. Teach breathing exercises.
	b. Develop schedule for client with progressively increasing amounts of exercises as tolerated.
10. Potential impaired skin integrity related to dryness secondary to excessive bathing	10a. Encourage client to decrease complete baths to every second or third day with daily partial baths.
	b. Instruct in use of moisturizers.

Nursing Diagnosis

11. Altered nutrition: more than body requirements related to excess carbohydrate intake; less than body requirements related to insufficient vitamin, mineral intake

12. Potential impaired skin integrity related to poorly fitting dentures

13. Potential altered nutrition: less than body requirements related to red, glossy tongue

14. Sensory-perceptual alterations (visual) related to farsightedness, decreased peripheral vision in right eye, and poor vision for depth and dimly lit areas

15. Sensory-perceptual alterations (auditory) related to decreased hearing ability

16. Sensory-perceptual alterations (auditory) and pain related to cerumen accumulation

17. Knowledge deficit and altered health maintenance related to lack of chest x-ray for more than 20 years

18. Decreased cardiac output related to irregular heart rate and systolic ejection murmur

Plan

11a. Refer to nutritionist for diet review and instruction.

b. Explore with client possibility of food stamps and congregate eating programs.

12a. Refer to local dental clinic offering services on sliding scale basis.

13a. Review blood chemistry for possible deficit of vitamin B_{12}, niacin, or iron.

14a. Review value of ophthalmologic examination.

b. Refer to ophthalmologist.

c. Instruct in safety measures (for example, stairways well lighted, hold on to rails when climbing stairs, color code medication containers).

15a. Encourage client to ask for communication to be repeated if not heard clearly.

b. Refer for audiometric evaluation.

16a. Perform ear irrigation to loosen cerumen.

b. Instruct client in proper method of managing cerumen problems.

17a. Refer to chest clinic for x-ray.

18a. Refer to cardiologist for evaluation.

b. Discuss ways to manage physical and emotional stress.

Nursing Diagnosis	Plan
19. Altered tissue perfusion (peripheral) related to varicosities in lower extremity	19a. Instruct client to elevate legs several times during the day. b. Review special attention needed for legs and feet (for example, avoidance of extreme temperatures and constricting clothing).
20. Pain related to severe hemorrhoids	20a. Refer to gastroenterology clinic for evaluation.
21. Altered patterns of urinary elimination related to frequency, burning, urgency, incontinence (recent)	21a. Obtain clean catch urine sample for microscopic evaluation.
22. Pain related to pelvic pressure, heaviness; knowledge deficit related to never having had gynecologic (GYN) exam	22a. Refer to gynecologist for complete exam, including evaluation of possible prolapsed uterus. b. Discuss importance of regular GYN exam and review what procedures she can expect during exam.
23. Knowledge deficit related to inability to examine breasts	23a. Instruct client in breast self-examination technique.
24. Altered health maintenance, potential for injury, potential noncompliance, and altered thought processes related to short-term memory deficit	24a. Develop medication chart with client for her use in recording medication administration. b. Put all instructions in written form (large enough for client to read). c. Review the use of checklists and other memory aids for her personal use.

Appendix A:
Samples of
Assessment
Tools

Nursing History for Older Adults

1. *Profile of Patient*
   Name _____ Sex _____ Race _____ Religion _____ Date of birth _____
   Address _____ Telephone _____
   Language spoken _____ Nearest contact person _____

2. *Profile of Family*

   Spouse   Children
   _____ Living   _____ Living
       Health status: Names and addresses:
       Age: _____ Deceased
       Occupation: Year deceased:
   _____ Deceased   Cause of death:
       Year deceased:
       Cause of death:
   Others in household:

3. *Occupational Profile*

   _____ Employed   _____ Unemployed
       Type of work: Reason:
       Length of employment: Length of unemployment:
       Working hours: Feelings about unemployment:
       Sources of income: Previous occupations:

Nursing History for Older Adults—(*Continued*)

4. *Home Profile*
   _____ Single dwelling
   _____ Multiple dwelling
   _____ Own
   _____ Rent
   _____ Telephone
   _____ Pets

   Number of levels:
   Location of bathroom:
   Location of bedroom:
   Nearest neighbor:
   Household responsibilities:

5. *Economic Profile*
   Sources of income:
   Monthly income:
   Monthly expenses:
   Financial concerns:

6. *Health Insurance*
   _____ Medicaid
   _____ Medicare
   _____ Blue Cross/Blue Sheild
   _____ Other:
   Policy number:

7. *Health and Social Resources Currently Utilized*
   _____ Private MD   _____ HMO   _____ Social worker
   _____ Hospital   _____ Visiting nurse   _____ Meals on
   _____ Clinic   _____ Public health nurse   wheels
                                                    Other:

8. *Social/Leisure Activities*
   Organization membership:
   Hobbies/Interests:

9. *Health History*
   _____ Allergies
       Food:
       Drug:
       Other:
   _____ Diabetes
   _____ Hypertension
   _____ Cancer

   _____ Hospitalizations:
   _____ Surgery:
   _____ Fractures:
   _____ Major health problems:

10. *Current Health Status*
    Knowledge and understanding of health problems:

    Limitations of function or
        performance of ADL:

    Management of limitations:

    Health goals:

11. *Medications*

Name	Dosage	How and when taken	How obtained	Knowledge and understanding of medication
_____	_____	_____	_____	_____
_____	_____	_____	_____	_____
_____	_____	_____	_____	_____
_____	_____	_____	_____	_____
_____	_____	_____	_____	_____
_____	_____	_____	_____	_____

12. *Physical Status*

T _____ (AOR)   Height _____   Urine:
P _____   Weight _____ (recent   S/A: _____
R _____   changes:)   Specific gravity:
                   BP _____ (sitting,   How obtained:
                        standing, lying)   Characteristics:

Skin condition
_____ Intact   _____ Rash (describe)   _____ Wounds (describe)
_____ Dry   _____ Discoloration (describe)

Hair condition:	Nail condition:

Mobility
_____ Ambulatory   _____ Able to rise from chair or
_____ Nonambulatory   toilet
_____ Ambulatory with assistance   _____ Able to climb stairs
       (specify):

Extremity function

	Location	Degree of limitation	Assistive/Relief measures
Contracture			
Arthritis			
Painful movement			
Paralysis			
Spasm			
Amputation			
Dominant hand			

Nursing History for Older Adults—(*Continued*)

Respiration

	Precipitating factors	Degree of limitation	Assistive/Relief measures
Orthopnea			
Dyspnea			
Shortness of breath			
Wheezing			
Asthma			
Coughing			

Sputum characteristics:
Smoking history: _____ Tracheostomy

Circulation

	Precipitating factors	Degree of limitation	Assistive/Relief measures
Chest pain			
Tachycardia			
Edema			
Cramping in extremities			

Equality of pulse, temperature, and color in extremities:

Nutrition

Teeth: Dentures: Chewing problems:
   Number: _____ Partial   Swallowing problems:
   Status: _____ Complete   Feeding tube:
Date last dental exam: Fit:

	Precipitating factors	Assistive/Relief measures
Indigestion		
Constipation		
Diarrhea		

Usual meal pattern:	Fluid intake:
	Alcohol use:
Food preferences:	Food restrictions:

Bladder

_____ Nocturia   _____ Burning   _____ Incontinence   _____ Catheter
_____ Frequency   _____ Urgency   _____ Stress   _____ Ostomy
Voiding pattern: incontinence
Urine
characteristics:

Bowel

_____ Hemorrhoids   _____ Pain during movement
_____ Straining   _____ Recent change in pattern

_____ Chronic constipation   _____ Incontinence
_____ Chronic diarrhea   _____ Ostomy

Stool

Bowel movement pattern:
Characteristics:

	Frequency of use	Results obtained
Laxatives		
Suppositories		
Enemas		

Sensory status

Hearing

All sounds:
High frequency:

Vision

Full vision:
Night vision:
Peripheral vision:
Reading:
Color discrimination:
Depth perception:

Taste

Smell

Touch

Feels pressure and pain:
Differentiates temperature:
Speech:
Pain:

_____ Hearing aid   _____ Eyeglasses   Date last vision exam:
Other sensory data: _____ Contact lenses   Date last hearing exam:

Rest and sleep

_____ Insomnia (describe)   Medicines and alcohol used to induce sleep:
_____ Night restlessness   Factors interfering with rest:
_____ Night confusion   Usual sleep and rest pattern:

Nursing History for Older Adults—(*Continued*)

Female reproductive factors:		Male reproductive factors:
_____ Vaginal discharge	_____ Nipple discharge	_____ Scrotal
_____ Itching	_____ Breast pain	swelling
_____ Lesions	_____ Mastectomy	_____ Lesions
_____ Breast mass	(indicate right or left)	_____ Discharge
_____ Other	_____ Prosthesis	_____ Impotency
Date last exam:		

Sexual profile

_____ Interest   _____ Dyspareunia   Attitude:
_____ Sexually active   _____ Limitations: Frequency:

13. *Mental Status*

     _____ Alert   Orientation
     _____ Rapid response to verbal stimuli   _____ Person
     _____ Slow response to verbal stimuli   _____ Place
     _____ Confused   _____ Time
     _____ Stuporous   Attention span:
     _____ Comatose
     Memory of recent events: Memory of past events:

14. *Emotional Status*

     _____ Anxious   _____ Hyperactive   _____ Disinterest in life
     _____ Fearful   _____ Hypoactive   _____ Emotionally labile
     _____ Depressed   _____ Suspicious   _____ Suicidal

     Self concept: Current stress factors:

     Attitude and concerns about death:

     Other data:

     Informant
     _____ Patient
     _____ Other (specify)

     _____
          Signature of Nurse   Date

Source: Eliopoulos C. *Gerontological Nursing*. New York: Harper and Row, 1979, pp 97–102.

Nursing Assessment of the Geriatric Lower Extremity

Patient number _____
Date _____
RN number _____

Instructions: For each item, circle the response in the appropriate column, unless directed otherwise.

1. Mobility (check one): ☐ Walks without assistance ☐ Walks with help of equipment ☐ Does not walk—uses wheelchair ☐ Bedfast
2. Ask the client, "Does the condition of your feet or legs limit your activity in any way?" ☐ Yes ☐ No ☐ If *yes*, describe: _____
3. Ask the client to walk approximately 10 feet. Is there any gait disturbance? ☐ Yes ☐ No

Remove the client's shoes and stockings
4. Cleanliness of feet: ☐ Acceptable ☐ Unacceptable
5. Are the stockings a good fit? ☐ Yes ☐ No
6. Does the client usually wear well-fitting, leather (synthetic) shoes that cover the feet completely? ☐ Yes ☐ No If *yes*, are they in good condition? ☐ Yes ☐ No
7. Does the client wear circular garters? ☐ Yes ☐ No

Dermatologic assessment
8. Skin lesions
   a. Fissure between the toes? ☐ Yes ☐ No
   b. Fissure on heel(s)? ☐ Yes ☐ No
   c. Excoriation on legs or feet? ☐ Yes ☐ No
   d. Corn(s)? (Figure A-1) ☐ Yes ☐ No
      (Corn—painful, circular area of thickened skin, appearing on skin that is normally thin)
   e. Callus(es)? ☐ Yes ☐ No
      (Callus—thickened skin, occurring on skin that is normally thick, such as soles)
   f. Plantar wart? ☐ Yes ☐ No
   g. Other? ☐ Yes ☐ No
      Describe: _____
9. Itching on legs or feet? ☐ Yes ☐ No
10. Rash on legs or feet? ☐ Yes ☐ No
11. Inspect pressure areas on the feet for localized areas of redness. Are any present? ☐ Yes ☐ No If *yes*, which foot? ☐ Right ☐ Left
12. Inspect legs, feet, and toes for localized swelling, warmth, tenderness, and redness. Is any present? ☐ Yes ☐ No If *yes*, specify location: ☐ R leg ☐ R foot ☐ L leg ☐ L foot

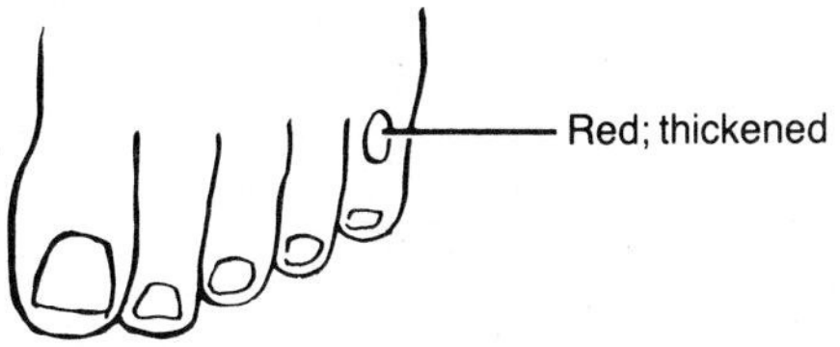

Red; thickened

Figure A-1
Corn

Source: King P. Nursing assessment of the geriatric lower extremity. In: *Confusion: Prevention and Care*. Wolanın MO, Phillips LRF (editors). St. Louis: Mosby, 1981. Illustrations by Thomas A. King.

Nursing Assessment of the Geriatric Lower Extremity—(*Continued*)

13. Toenails
    a. Ingrown? ☐ Yes ☐ No
       (Ingrown toenail—a sensitive and tender overhanging nail fold)
    b. Overgrown (long)? ☐ Yes ☐ No
    c. Thickened? ☐ Yes ☐ No
    d. Yellow discoloration? ☐ Yes ☐ No
    e. Black discoloration? ☐ Yes ☐ No

Circulatory status
Questions 14 to 18 relate to feet only.
14. Do the feet have any red, reddish blue, or bluish discoloration? ☐ Yes ☐ No
15. Is there any brownish discoloration around the ankles? ☐ Yes ☐ No
16. Is the dorsalis pedis pulse present? (Figure A-2) ☐ Yes ☐ No If *no*, which foot? ☐ Right ☐ Left
17. Is the posterior tibial pulse present? (Figure A-3) ☐ Yes ☐ No If *no*, which foot? ☐ Right ☐ Left
18. Is the skin dry? ☐ Yes ☐ No

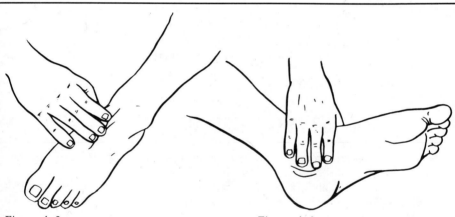

Figure A-2
Dorsalis pedis pulse. Use three fingers on the dorsum of the foot, usually just lateral to the extensor tendon of the great toe.

Figure A-3
Posterior tibial pulse. Curve your fingers behind and slightly below the medial malleolus of the ankle.

Questions 19–23 relate to both feet and legs.
19. Is edema present? ☐ Yes ☐ No

Check the temperature of the legs and the feet with the backs of your fingers, comparing one extremity with the other
20. Are the feet the same temperature? ☐ Yes ☐ No
21. Are the legs the same temperature? ☐ Yes ☐ No
22. Does the client have any pain in legs or feet? ☐ Yes ☐ No If *yes*, describe:

_____

Inspect the legs, sides of ankles, soles, and toes for ulceration
23. Is any ulceration present? ☐ Yes ☐ No If *yes*, specify location: ☐ R leg ☐ R foot ☐ L leg ☐ L foot

Structural deformities
24. Hallux valgus (bunion)? (Figure A-4) ☐ Yes ☐ No
25. Hammertoes? (Figure A-5) ☐ Yes ☐ No
26. Overlapping digits? ☐ Yes ☐ No

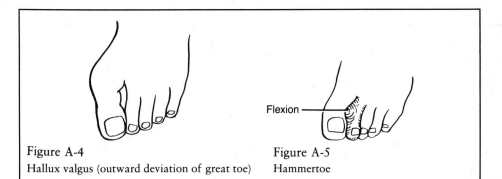

Figure A-4
Hallux valgus (outward deviation of great toe)

Figure A-5
Hammertoe

Ask the client to stand
27. Are the legs the same relative size? ☐ Yes ☐ No
28. Are the legs the same relative length? ☐ Yes ☐ No
29. Are varicosities present? ☐ Yes ☐ No

Additional notes

Items of Mini-Mental State Examination

Maximum score	
	Orientation
5	What is the (year) (season) (date) (day) (month)?
5	Where are we (state) (county) (hospital) (floor)?
	Registration
3	Name three objects: One second to say each. Then ask the patient all three after you have said them. Give one point for each correct answer. Repeat them until patient learns all three. Count trials and record number.
	Number of trials
	Attention and calculation
5	Begin with 100 and count backwards by 7 (stop after five answers). Alternatively, spell "world" backwards.
	Recall
3	Ask for the three objects repeated above. Give one point for each correct answer.

Items of Mini-Mental State Examination (*Continued*)

Maximum score	
	Language
2	Show a pencil and a watch and ask subject to name them.
1	Repeat the following: "No 'ifs,' 'ands,' or 'buts.'"
3	A three-stage command, "Take a paper in your right hand; fold it in half and put it on the floor."
1	Read and obey the following (show subject the written item): CLOSE YOUR EYES.
1	Write a sentence.
1	Copy a design (complex polygon as in Bender-Gestalt).
30	Total score possible

Source: Adapted from Folstein MF, Folstein S, and McHugh PR. Mini-mental state: A practical method for grading the cognitive state of patients for the clinician. *Journal of Psychiatric Research* 1975; (12):189–198. Reprinted with permission from Pergamon Press, Ltd.

OARS Mental Health Screening Questions

1. Do you wake up fresh and rested most mornings?
2. Is your daily life full of things that keep you interested?
3. Have you at times very much wanted to leave home?
4. Does it seem that no one understands you?
5. Have you had periods of days, weeks, or months when you couldn't take care of things because you couldn't "get going"?
6. Is your sleep fitful and disturbed?
7. Are you happy most of the time?
8. Are you being plotted against?
9. Do you certainly feel useless at times?
10. During the last few years, have you been well most of the time?
11. Do you feel weak all over much of the time?
12. Are you troubled by headaches?
13. Have you had difficulty in keeping your balance in walking?
14. Are you troubled by your heart pounding and a shortness of breath?
15. Even when you are with people, do you feel lonely much of the time?

Source: Duke University Center for the Study of Aging. *Multidimensional Functional Assessment: The OARS Methodology.* Durham, NC: Duke University, 1978.

Short Portable Mental Status Questionnaire (SPMSQ)

1. What is the date today (month/day/year)?
2. What day of the week is it?
3. What is the name of this place?
4. What is your telephone number? (If no telephone, what is your street address?)
5. How old are you?

6. When were you born (month/day/year)?
7. Who is the current president of the United States?
8. Who was the president just before him?
9. What was your mother's maiden name?
10. Subtract 3 from 20 and keep subtracting each new number you get, all the way down.

0-2 errors = intact
3-4 errors = mild intellectual impairment
5-7 errors = moderate intellectual impairment
8-10 errors = severe intellectual impairment

Allow one more error if subject had only grade school education.
Allow one fewer error if subject has had education beyond high school.

Source: Adapted from Duke University Center for the Study of Aging. *Multidimensional Functional Assessment: The OARS Methodology*. Durham, NC: Duke University, 1978.

Zung Self-rating Depression Scale

1. I feel downhearted and blue.
2. Morning is when I feel the best.
3. I have crying spells or feel like it.
4. I have trouble sleeping at night.
5. I can eat as much as I used to.
6. I still enjoy sex.
7. I notice that I am losing weight.
8. I have trouble with constipation.
9. My heart beats faster than usual.
10. I get tired for no reason.
11. My mind is as clear as it used to be.
12. I find it easy to do the things I used to.
13. I am restless and can't keep still.
14. I feel hopeful about the future.
15. I am more irritable than usual.
16. I find it easy to make decisions.
17. I feel that I am useful and needed.
18. My life is pretty full.
19. I feel that others would be better off if I were dead.
20. I still enjoy the things I used to do.

Source: Zung WWK. A self-rating depression scale. *Archives of General Psychiatry* 1965; (12):63–70. Copyright 1965, American Medical Association.

Philadelphia Geriatric Center Mental Status Questionnaire

1. What is your name?
2. Who am I (point to self)?
3. Who is that (point to nurse)?
4. Are you married or single?
5. If married, do you have children?
6. If yes, what are their names? (incorrect if not known)

Philadelphia Geriatric Center Mental Status Questionnaire—(*Continued*)

7. Where is your room?
8. What is your room number?
9. What is the name of this place?
10. What floor is this?
11. Where is the bathroom?
12. Where do you eat your meals?
13. What meal did you eat last?
14. What is today and what is the date?
15. What month is it now?
16. What year is this?
17. What season is this? (accept either if season is changing)
18. What is the weather outdoors now?
19. How old are you?
20. When were you born (month)?
21. What year were you born?
22. What is your mother's first name?
23. What is your father's first name?
24. Who is the president of the United States?
25. Who was the president of the United States before him?
26. Do you wear glasses?
27. Where are they now?
28. Do you have your own teeth?
29. If not, do you have plates or dentures?
30. Where are they now?
31. Do you dress yourself? (Note if capable.)
32. Do you feed yourself? (Observe if patient uses cutlery or fingers.)
33. Bladder and bowel continence (ask nurse).
34. Family recognition (ask nurse).
35. Is it now morning or afternoon?

One point for each correct answer

0 = total loss	21–33 = mild
1–10 = severe loss	34–35 = not impaired
11–20 = moderate	

Source: Fishback DB. Mental status questionnaire for organic brain syndrome, with a new visual counting test. *Journal of the American Geriatrics Society* 1977; (25):167–170.

Katz Index of Independence in ADL

INDEX OF INDEPENDENCE IN ACTIVITIES OF DAILY LIVING

The Index of Independence in Activities of Daily Living is based on an evaluation of the functional independence or dependence of patients in bathing, dressing, going to the toilet, transferring, continence, and feeding. Specific definitions of functional independence and dependence appear below the index.

A   Independent in feeding, continence, transferring, going to toilet, dressing, and bathing.

B   Independent in all but one of these functions.

C   Independent in all but bathing and one additional function.

D   Independent in all but bathing, dressing, and one additional function.

E   Independent in all but bathing, dressing, going to toilet, and one additional function.

F   Independent in all but bathing, dressing, going to toilet, transferring, and one additional function.

G   Dependent in all six functions.

Other   Dependent in at least two functions, but not classifiable as C, D, E, or F.

Independence means without supervision, direction, or active personal assistance, except as specifically noted on the next page. This is based on actual status and not on ability. A patient who refuses to perform a function is considered as not performing the function, even though he is deemed able.

BATHING (Sponge, shower or tub)

Independent: assistance only in bathing a single part (as back or disabled extremity) or bathes self completely

Dependent: assistance in bathing more than one part of body; assistance in getting in or out of tub or does not bathe self

TRANSFER

Independent: moves in and out of bed independently and moves in and out of chair independently (may or may not be using mechanical supports)

Dependent: assistance in moving in or out of bed and/or chair; does not perform one or more transfers

DRESSING

Independent: gets clothes from closets and drawers; puts on clothes, outer garments, braces; manages fasteners; act of tying shoes is excluded

Dependent: does not dress self or remains partly undressed

CONTINENCE

Independent: urination and defecation entirely self-controlled

Dependent: partial or total incontinence in urination or defecation; partial or total control by enemas, catheters, or regulated use of urinals and/or bedpans

GOING TO TOILET

Independent: gets to toilet; gets on and off toilet; arranges clothes, cleans organs of excretion; (may manage own bedpan used at night only and may not be using mechanical supports)

Dependent: uses bedpan or commode or receives assistance in getting to and using toilet

FEEDING

Independent: gets food from plate or its equivalent into mouth; (precutting of meat and preparation of food, as buttering bread, are excluded from evaluation)

Dependent: assistance in act of feeding (see above); does not eat at all or parenteral feeding

EVALUATION FORM

Name _____ Date of Evaluation _____

For each area of functioning listed below, check description that applies. (The word *assistance* means supervision, direction of personal assistance.)

BATHING—either sponge bath, tub bath, or shower

☐   ☐   ☐

Receives no assistance (gets in and out of tub by self if tub is usual means of bathing)	Receives assistance in bathing only one part of body (such as back or a leg)	Receives assistance in bathing more than one part of body (or not bathed)

Katz Index of Independence in ADL (*Continued*)

INDEX OF INDEPENDENCE IN ACTIVITIES OF DAILY LIVING

DRESSING—gets clothes from closets and drawers—including underclothes, outer garments, and using fasteners (including braces, if worn)

☐

Gets clothes and gets completely dressed without assistance

☐

Gets clothes and gets dressed without assistance except for assistance in tying shoes

☐

Receives assistance in getting clothes or in getting dressed, or stays partly or completely undressed

TOILETING—going to the "toilet room" for bowel and urine elimination; cleaning self after elimination and arranging clothes

☐

Goes to "toilet room," cleans self and arranges clothes without assistance (may use object for support such as cane, walker, or wheelchair and may manage night bedpan or commode, emptying same in morning)

☐

Receives assistance in going to "toilet room" or in cleansing self or in arranging clothes after elimination or in use of night bedpan or commode

☐

Doesn't go to room termed "toilet" for the elimination process

TRANSFER—

☐

Moves in and out of bed as well as in and out of chair without assistance (may be using object for support such as cane or walker)

☐

Moves in or out of bed or chair with assistance

☐

Doesn't get out of bed

CONTINENCE—

☐

Controls urination and bowel movement completely by self

☐

Has occasional "accidents"

☐

Supervision helps keep urine or bowel control; catheter is used or is incontinent

FEEDING—

☐

Feeds self without assistance

☐

Feeds self without getting assistance in cutting meat or buttering bread

☐

Receives assistance in feeding or is fed partly or completely by using tubes or intravenous fluids.

Source: Katz S et al. Studies of illness in the aged. The index of ADL: A standardized measure of biological and psychosocial function. *Journal of the American Medical Association* 1963; (185):914. Copyright 1963, American Medical Association.

OARS Social Resource Scale

Now I'd like to ask you some questions about your family and friends.
Are you single, married, widowed, divorced or separated?

1 Single
2 Married
3 Widowed
4 Divorced
5 Separated
− Not answered
(Inst.)
(If "2" ask a)
a. *Does your spouse live here also?*
   1 Yes
   2 No
   − Not answered

Who lives with you? (Ask each of the following and check accordingly)

Yes	No	
_____	_____	No one
_____	_____	Husband or wife
_____	_____	Children
_____	_____	Grandchildren
_____	_____	Parents
_____	_____	Grandparents
_____	_____	Brothers and sisters
_____	_____	Other relatives (does not include in-laws covered in the above categories)
_____	_____	Friends
_____	_____	Nonrelated paid help (includes free room)
_____	_____	Others (specify) _____

(Inst.): In the past year about how often did you leave here to visit your family and/or friends for weekends or holidays, or to go on shopping trips or outings?
   1 Once a week or more
   2 1–3 times a month
   3 Less than once a month or only on holidays
   4 Never
   − Not answered

How many people do you know well enough to visit with in their homes?

3 Five or more
2 Three to four
1 One to two
0 None
− Not answered

About how many times did you talk to someone—friends, relatives or others—on the telephone in the past week (either you called them or they called you)? [IF SUBJECT HAS NO PHONE, QUESTION STILL APPLIES.]

Note: Italicized questions apply to those living in institutions.

OARS Social Resource Scale—(*Continued*)

---

    3 Once a day or more
    2 2 times
    1 Once
    0 Not at all
    − Not answered
(Inst.): Do not ask following. Ask following (Inst.) instead.

How many times during the past week did you spend some time with someone who does not live with you: that is, you went to see them, or they came to visit you, or you went out to do things together?

How many times in the past week did you visit with someone, either with people who live here or people who visited you here?
    3 Once a day or more
    2 2–6 times
    1 Once
    0 Not at all
    − Not answered

Do you have someone you can trust and confide in?
    2 Yes
    0 No
    − Not answered

Do you find yourself feeling lonely quite often, sometimes, or almost never?
    0 Quite often
    1 Sometimes
    2 Almost never
    − Not answered

Do you see your relatives and friends as often as you want to, or are you somewhat unhappy about how little you see them?
    1 As often as wants to
    2 Somewhat unhappy about how little
    − Not answered

Is there someone (*Inst.: Outside this place*) who would give you any help at all if you were sick or disabled; for example, your husband/wife, a member of your family, or a friend?
    1 Yes
    0 No one willing and able to help
    − Not answered

If "yes" ask a and b.
  a. Is there someone (*Inst.: Outside this place*) who would take care of you as long as needed, or only for a short time, or only someone who would help you now and then (for example, taking you to the doctor, or fixing lunch occasionally, etc)?
     1 Someone who would take care of subject indefinitely (as long as needed)
     2 Someone who would take care of subject for a short time (a few weeks to six months)
     3 Someone who would help subject now and then (taking him to the doctor or fixing lunch, etc.)
     − Not answered

b. Who is this person?
Name _____
Relationship _____

Rating Scale

Rate the current social resources of the person being evaluated along the six-point scale presented below. Circle the *one* number that best describes the person's present circumstances.

1. *Excellent social resources*: Social relationships are very satisfying and extensive; at least one person would take care of him (her) indefinitely.

2. *Good social resources*: Social relationships are fairly satisfying and adequate and at least one person would take of him (her) indefinitely, *or*
Social relationships are very satisfying and extensive, and only short-term help is available.

3. *Mildly socially impaired*: Social relationships are unsatisfactory, of poor quality, few; but at least one person would take care of him (her) indefinitely, *or*
Social relationships are fairly satisfactory and adequate, and only short-term help is available.

4. *Moderately socially impaired*: Social relationships are unsatisfactory, of poor quality, few; and only short-term care is available, *or*
Social relationships are at least adequate or satisfactory, but help would only be available now and then.

5. *Severely socially impaired*: Social relationships are unsatisfactory, of poor quality, few; and help would be available only now and then, *or*
Social relationships are at least satisfactory or adequate, but help is not available even now and then.

6. *Totally socially impaired*: Social relationships are unsatisfactory, of poor quality, few; and help is not available even now and then.

Source: Adapted from Duke University Center for the Study of Aging and Human Development. *Multidimensional Functional Assessment: The OARS Methodology*. Durham, NC: Duke University, 1978.

Appendix B: Reference for Laboratory Values

Hematocrit

Men	*Women*
38%–54%	35%–47%

Hemoglobin

Men	*Women*
10.5–18 g/100 mL	11.4–17 g/100 mL

Sedimentation Rate

Men	*Women*
<20 mm/h	<30 mm/h

Blood Cells

Constituent	*Normal Values*	*Deviations*
Red blood cells		Increase:
Men	4,600,000–6,200,000/mm^3	Acute poisoning
Women	4,200,000–5,400,000/mm^3	Bone marrow hyperplasia
		Dehydration
		Diarrhea
		Polycythemia
		Pulmonary fibrosis

		Decrease:
		  Anemias
		  Hemorrhage
		  Hypothyroidism
		  Thalassemia
		  Toxicity

White blood cells	3,100–9,000 mm^3	Increase:
		  Acute bacterial infection
		  Leukemia
		  Polycythemia

		Decrease:
		  Acute alcohol ingestion
		  Acute viral infection
		  Agranulocytosis
		  Bone marrow depression

Neutrophils	50%–70% of total WBC Count	Increase:
		  Acute hemorrhage
		  Bacterial infections
		  Carcinoma
		  Cushing's disease
		  Diabetes mellitus
		  Gout
		  Hemolytic anemia
		  Increased corticosteroids
		  Lead poisoning
		  Pancreatitis
		  Rheumatic fever
		  Rheumatoid arthritis
		  Thyroiditis
		  Stress

		Decrease:
		  Acute viral infection
		  Bone marrow damage
		  Folic acid deficiency
		  Vitamin B$_{12}$ deficiency

Eosinophils	1%–4% of total WBC Count	Increase:
		  Allergy
		  Colitis
		  Collagen diseases
		  Eosinophilic granulomatosis
		  Eosinophilic leukemia
		  Parasitosis

Basophils	0%–1% of total WBC Count	Increase:
		  Myelofibrosis
		  Polycythemia vera

		Decrease: Anaphylactic reaction

Lymphocytes	20%–40% of total WBC Count	Increase:
		  Cushing's disease
		  Infectious diseases
		  Leukemia
		  Thyrotoxicosis

(Continued)

Constituent	Normal Values	Deviations

Monocytes	0%–6% of total WBC Count	Increase:
		    Malaria
		    Subacute bacterial endocarditis
		    Tuberculosis
		    Typhoid fever

Platelets	150,000–350,000 mm^3	Increase:
		    Chronic granulocytic leukemia
		    Hemoconcentration
		    Polycythemia
		    Splenectomy
		
		Decrease:
		    Acute leukemia
		    Aplastic anemia
		    Bone marrow depression
		    Chemotherapy
		    Thrombocytopenic purpura

Blood Chemistry

Constituent	Normal Values	Deviations

Bilirubin, Total	0.1–1.2 mg/100 mL	Increase:
		    Liver disease
		    Hemolysis posttransfusion
		    Pernicious anemia
		    (Jaundice present when
		        bilirubin level exceeds
		        1.5 mg/100 mL)
		
		Decrease:
		    Carcinoma
		    Chronic renal disease

Calcium	9–11 mg/100 mL
	(4.5–5.5 mEq/L)
		Increase:
		    Addison's disease
		    Hyperparathyroidism
		    Malignant bone tumors
		
		Decrease:
		    Chronic renal disease
		    Hypoparathyroidism
		    Vitamin D deficiency

Bicarbonate	(24–32 mEq/L)	Increase:
		    Metabolic alkalosis
		    Intestinal obstruction
		    Respiratory disease
		    Tetany
		    Vomiting
		
		Decrease:
		    Metabolic acidosis
		    Diarrhea
		    Nephritis

Chloride	350–390 mg/100 mL (95–105 mEq/L)	Increase: Renal tubular acidosis

		Decrease:
		  Diuretics that save potassium
		  Hypokalemic alkalosis
		  Ingestion of potassium without
		    chloride
		  Loss of gastric secretions

Cholesterol
  Total
  Free
  Esterified
	120–220 mg/100 mL
	40–50 mg/100 mL
	75–210 mg/100 mL
		Increase:
		  Chronic renal disease
		  Diabetes mellitus
		  Hypothyroidism
		  Liver disease with jaundice
		  Pancreatic dysfunction

		Decrease:
		  Fasting state
		  Hemolytic anemia
		  Hypermetabolic states
		  Hyperthyroidism
		  Intestinal obstruction
		  Liver disease
		  Malnutrition
		  Pernicious anemia
		  Tuberculosis

Creatinine	0.6–1.9 mg/100 mL	Increase:
		  Chronic glomerulonephritis
		  Nephrosis
		  Pyelonephritis
		  Other renal dysfunctions

Fibrinogen	150–300 mg/100 mL	Increase: Infection

		Decrease:
		  Liver disease
		  Malnutrition

Glucose	70–145 mg/100 mL	Increase:
		  Cerebral lesions
		  Cushing's disease
		  Diabetes mellitus
		  Emotional stress
		  Exercise
		  Hyperthyroidism
		  Infections
		  Pancreatic dysfunctions
		  Steroid therapy
		  Thiazide diuretic
		    therapy

		Decrease:
		  Addison's disease
		  Beta cell neoplasm
		  Hyperinsulinism
		  Hypothyroidism
		  Starvation

Iodine,
  protein-bound
	4–8 μg/100 mL	Increase:
		  Hyperthyroidism

(Continued)

Constituent	Normal Values	Deviations

Iron	60–150 μg/100 mL	Decrease:
		  Hypothyroidism
		Increase:
		  Aplastic anemia
		  Hemolytic anemia
		  Hemochromatosis
		  Hepatitis
		  Pernicious anemia
		Decrease:
		  Iron deficiency anemia

Lead	≤40 μg/100 mL	Increase: Lead poisoning

Lipids, Total	400–1000 mg/100 mL	Increase:
		  Diabetes mellitus
		  Glomerulonephritis
		  Hypothyroidism
		  Nephrosis
		Decrease:
		  Hyperthyroidism

pCO_2 (arterial)	35–45 mm Hg	Increase:
		  Metabolic alkalosis
		  Respiratory acidosis
		Decrease:
		  Metabolic acidosis
		  Respiratory alkalosis

pH (arterial)	7.35–7.45	Increase:
		  Fever
		  Hyperapnea
		  Intestinal obstruction
		  Vomiting
		Decrease:
		  Diabetic acidosis
		  Hemorrhage
		  Nephritis
		  Uremia

Phosphatase
  Acid
  Alkaline
	
	0.5–3.5 units
	2–4.5 units
		Increase:
		  Bony metastasis
		  Carcinoma of the prostate

pO_2 (arterial)	95–100 mm Hg	Increase:
		  Administration of pure O_2
		Decrease:
		  Circulatory disorders
		  Decreased hemoglobin
		  Decreased O_2 supply
		  High altitudes
		  Poor O_2 uptake and utilization
		  Respiratory exchange problems

Potassium	18–22 mg/100 mL
	(3.5–5.5 mEq/L)
		Increase:
		  Addison's disease
		  Anuria
		  Bronchial asthma
		  Burns
		  Renal disease
		  Tissue breakdown
		  Trauma
		Decrease:
		  Cirrhosis
		  Cushing's disease
		  Diabetic acidosis
		  Diarrhea
		  Diuretic therapy
		  Potassium-free intravenous
		    therapy
		  Steroid therapy
		  Vomiting

Protein, Total	6–8 g/100 mL	Increase:
		  Infections
		Decrease:
		  Intestinal tract disease
		  Liver disease
		  Malnutrition
		  Renal disease

Protein, Albumin	3.2–4.5 g/100 mL	Increase:
		  Multiple myeloma
		Decrease:
		  Acute stress
		  Chronic infection
		  Chronic liver disease
		  Loss of plasma
		  Malabsorption of protein
		  Malnutrition
		  Nephrotic syndrome

Protein, Globulin	2.3–3.5 g/100 mL	Increase:
		  Chronic hepatitis
		  Chronic infections
		  Collagen disease
		  Leukemia
		  Liver disease
		  Multiple myeloma
		  Sarcoidosis
		Decrease:
		  Proteinuria

Sodium	310–340 mg/100 mL
	(135–154 mEq/L)
		Increase:
		  Cardiac disease
		  Cushing's disease
		  Excessive water loss
		  Insufficient water intake
		  Renal disease

(Continued)

Constituent	Normal Values	Deviations

		Decrease:
		    Addison's disease
		    Chronic renal insufficiency
		    Cirrhosis
		    Congestive heart failure
		    Dehydration
		    Diabetic acidosis
		    Diarrhea
		    Diuretic therapy
		    Excessive ingestion of water
		    Overhydration intravenously
		    Starvation

Urea nitrogen
    (BUN)
	9–33 mg/100 mL	Increase:
		    Acute glomerulonephritis
		    Burns
		    Dehydration
		    Gastrointestinal hemorrhage
		    High protein intake
		    Intestinal obstruction
		    Mercury poisoning
		    Prostatic hypertrophy
		    Protein catabolism
		    Renal disease

		Decrease:
		    Cirrhosis
		    Liver disease
		    Low protein intake
		    Starvation

Uric acid
    Men
    Women
	
	2.1–8.5 mg/100 mL
	2.7–7.3 mg/100 mL
		Increase:
		    Chronic lymphocytic and
		        granulocytic leukemia
		    Chronic renal failure
		    Fasting
		    Gout
		    High salicylate intake
		    Leukemia
		    Multiple myeloma
		    Pneumonia
		    Thiazide diuretic therapy

		Decrease: Allopurinol therapy

Urine Chemistry

Constituent	Normal Values	Deviations

Acetone; Acetoacetate	0	Increase:
		    Starvation
		    Uncontrolled diabetes

Creatine	0–200 mg/24 hr	Increase:
		  Fever
		  Hyperthyroidism
		  Liver cancer

Creatinine	0.8–2 g/24 hr	Increase:
		  Salmonella infections
		  Tetanus
		  Typhoid fever
		Decrease:
		  Anemia
		  Leukemia
		  Muscular atrophy
		  Renal failure

Creatinine clearance	100–150 mL/min	Decrease: Renal disease

Glucose	Negative
	(1+ not unusual
	finding in older adults)
		Increase:
		  Diabetes mellitus
		  Increased intercranial
		    pressure
		  Pituitary disorder

Lead	≤150 μg/24 hr	Increase: Lead poisoning

pH	4.6–8	Increase:
		  Metabolic alkalemia
		  Proteus infections
		  Stale specimen

Phenolphthalein
  (PSP)
	25% excreted: 15 min
	40% excreted: 30 min
	60% excreted: 120 min
		Decrease:
		  Congestive heart failure
		  Renal disease

Protein	0.1 g/24 hr	Increase:
		  Fever
		  Infection
		  Kidney disease
		  Strenuous exercise

Specific gravity	1.0179–1.0327	Increase:
		  (Urine less concentrated)
		  Dehydration
		Decrease:
		  (Urine less concentrated)
		  Diuretic therapy
		  Renal tubular dysfunction

Urea nitrogen	9–16 g/24 hr	Increase:
		  Excessive protein catabolism
		Decrease:
		  Renal disease

Uric acid	250–750 mg/24 hr	Increase:
		  Gout
		Decrease:
		  Nephritis

Appendix C: Additional Bibliographic Resources

This appendix contains *additional* resources. For specific topics, refer to the periodical and book references listed at the end of each chapter.

BOOKS

Bates B. *A Guide to Physical Examination*, 4th ed. Philadelphia: Lippincott, 1987.

Calkins E, Davis PJ, Ford AB (editors). *The Practice of Geriatrics*. Philadelphia: Saunders, 1986.

Carnevali DL, Patrick M (editors). *Nursing Management for the Elderly*, 2nd ed. Philadelphia: Lippincott, 1986.

Ebersole P, Hess P. *Toward Healthy Aging: Human Needs and Nursing Response*, 2nd ed. St Louis: Mosby, 1985.

Eliopoulos C. *Gerontological Nursing*, 2nd ed. Philadelphia: Lippincott, 1987.

Gambert SR (editor). *Handbook of Geriatrics*. New York: Plenum, 1987.

Gioiella E, Bevil C. *Nursing Care of the Aged Client*. Norwalk, CT: Appleton-Century-Crofts, 1984.

Henry JB. *Clinical Diagnosis and Management*, 17th ed. Philadelphia: Saunders, 1984.

Rogers CS, McCue JD (editors). *Managing Chronic Disease*. Oradell, NJ: Medical Economics Books, 1987.

Steffl BM (editor). *Handbook of Gerontological Nursing*. New York: Van Nostrand Reinhold, 1984.

Yurick AG et al. *The Aged Person and the Nursing Process*, 2nd ed. Norwalk, CT: Appleton-Century-Crofts, 1984.

Appendix D: Audiovisual Resources

This appendix offers audiovisual resources that can enhance your assessment skills. To obtain or learn more about the individual programs, please contact the appropriate distributor whose address is listed at the end of the section.

PROGRAMMED INSTRUCTION

PROFILES OF AGING

Communication with the Aging
Death and Dying
Demography of Aging
Health Care Law and Aging
Human Behavior and Aging
Institutionalization: Issues and
  Challenges

Nutrition and Aging
Psychology of Aging
Sexuality and Aging
Social Programs and the Aging
Sociological Aspects of Aging

Physician's Assessment Program, University of Nebraska

PATIENT ASSESSMENT

Taking a Patient's History
Examination of the Abdomen
Examination of the Chest and Lungs
Examination of the Ear
Examination of the Eye, Part I, II
Examination of the Female Pelvis,
  Part I, II
Examination of the Head and Neck

The Neurological Examination, Part I,
  II, III
Abnormalities of the Heartbeat
Blood-Gas and Acid-Base Concepts in
  Respiratory Care
Examination of the Heart and Great
  Vessels, Part I
Examination of the Heart,
  Auscultation, Part II
Pulses
Examination of the Male Genitalia

American Journal of Nursing Co., New York

AUDIOVISUAL TITLES

General Assessment

Aging: An Individual Matter
30 min, color, 16 mm, videocassette,
videotape
American Journal of Nursing Co.

Aging: The Losses
30 min, color, 16mm, videocassette,
videotape
American Journal of Nursing Co.

*Cancer: Early Diagnosis and
Management*
20 min, color, super 8mm
University of Oklahoma Health
Sciences Center

Cancer of the Skin
18 min, color, regular 8mm or 16mm
American Cancer Society

*Danowski on Special Problems in the
Older Diabetic*
7 min, color, super 8mm or 16mm
Upjohn Co.

Examination of the Mouth
8 min, color, super 8mm or 16mm
National Audiovisual Center

Functional Assessment of the Elderly
2 part, color, videocassette
American Journal of Nursing Co.

*The Head and the Neck (Physical
Examination Series)*
14½ min, color, super 8mm or 16mm
J. B. Lippincott Co.

*Inspection and Palpation of the
Anterior Chest*
52 min, black and white, super 8mm
or 16mm
National Audiovisual Center

Jaundice: Medical or Surgical
40 min, black and white, super 8mm
or 16mm
National Audiovisual Center

*Krall on Special Problems in the Older
Diabetic*
7 min, color, super 8mm or 16mm
Upjohn Co.

Life Stress on the Elderly
Color, super 8mm or 16mm,
videocassette
Medi-Tel Communications

*Medical Management: Role of the
Nurse in Establishing a Diagnosis
(Coronary Artery Disease)*
28 min, color, videocassette
American Journal of Nursing Co.

The Mental Status Examination
34 min, black and white, super 8mm
or 16mm
National Audiovisual Center

The Mental Status Examination
8 min, color, super 8mm or 16mm
University of Nebraska Medical
Center, Biomedical
Communications

*Miller on Special Problems in the
Older Diabetic*
6 min, color, super 8mm or 16mm
Upjohn Co.

Nursing Assessment
24 min, color, 16mm, videocassette,
videotape
American Journal of Nursing Co.

Oral Cancer: Intra-oral Examination
6 min, color, regular 8mm or super 8mm
National Audiovisual Center

The Phenomenon of Depression
Color, super 8mm or 16mm,
videocassette
Medi-Tel Communications

*Physical Examination Series (produced
by Barbara Bates)*
1) The Head and the Neck; 2) The
Thorax; 3) The Heart; 4) Pressures
and Pulses; 5) The Breasts and
Axillae; 6) The Abdomen; 7) The
Male Genitalia, Anus and Rectum;
8) The Female Genitalia, Anus and
Rectum; 9) The Peripheral Vascular
System; 10) The Musculoskeletal
System; 11) The Neurologic System,
Part I; 12) The Neurologic System,
Part II
Color, super 8mm or 16mm
J. B. Lippincott Co.

Psychogeriatrics
40 min, color, 16mm, videocassette,
 videotape, audiocassette
American Journal of Nursing Co.

Recognizing Depression Series
Color, super 8mm
Camera Talks, Ltd.

*A Seventy-three Year Old Female with
 a Neck Mass*
10 min, color, super 8mm
Instructional Systems for the Health
 Sciences

Sex and Aging
Color, super 8mm or 16mm
Edcoa Productions, Inc.

*Symptoms of Senility: Recognition
 and Management*
18 min, color, super 8mm
Sandoz Pharmaceuticals

*Techniques of Laboratory Diagnosis
 of Influenza*
17 min, black and white, super 8mm
 or 16mm
National Audiovisual Center

*Understanding the Older Adult:
 Nursing Assessment and Diagnosis
 in Geriatric Care*
 1) Older Population: Realities
 and Myths, 2) Interview and
 Mental Status Evaluation,
 3) Cardiovascular and Respiratory
 Systems, 4) Gastrointestinal and
 Genitourinary Systems,
 5) Musculoskeletal and Sensory
 Organs
5-part series, color, videocassette
Chesapeake Video Education

Urinalysis: Physical Examination
4 min, color, super 8mm
Harper & Row Publishers

Urinalysis: Test for Protein
4 min, color, super 8mm
Harper & Row Publishers

*Urinalysis: Tests for Ketones and
 Diacetic Acid*
4 min, color, super 8mm
Harper & Row Publishers

Urinary Tract Infections
32 min, color, super 8mm or 16mm
Eaton Laboratories

*Verbal Impairment Associated with
 Brain Damage*
16 min, color, super 8mm or regular
 8mm
National Audiovisual Center

Cardiovascular System

*An Approach to Peripheral Vascular
 Disease*
40 min, black and white, super 8mm
National Audiovisual Center

*Arteriosclerosis Obliterans: Its Early
 Recognition in the Lower
 Extremities, Parts I and II*
16 min, color, regular 8mm or super
 8mm
Institute for Dermatologic
 Communication and Education

Auscultation and the Normal Heart
Color, super 8mm or 16mm
J. B. Lippincott Co.

Blood Pressure
4 min, color, super 8mm
Prentice-Hall, Inc.

Blood Pressure Readings
29 min, black and white, super 8mm
 or 16 mm
National Audiovisual Center

Blood Pressure Readings
19 min, color, super 8mm or 16mm
National Audiovisual Center

Central Venous Pressure Measurement
10 min, color, super 8mm or 16mm,
 videocassette
American College of Physicians

Congestive Heart Failure
40 min, black and white, super 8mm
 or 16mm
National Audiovisual Center

Electrocardiographic Monitoring
12 min, color, super 8mm
Sutherland Learning Assoc.

Electrocardiography and Arrhythmias
22 min, color, super 8mm
Sutherland Learning Assoc.

The Heart (Physical Examination Series)
See *Physical Examination Series* under General Assessment

Inspection and Palpation of the Anterior Chest
52 min, black and white, super 8mm or 16mm
National Audiovisual Center

Interpretation of Arrhythmias and their Treatment
13 min, color, super 8mm
Sutherland Learning Assoc.

Introduction to the Neurovascular Examination
Color, super 8mm
National Audiovisual Center

Medical Management: Role of the Nurse in Establishing a Diagnosis (Coronary Artery Disease)
28 min, color, videocassette
American Journal of Nursing Co.

The Peripheral Vascular System
See *Physical Examination Series* under General Assessment

Physiological and Clinical Aspects of Cardiac Auscultation Series
Color, super 8mm or 16mm
J. B. Lippincott Co.

The Warning Arrhythmias
22 min, color, super 8mm
Sutherland Learning Assoc.

Gastrointestinal System

The Abdomen
See *Physical Examination Series* under General Assessment

Cancer of the Stomach
21 min, color, regular 8mm
American Cancer Society

Danowski on Special Problems in the Older Diabetic
7 min, color, super 8mm or 16mm
Upjohn Co.

Dental Care for the Chronically Ill and Aged
19 min, color, super 8mm
Upjohn Co.

The Dentist and Cancer
21 min, color, super 8mm
American Cancer Society

Diagnosis and Management of Cancer of the Colon and Rectum
17 min, color, regular 8mm
American Cancer Society

Diagnosis of Pancreatic Disease
50 min, black and white, super 8mm or 16mm
National Audiovisual Center

Esophagoscopy and Bronchoscopy
5 min, color, regular 8mm or 16mm
Upjohn Co.

Examination of the Mouth
8 min, color, super 8mm or 16mm
National Audiovisual Center

Fecal Smears for Parasitological Examination
8 min, color, regular 8mm or super 8mm
National Audiovisual Center

The Female Genitalia, Anus and Rectum
See *Physical Examination Series* under General Assessment

The Head and the Neck
See *Physical Examination Series* under General Assessment

Jaundice: Medical or Surgical
40 min, black and white, super 8mm or 16mm
National Audiovisual Center

Krall on Special Problems in the Older Diabetic
7 min, color, super 8mm or 16mm
Upjohn Co.

The Male Genitalia, Anus and Rectum
See *Physical Examination Series* under General Assessment

Miller on Special Problems in the Older Diabetic
6 min, color, super 8mm or 16mm
Upjohn Co.

Oral Cancer: Intra-oral Examination
6 min, color, regular 8mm or super 8mm
National Audiovisual Center

Genitourinary System

The Breasts and Axillae
See *Physical Examination Series* under General Assessment

Breast Self-Exam
15 min, color, super 8mm
Omni Education

Cancer of the Urinary System
20 min, color, super 8mm
American Cancer Society

Detecting Breast Cancer Earlier
18 min, color, super 8mm
American Cancer Society

Diagnosis and Treatment of Cancer of the Prostate
18 min, color, super 8mm
American Cancer Society

The Female Genitalia, Anus and Rectum
See *Physical Examination Series* under General Assessment

The Male Genitalia, Anus and Rectum
See *Physical Examination Series* under General Assessment

Self-Examination of the Breasts
7 min, color, regular 8mm
Professional Research, Inc.

Sex and Aging
Color, super 8mm or 16mm
Edcoa Productions, Inc.

Sexual Anatomy
Color, super 8mm
Edcoa Productions, Inc.

Urinalysis: Physical Examination
4 min, color, super 8mm
Harper & Row Publishers

Urinalysis: Test for Protein
4 min, color, super 8mm
Harper & Row Publishers

Urinalysis: Tests for Ketones and Diacetic Acid
4 min, color, super 8mm
Harper & Row Publishers

Urinary Tract Infections
32 min, color, super 8mm or 16mm
Eaton Laboratories

Integumentary System

Cancer of the Skin
18 min, color, regular 8mm or 16mm
American Cancer Society

Diagnosis of Latent Psoriasis
6 min, color, regular 8mm or super 8mm
Institute for Dermatologic Communication and Education

Physical Assessment: The Skin and Extremities
18 min, color, slide-tape
Trainex Corporation

Mental Health Assessment

The Mental Status Examination
34 min, black and white, super 8mm or 16mm
National Audiovisual Center

The Mental Status Examination
8 min, color, super 8mm or 16mm
University of Nebraska Medical Center, Biomedical Communications

The Phenomenon of Depression
Color, super 8mm or 16mm, videocassette
Medi-Tel Communications

Physical Examination Series
See under General Assessment

Psychogeriatrics
40 min, color, 16mm, videocassette, videotape, audiocassette
American Journal of Nursing Co.

Recognizing Depression Series
Color, super 8mm
Camera Talks, Ltd.

Symptoms of Senility: Recognition and Management
18 min, color, super 8mm
Sandoz Pharmaceuticals

Verbal Impairment Associated with Brain Damage
16 min, color, super 8mm or regular 8mm
National Audiovisual Center

Musculoskeletal System

Breast Self-Exam
15 min, color, super 8mm
Omni Education

The Breasts and Axillae
7 min, color, super 8mm or 16mm
J. B. Lippincott Co.

Detecting Breast Cancer Earlier
18 min, color, super 8mm
American Cancer Society

Fractures, Dislocations, and Sprains
40 min, color, super 8mm or 16mm
National Audiovisual Center

The Head and the Neck
See *Physical Examination Series* under
  General Assessment

*The Hip (Physical Examination of the
  Joints and Examination of the
  Peripheral Joints Series)*
8 min, color, super 8mm
University of Minnesota, Audiovisual
  Library Service

*The Knee (Physical Examination of
  the Joints and Examination of the
  Peripheral Joints Series)*
8 min, color, super 8mm
University of Minnesota, Audiovisual
  Library Service

The Musculoskeletal System
See *Physical Examination Series* under
  General Assessment

*Osteoporosis: Diagnosis and
  Treatment*
30 min, color, super 8mm or 16mm
Professional Research, Inc.

Self-Examination of the Breasts
7 min, color, regular 8mm
Professional Research, Inc.

Neurologic System

Aging: Sensory Losses
30 min, color, 16mm, videocassette,
  videotape
American Journal of Nursing Co.

Anatomy of the Eye Series
  1) The Orbit; 2) The Extraocular
  Muscles; 3) The Visual System: The
  Globe; 4) The Visual System: The
Visual Pathway; 5) The Anterior
  Adnexa; 6) The Circulation; and
  7) The Nerves.
15 min each, color, super 8mm or
  16mm, videocassette
Teaching Films, Inc.

Auditory Process
4 min, color, super 8mm
Hubbard

Cataracts
8 min, color, regular 8mm
Professional Research, Inc.

The Ear: Its Structure and Function
2 min, color, regular 8mm or super
  8mm
Encyclopedia Brittanica Educational
  Corp.

Field of View
3 min, black and white, regular 8mm
  or super 8mm
Gateway Educational Media

Glaucoma
14 min, color, regular 8mm
Professional Research, Inc.

The Head and the Neck
See *Physical Examination Series* under
  General Assessment

*Introduction to the Neurovascular
  Examination*
Color, super 8mm
National Audiovisual Center

The Neurologic System: Parts I and II
35 min, color, super 8mm or 16mm
J. B. Lippincott Co.

*Verbal Impairment Associated with
  Brain Damage*
16 min, color, super 8mm or regular
  8mm
National Audiovisual Center

Respiratory System

*Collection and Processing of
  Specimens for Respiratory Virus
  Isolation*
4 min, color, super 8mm or 16mm
National Audiovisual Center

Esophagoscopy and Bronchoscopy
5 min, color, regular 8mm or 16mm
Upjohn Co.

The Head and the Neck
See *Physical Examination Series* under
    General Assessment

*Inspection and Palpation of the
    Anterior Chest*
52 min, black and white, super 8mm
    or 16mm
National Audiovisual Center

*Lung Cancer: Early Diagnosis and
    Management*
18 min, color, super 8mm
American Cancer Society

Obstructive Lung Disease
15 min, color, super 8mm
Professional Research, Inc.

*Physiologic Manifestations of
    Emphysema*
11 min, color, super 8mm or regular
    8mm
National Audiovisual Center

Physical Assessment: The Chest
22 min, color, slide-tape
Trainex Corporation

*Techniques of Laboratory Diagnosis
    of Influenza*
17 min, black and white, super 8mm
    or 16mm
National Audiovisual Center

Tests for Bronchitis and Emphysema
7 min, color, super 8mm or regular
    8mm
National Audiovisual Center

DISTRIBUTOR ADDRESS LIST

American Cancer Society
777 Third Avenue
New York, NY 10017

American College of Physicians
4200 Pine Street
Philadelphia, PA 19104

American Journal of Nursing Co.
Educational Services Division
555 West 57th Street
New York, NY 10019

Biomedical Communications
University of Nebraska Medical
    Center
42nd and Dewey
Omaha, NB 68105

Camera Talks, Ltd.
31 North Row (Park Lane)
London W1 Hyde Park,
England

Chesapeake Video Education
The Grempler Building
Suite 200
Columbia, MD 21044

Eaton Medical Film Library
Eaton Laboratories Division
Morton-Norwich Products, Inc.
Norwich, NY 13815

Edcoa Productions, Inc.
520 South Dean Street
Englewood, NJ 07631

Encyclopedia Brittanica Educational
    Corp.
425 North Michigan Avenue
Chicago, IL 60611

Gateway Educational Films, Ltd.
E.S.L. Bristol
St. Lawrence House
29/31 Broad Street
Bristol, BSI 2HF England

Harper & Row Publishers
10 East 53rd Street
New York, NY 10022

Hubbard Scientific Co.
P.O. Box 105
2855 Shermer Road
Northbrook, IL 50062

Institute for Dermatologic
    Communication and Education
2785 Jackson Street
San Francisco, CA 94115

Instructional Systems for the Health
    Sciences
11899 West Pico Boulevard
West Los Angeles, CA 90064

J. B. Lippincott Co.
East Washington Square
Philadelphia, PA 19105

Medi-Tel Communications
652 First Avenue
New York, NY 10016

National Audiovisual Center
General Services Administration
Washington, DC 20409

Omni
190 West Main Street
Somerville, NJ 08876

Physician's Assistant Program
4014 Conkling Hall
University of Nebraska Medical
   Center
42nd and Dewey Avenue
Omaha, NB 68105

Prentice-Hall, Inc.
Sylvan Avenue
Englewood Cliffs, NJ 07632

Professional Research, Inc.
660 South Bonnie Brae
Los Angeles, CA 90057

Sandox Pharmaceuticals
Division of Sandoz-Wander, Inc.
East Hanover, NJ 07936

Sutherland Learning Assoc.
8425 West Third Street
Los Angeles, CA 90048

Teaching Films, Inc.
Division of A-V Corp.
2518 North Boulevard
P.O. Box 66824
Houston, TX 77006

Trainex Corporation
P.O. Box 116
Garden Grove, CA 92642

University of Minnesota
Audiovisual Library Service
3300 University Avenue S.E.
Minneapolis, MN 55414

Upjohn Co.
Professional Communications
7000 Portage Road
Kalamazoo, MI 49001

Index